Film Festivals, Ideology and Italian Art Cinema

Film Festivals, Ideology and Italian Art Cinema

Politics, Histories and Cultural Value

Rachel Johnson

Routledge
Taylor & Francis Group
LONDON AND NEW YORK

This book was made possible through various grants, and I am grateful to the Arts and Humanities Research Council, White Rose College of the Arts and Humanities, Leeds Arts and Humanities Research Institute, and University of Leeds School of Languages, Cultures and Societies for their support.

First published in 2024 by Amsterdam University Press Ltd.

Published 2025 by Routledge
4 Park Square, Milton Park, Abingdon, Oxon OX14 4RN
605 Third Avenue, New York, NY 10158

Routledge is an imprint of the Taylor & Francis Group, an informa business

ISBN: 9789463720366 (hbk)
ISBN: 9781041179337 (pbk)
ISBN: 9781003695523 (ebk)
NUR 670

Cover illustration: Director Gianfranco Rosi poses with his award after winning the Golden Bear for his film *Fuocoammare*. Berlin, 2016. Tania Volobueva. ShutterStock.com.

Cover design: Coördesign, Leiden

DOI: 10.5117/9789463720366

Table of Contents

List of Illustrations

Acknowledgements

Thank you to those who have been there since the beginning: my mother, for your unconditional love, support and pedantry; my father, for the same love and support, and unquenchable curiosity; my brother, for reminding me not to take myself too seriously. Each of you contributed to this book, in often invisible but ever invaluable ways.

Thank you to my mentor and friend, Alan O'Leary: this book would not be what it is, and I would not be the scholar I am, without your guidance, honesty and willingness to indulge my fascination with psychoanalysis. Thank you for reading countless drafts of this and other writings; for helping me find my courage and my voice.

Thank you to everyone who has read part or all of the many iterations of this book, who have shared feedback and reassurance when it was most needed. Mani Sharpe, whose reading of the film festivals and ideology chapter helped me see what I was really writing about; Catherine O'Rawe, who not only provided the inspiration for but offered helpful feedback on, the chapter about gender; Rebecca Macklin, for reading early drafts about Orientalism and ecocinema, and for sitting alongside me in numerous cafés while I muddled through the introduction. Hayley Toth, for her encouragement and incisive feedback on chapters about colonialism. Nathan Brand, for his continuous advice while I worked through the political implications of my arguments. Thank you to all the friends who lent their eyes, ears and support over the last few years. Special thanks to Sam Coveney for turning me onto ideology in the first place, and to Maddalena Moretti—my forever partner in cinematic crime.

My final and heart-filled thanks go to Adrienne Mortimer, for more than these acknowledgements could express. For being there, always; for nourishing me, all ways.

Introduction

Abstract: The Introduction discusses the main relationships this book investigates: art cinema and film festivals, film festivals and Europe, and Italian cinema and film festivals. I consider the various terms through which we might taxonomise films celebrated at festivals—world cinema, global art cinema, peripheral cinema—before outlining the Eurocentric histories of the film festival network and dominant canons of art cinema. I show how the meaning of terms such as art cinema is contingent upon the flows of prestige, geopolitical relations and economic structures in which film festivals participate. The introduction then focuses on Italian cinema's status as emblematic of filmmaking dependent on festivals for circulation and its centrality to the historical development of the European film festival circuit.

Keywords: art cinema, film festivals, Italian cinema, film circulation, European cinema

The central premise of this book is that art cinema does not exist. It is a fantasy that is brought into being again and again through rituals that take place at film festivals—rituals such as film selections and screenings, prize-giving, red carpet parades, as well as the production of endless pronouncements on each film, from festival programmes to jury statements, interviews, critics' reviews, social media posts and, of course, the excited exchange of opinions between audience members after (and sometimes during) a screening.

Yet these rituals, and the sites in which they take place, are not pure: they are constituted by and reproduce economic and geopolitical interests. Film festivals' construction of that which we call art cinema not only serves the dictates of some rarefied aesthetic value, but, to bring things abruptly back down to earth, it also serves "the interests of nation states and global capital" (Rhyne, 2009, p. 10). Art cinema is a fantasy, yes, but one produced under material conditions, and with material consequences. This book is

Johnson, R., Film Festivals, *Ideology and Italian Art Cinema: Politics, Histories and Cultural Value*. Taylor & Francis Group, 2024
DOI 10.5117/9789463720366_INTRO

an investigation of those conditions and consequences—in other words, the ideology of art cinema reproduced through film festivals.

Through the case of new millennium Italian cinema, this book seeks to develop our understanding of which films are permitted international attention and legitimation at European competitive film festivals. It interrogates received notions of artistic value, political legitimacy and cultural relevance, notions that circulate through festivals, through the wider film industry and through academic film canons. Treating such notions as constructed, underpinned by unspoken and sometimes unspeakable values, this book proposes a methodology of ideology critique adapted for the study of film festivals and other cultural institutions involved in the legitimation of artworks.

I focus on the ideological functioning of European A festivals, European film festivals that run an international competition and are accredited as "A-list" by the International Federation of Film Producers Associations (FIAPF). A full list of these festivals can be found in the appendix. I identify several values that characterise such festivals' ideological functioning, including notions of the auteur, deployed as a signifier of anti-commercial purity, and a structural preoccupation with difference. While I interrogate these constructions of art cinema in general, I also investigate the specificities of the ideological representation and circulation of Italian film since the year 2000.

This book aspires to contribute to debates surrounding film festivals and the construction of value, the international circulation of Italian cinema, and the continuing relevance of ideology critique as a method. In this chapter and the next, I explore each of these debates, outlining their coordinates and highlighting the intersections between them. Below, I discuss the role of film festivals in reproducing the contested category of art cinema, before highlighting similar processes of contestation in the valorisation of a certain kind of Italian cinema by both scholars and cinematic institutions. Italian cinema and art cinema find intersection in shared institutional histories such as the founding of the Venice International Film Festival, the first of its kind, and the positioning of postwar neorealism as one of art cinema's central traditions (Pisu, 2018; Galt & Schoonover, 2012). I conclude with an outline of the book's chapters, each one exploring a figure or fantasy within the ideology of European A festivals through an award-winning Italian film.

Film Festivals and Art Cinema

In the first *Film Festival Yearbook*, Dina Iordanova and Ragan Rhyne (2009, p. 1) argue that film festivals are "the driving force behind the global circulation of cinema." The range of cinemas with which film festivals engage cannot be overstated. Film festivals have long been considered crucial to the exhibition, distribution and ideological construction of a variety of films mostly produced outside the Hollywood film industry, encompassing a broad range of cinematic traditions. For example, scholars have analysed the international distribution and prestige that festivals afford queer cinema (Damiens, 2018), their exhibition and cultivation of migration cinema (de Valck, 2013), and their discursive construction of numerous national cinemas, such as Chilean (Paz Peirano, 2021), French (Mazdon, 2006), Iranian (Nichols, 1994) and Senegalese (Sendra, 2021).

The range of cinemas that film festivals have helped to cultivate is facilitated by the enormous, and still growing, number of festivals currently in operation: over 11,000 according to the industry festival directory, *Film Freeway*. These vary from major competitive film festivals such as Cannes, through international NGO-funded human rights festivals such as the Human Rights Watch Film Festival, to local, volunteer-run queer film festivals such as the Leeds Queer Film Festival. Such events tend to exhibit a certain kind of filmmaking according to a specific set of aims, be they industry-led, advocacy-based, community-focused or otherwise.

In the case I consider, European A festivals, we find a generalist approach to film programming that seeks to encompass many of the cinematic modes, and some of the aims, discussed above. This raises the question of which term or terms these festivals organise the diversity of their curation around. Broadly speaking, which "cinema" do A festivals reproduce? Aida Vallejo (2020) suggests that this may be "world cinema." Yet this is grounded in her concern with the canonisation of films reproduced in academia, "world cinema" being an appellation largely favoured by (and hotly debated among) academics. Considering the broad film festival phenomenon, Maria Paz Peirano (2021, p. 48) suggests another set of terms, by no means mutually exclusive from Vallejo's: "peripheral cinemas," "independent world cinema" and "global art cinema." In both cases, we find conceptions of a cinema that is aside from an implied or "missing" centre of the global film industry, Hollywood (Jeong, 2021, p. 32). Festivals' cinema is transnational—a "global" or "world" cinema—although it is unclear whether this globality is set within or against a world system in which the USA, and possibly Europe, are once again positioned at the centre, with "global" functioning as a marker of difference. Paz Peirano also introduces the notion of "art," which we might assume to be a reference to Rosalind Galt and Karl Schoonover's (2010) edited collection, *Global Art Cinema*. While each of these terms offer a sense of the kinds of films that A-list festivals exhibit and legitimate, their proliferation also underlines that no definition of the cinemas that such festivals cultivate is neutral. Each combination of words—global, world, art, and so on—brings with it a particular understanding of geopolitical space and, in some instances, aesthetic value.

This book centres on the term "art cinema" and, in particular, "Italian art cinema." The book's title posits the study of art cinema *through* Italian cinema. The replacement of "global" registers the tension between the local and transnational that such a project necessitates. I treat festivals' construction of Italian cinema as a heuristic through which to apprehend the dominant values through which such festivals legitimate art cinema more broadly. Simultaneously, I aim to situate Italian cinema within global structures of exhibition, circulation and canonisation. Yet the very possibility of reading art cinema through Italian cinema highlights the particularity of the dominant values driving festival legitimation, their rootedness in those European traditions of filmmaking in which Italian production has historically been foregrounded, and which I discuss at length below. In short, while situating this study, this book's focus on Italian art cinema also hones in on the situatedness of dominant conceptions of art cinema, the contestation underlying appellations such as "global."

I emphasise "art," moreover, as this is one of the central values around which A-list festivals have traditionally been organised (de Valck, 2007; Andrews, 2010). It is also a term that this book is intent on interrogating. While the ideologies that may underpin some instances of popular cinema have been apprehended extensively within film scholarship over the last fifty years, research has been somewhat less attentive to the ideological aspects of art cinema—the structures of exhibition and value through which art cinema, too, has come to be reproduced, and their embeddedness in the circulation of global capital.[1] This line of interrogation has been suggested recently in calls for a "new cinephilia" (Shambu, 2019), which highlight the fact that some of the most cherished tenets of cinematic and aesthetic value remain rooted in largely Eurocentric film histories, organised around a select few white male auteurs, from the leading figures of Italian neorealism to the French New Wave.

We find early suggestions of film festivals' role in constructing categories of "art cinema" in foundational texts such as Andrew Higson's (1989) "The Concept of National Cinema" and Steve Neale's (1981) "Art Cinema as Institution." Both acknowledge the role of structures of production, exhibition,

1 For an exception to this rule, see King (2022).

distribution and representation in constituting art cinema as precisely a "cinema," or institutional paradigm. They underline the importance of film festivals in defining art cinema and facilitating the circulation of the seemingly disparate films grouped under this term. In a brief note on the paradox of art cinema often being considered in terms of national cinemas, Higson (1989, p. 41) describes the "network of film festivals and reviewing practices" as the "means of achieving a critical reputation and both a national and an international cultural space for such films" (that is, art films). More than securing international distribution, however, films shown at film festivals achieve a discursive currency: their "status as 'Art' [...] [is] confirmed and re-stated through the existence of prizes and awards" (Neale, 1981, p. 35).

While festivals receive only a passing mention in Neale's and Higson's essays, their importance to the exhibition, distribution and creation of meaning for art cinema has become clearer in recent years. David Andrews (2010, pp. 7–9), explicitly builds on Neale's argument, positing that film festivals have become "art cinema's central institution" and "the primary mechanism through which art cinema has sustained through time the ideas of high-art value that have bound it together." Film festivals not only maintain these ideals of high art, however; festivals have a "generative function," producing the key terms and tropes through which art cinema comes to be defined (Andrews, 2010, p. 6).

Given their significance, it is fundamental to understand the processes by which film festivals construct art cinema. Many of the studies cited above frame these processes of construction in a way that indicates the influence of different factors—the two main ones being notions of artistic worth and potential for commercial success. These culminate to produce a homogenising definition (art cinema) for a body of films that can differ enormously in style, theme, site of production and so on. Returning to Neale (1981, p. 15), we find a thrust towards a homogenisation of meaning in the institutional construction of art cinema, in this case via auteurist conceptions of film:

> Even where the marks of enunciation themselves are heterogeneous, they tend to be unified and stabilised within the space of an institution which reads and locates them in a homogeneous way (each mark serving equally as the sign of the author) and which mobilises that meaning in accordance with commodity-based practices of production, distribution and exhibition (the mark of the author is used as a kind of brand name, to mark and to sell the filmic product).

This not only occurs through festivals' preoccupation with the figure of the auteur (which I analyse in chapters 2 and 3). At the most fundamental level, film festivals should be understood as unifying and stabilising the heterogeneous production of art cinema: their construction of films entails reading "marks of enunciation"—in this case, aspects of a film text—in "a homogeneous way" and, crucially, the mobilisation of their meaning "in accordance with commodity-based practices of production, distribution and exhibition."

Meaning is mobilised in a way that serves certain interests. This is necessitated by the very structure of film festivals and their own embeddedness in geopolitical networks and flows of capital. As third-sector cultural events, film festivals rely upon a mixture of public and private investment, and their success in securing this depends upon their ability to present themselves as culturally important and commercially viable (Rhyne, 2009, p. 20). Film festivals are required to present themselves under a common identity as a "discrete cultural sector," meanwhile differentiating themselves from each other in order to attract investment from public and private organisations (Rhyne, 2009, pp. 9–10). Rhyne (2009, p. 19) underlines the relationship between film festivals and their economic functioning, arguing that, while they may appear "discursively independent," they are "financially dependent" on state, public and corporate bodies. These bodies can include ministries of culture, local authorities, and multi-national corporations. Film festivals have thus developed models for managing diverse stakeholders and, crucially, for "channeling their diverse interests towards the goals of nation-states and global capital" (Rhyne, 2009, p. 10). Yet the discursive independence to which Rhyne refers has also been questioned, with a wealth of recent scholarship demonstrating the link between festivals' promotion of certain films and their management of political and economic interests (Chan, 2011; Ahn, 2012; Cheung, 2016). Several of these studies—from Chan's (2011) "Making of a National Cinema" to Ahn's (2012) analysis of the Pusan International Film Festival—focus on individual festivals and their construction of certain national cinemas. To what extent, then, do geopolitical and commercial interests condition the construction of categories of art cinema across several festivals?

Marijke de Valck (2014) highlights the generalised flows of prestige and capital across the global network of film festivals in a way that is particularly apposite to our study of their role in the institutional construction of art cinema. Due to the increasing commercialisation of major, competitive festivals in the new millennium, cultural legitimisation is contingent upon selection committees' and juries' perceptions of not only the artistic worth but the commercial viability of a film. De Valck (2014, p. 76) concludes that global art cinema has moved on from being a "loser takes all game" in which financial success is detrimental to a film's symbolic success as a piece of art. Rather, a film's chances of being selected or receiving an award at a film festival are determined as much by its expected viability in the global marketplace as its perceived artistic integrity (de Valck, 2014, p. 81). Thus, not only the selection of films, but the additional prestige afforded by awarding prizes to some films within that selection is motivated by commercial as well as aesthetic judgments. The legitimisation of some films as "art," and therefore art cinema, is achieved through processes of selection and awarding that have become more intensely influenced by commercial interests in recent years.

The European A Circuit

Film festivals' practices constitute a long-standing process of contestation for the meaning(s) of art cinema. Such practices, and thus the process of contestation, are underpinned by commercial and sometimes geopolitical pressures. The influence of these factors is clearest within a particular sub-set of film festivals: the A circuit, festivals that have been accredited by FIAPF as "competitive feature film festivals"—annual, non-specialised festivals that hold an international competition, such as Cannes or Karlovy Vary (FIAPF, 2019). While film festival scholars have long manifested suspicion towards the notion of the "circuit" due to its unreflexive use to refer to *all* film festivals (Elsaesser, 2005; de Valck, 2007; Iordanova, 2009; Loist, 2016), European A festivals present several common features that justify not only their grouping as a circuit, but also their treatment as exemplary sites for the institutional construction of art cinema.

The A-list is archetypal of a festival circuit both in its organisation and its status in the imaginary of the film industry. This circuit is, in fact, the one that many scholars and industry professionals implicitly refer to when they speak of the film festival circuit in general: as Skadi Loist (2016) notes, "'circuit' is often used synonymous[ly] with the elite A-list" (p. 60). A-list festivals may also underpin the notion of the circuit itself: "as soon as FIAPF started to regulate the festivals and create the "A-list" festivals, the idea of a circuit became visible" (Loist, 2016, p. 55). Moreover, in a very practical sense, A festivals can be distinguished and grouped together due to their common subscription to the regulations that FIAPF imposes on them; their shared accreditation by FIAPF requires them to meet the federation's "minimum standards" of organisational infrastructure, inclusion of international premieres (at least fifteen) in each annual competition, and commitment to serving the film industry.

The features that secure such festivals' accreditation make them not only typical as a festival circuit, but render them particularly relevant to a study of the dominant notions of cinema that film festivals (re)produce. A-list festivals are at once particularly commercialised and particularly influential in the film industry. In part, this is a result of FIAPF's role in managing festivals, since accreditation as A-list is influenced by the association's mediation of industrial and commercial interests. FIAPF (2016) is a regulatory body whose aim is to "facilitate the job of the producers, sales agents and distributors in the management of their relationships with the festivals." Moreover, its accreditation and regulations "constitute a trust contract between those festivals and the film industry at large. Accredited festivals are expected to implement quality and reliability standards that meet industry expectations" (FIAPF, 2016). In other words, FIAPF functions as a mediator between festivals and the film industry, with its accreditation guaranteeing certain standards for film professionals. An accredited film festival must meet certain requirements in order to attract the sales agents, distributors and producers that, in turn, secure the festival's influence. Indeed, the strong commercial presence at A festivals has led to them being dubbed "business festivals," events aimed primarily at facilitating the business of the film industry (Peranson, 2008, p. 38).

While it is reasonable to assume that simply being present in a festival's programme has a positive effect on a film's international success, it is winning awards at A festivals that has a demonstrable impact on a film's distribution.[2] Stephen Mezias et al. (2008, 2011) have shown that winning top prize at Cannes, Venice or Berlin significantly increases the number of countries that a film is distributed in, making entering and winning the main competition at such festivals an attractive strategy for sales agents and distributors. Their study suggests that Best Picture winners are among the most significant cases of films that come to represent a cinema worldwide, achieving the widest global distribution. While there are likely to be exceptions to this rule, Mezias et al.'s findings suggest the value of studying top prize-winning films as a means of identifying and interrogating the dominant notions of art cinema most likely to circulate widely around the globe.

2 For further research on the role of major competitive film festivals in film circulation, see Skadi Loist's project *Film Circulation on the International Film Festival Network and the Impact on Global Film Culture* (2017–2022).

The festivals Mezias et al. use for their analysis are all European A festivals. In fact, even within the "top tier" of the festival hierarchy lies another hierarchy, one that underscores the geopolitical fault lines with which global film culture is riven. Whether in film festivals or the academy, to speak of art cinema is to evoke a struggle to define a certain kind of cinema that has historically taken place through largely Eurocentric structures of film exhibition—including the European A festival circuit. This echoes Galt and Schoonover's (2010) discussion of art cinema as a profoundly politicised "discursive field," inflected by geopolitical power relations and "enmeshed in an imperialist and Eurocentric history" (p. 4). The development of both the film festival phenomenon itself, and the accreditation of film festivals by FIAPF, are expressive of a persistent Eurocentrism in both the industry and the academy.

Julian Stringer's (2001) assessment of film historiography underscores the influence of a select few North-Western competitive film festivals over the canonisation of certain films. Stringer (2001, p. 137) argues that the organisation of the festival circuit is "a metaphor for the geographically uneven development that characterises the world of international film culture." He identifies film scholarship's reproduction of these structures of value, canonising only films that have been recognised by "the apex of international media power, the center of which is located, by implication, at Western film festivals" (p. 135). Vallejo (2020) continues Stringer's argument, drawing our attention to the continuing "cultural hegemony" of specifically European competitive film festivals, as well as the "cultural hierarchies" that this produces within film canons (p. 158). Crucially, Vallejo argues for the need to take a situated approach to the study of film festivals and film canons rather than collapsing the distinctions between national and regional film cultures and reproducing notions of European film culture as universal. Building on Vallejo's proposition, this book explicitly engages with a limited, and situated, circuit of film festivals: European A festivals. I treat these festivals, and their influence, as not universal but contingent and proceed throughout the book to examine the effects of this contingency on institutional meanings of art cinema.

FIAPF's accreditation of film festivals as "A-list" is itself rooted in historical Eurocentrism: the festivals it recognises and standards it requires for recognition were borne of the "Cannes-Venice duopoly" that dominated both European film culture and FIAPF in the postwar years (Pisu, 2018, p. 110). We thus cannot understand the A festival phenomenon without considering the period of postwar European reconstruction in which Cannes and Venice became the circuit's two main nodes of power. As Janet Harbord (2002) argues, the film festival phenomenon was driven by the "broad historical project of rebuilding Europe [...] the consolidation of Europe as a significant player in a global economy" (p. 64). This project gave rise to a proliferation of accredited, European film festivals, starting with Cannes and Venice in 1951, which were recognised immediately following FIAPF's decision to begin accrediting festivals (Strandgaard Pederson & Mazza, 2011, p. 147). Soon after, FIAPF-accredited festivals such as the Berlinale and Karlovy Vary, in a move that was deeply influenced by the diplomatic project of promoting capitalist democracy synonymous with Western Europe and the US (de Valck, 2007; Iordanova, 2009; Cordoba, 2022). As I show in later chapters, these projects continue today through European A festivals' advocation of ideals of cinematic value rooted in traditional notions of European art cinema, and political progressiveness rooted in traditions of European humanism. In promoting such ideals, and legitimising films in relation to them, these festivals maintain Europe's position as central in global film culture and the production of meanings for art cinema.

FIAPF continues to manifest a bias towards European and, more broadly, Global Northern film festivals. This "A-list" is currently comprised of fourteen competitive feature film festivals, of which eight are based in Europe.[3] These include the European "early adopters" of the film festival model, such as Cannes, Venice and Berlin, which established norms that other festivals face "isomorphic pressure" to follow (Standgaard Pederson & Mazza, 2011, p. 145).[4] Since the aim of this book is to analyse and critique the most dominant representations of art cinema by film festivals, I have chosen to focus on films that have won top prize at an A festival within the European sub-section of the A circuit. This has been narrowed down to European A festivals due to their ongoing dominance in the circuit and as a means of limiting this book's corpus to a manageable size. It must be acknowledged, however, that in centring its analysis on European A festivals, this book risks reproducing the uneven structures of power that have materially

3 Of the remaining seven, two are based in the Middle East, two in East Asia, one in South America and one in South Asia. A full list of FIAPF-accredited A festivals can be found in Appendix 1.

4 Strandgaard Pederson and Mazza (2011) list Venice, Moscow, Cannes, Karlovy Vary, Locarno and Berlin. They also discuss Indian, Argentinian and Australian festivals but situate these in relation to the forerunners just mentioned. More detailed research into the extent to which festivals such as the International Film Festival of India straightforwardly adopted the model set out by Venice and others would illuminate or perhaps challenge these scholars' argument. IFFI was founded in 1952, early in the history of film festivals' development and shortly after India's formal decolonisation in 1949.

and discursively placed such festivals in a hegemonic position. As scholars such as Antoine Damiens (2020) have argued, there is a need to undo the demarcations between different festival types, above all between this "top tier" of international, competitive feature film festivals and specialised or identity-based film festivals. Robbins and Saglier (2015, p. 4), for example, seek to put all film festivals on an equal footing of attention, and acknowledge the "porosity" of the film festival network. Although taking European A festivals as its case study, this book aims to open a conversation about the ideological functioning—the mechanisms of meaning creation and legitimisation—of film festivals in general, as well as the possible flows of prestige between them.

Moreover, it is impossible to ignore the many calls to decolonise film studies, including film festival studies, calls in which I have participated elsewhere (Johnson & O'Leary, 2022; Johnson, forthcoming). Scholars such those cited above, as well as Lindiwe Dovey, Joshua McNamara and Federico Olivieri (2013; Dovey, 2015), and Abé Marcus Nornes (2013) have rightly challenged the Eurocentric model through which film festivals have often been researched. This book at once replicates and aims to undermine this model: it situates the European A festival phenomenon in a way that challenges the uncritical positioning of European film cultures as universal or central. (I directly challenge such positioning, effected by European A festivals themselves, throughout the book.) To be clear: decolonisation is a distinct project, the appropriation of which has been warned against by Indigenous scholars such as Eve Tuck and K. Wayne Wang (2012). This book, in its focus on European film festivals and Italian cinema, as well as its use of Anglo-French psychoanalytic theory (see the following chapter), is not decolonial. However, it aims to support ongoing, vital calls for decolonisation by making explicit the structures of imperialist power where they would otherwise remain implicit (Bhambra et al. 2018). I seek to offer a modest contribution to scholarship that highlights the stakes of decolonisation by tracing such imperialist histories via European film festivals and Italian cinema, as well as by identifying and critiquing the values, norms and ideological structures that constitute hegemonic ideas of "art cinema" today. While focusing on Italian cinema, I aim to draw attention to systems of value that may pertain to the institutional legitimisation of a range of cinemas, including those associated with Asia, South America and Africa. In making such values—the "unwritten rules" of European A-list film festivals—explicit, I hope to provide a basis for further analyses of the discursive power that film festivals wield; in interrogating them, I seek to further support demands for the decolonisation of global film culture.

Film Festivals and Italian Cinema

Italian cinema is a central pillar of dominant conceptions of art cinema and its sites of exhibition. While the concept of national cinema has been problematised down to its most basic meanings, signifiers of nationality continue to carry weight in the institutional construction of film (Hjort & Mackenzie, 2000; Bergfelder, 2005; Higson, 2020). European A festivals continue to highlight films' supposed nationalities in their programmes and, as will become clear throughout this book, also tend to situate films within national cinematic traditions either explicitly or implicitly through their marketing copy. Although I acknowledge the risk of homogenising the idea of art cinema by attempting to view it through one case of a national cinema, I treat the study of European A festivals and art cinema *through* Italian cinema as a largely experimental iteration that offers a starting point rather than an end point for inquiry. I have chosen to use a relatively small unit of art cinema (a singular national cinema) as a means to test out the hypotheses I put forward above, and a particular methodology—ideology critique—that I discuss in detail in the next chapter. In other words, I have chosen to use something relatively small (Italian cinema) as a means of looking at some very big things (film festivals, art cinema and ideology), with the ultimate aim of stimulating discussion rather than offering a definitive statement on either. The case of Italian cinema was selected for its historical centrality to the film festival phenomenon as well as the roles of Italian neorealism and auteur cinema in producing dominant notions of art cinema: both afford a productive significance to the study of art cinema's institutional construction. The Italian film industry is, too, representative as one whose films depend on exposure at film festivals for access to the international film market. My hope, then, is that an investigation of European A festivals' construction of a representative case such as Italian cinema can offer a place from which future inquiries into A festivals' ideological construction of films might begin.

National cinemas, like art cinema, must be treated as contested categories: they are part of taxonomies of filmmaking produced and reproduced at film festivals and in the academy. Italian film scholars have underscored the role of institutions in constructing a narrow canon of "legitimate" films. This institutional legitimisation is usually conditioned by a film's perceived relationship to certain traditions of Italian filmmaking—again, neorealism and auteur cinema (Hipkins & Renga, 2016). Working through this perspective, several studies have questioned the unacknowledged aspects of these national cinematic legacies in relation to gender, sexuality, post-colonialism and notions of "worthy" cinema.[5] However, the institution that Italian film studies has thus far been most attentive to is the academy itself, notwithstanding some investigations into journalistic film criticism (O'Rawe, 2008) and state funding (Manzonli & Minuz, 2017). While focusing on higher education, Hipkins and Renga (2016) identify several institutions that contribute to the process of canon-making, including the Italian Ministry of Cultural Heritage and Activities (Ministero per i beni e le attività culturali, MiBACT), universities and film festivals. Considering these together as a network from which the "new canon" of contemporary Italian film emerges, Hipkins and Renga point to the importance of taking a holistic approach to the construction of Italian film and the need to begin researching each of the institutions involved in such a process.

We find a focus on film festivals in one study of Italian film circulation, Damiano Garofalo's "Italian Cinema in the Shadow of the Film Festival Crisis" (2018). Garofalo highlights the importance of Italian cinema to film festivals, observing the "notably high presence" of Italian films at ten major international film festivals in 2008–2017.[6] While this indicates the continuing relevance of Italian cinema to these institutions, Garofalo also shows that film festivals maintain influence over the circulation of Italian cinema. Many of the Italian films selected at these events have since secured international distribution, and every prizewinner was distributed in at least ten countries beyond Italy. This confirms Mezias et al.'s (2011) claim that winning top prize leads to greater international circulation for films.

However, Garofalo (2018) identifies a decline in the presence of Italian cinema at these festivals between 2011 and 2017, and suggests that film festivals themselves are waning in influence. We should be wary of drawing conclusions about the importance of festivals to the construction of Italian cinema from this data alone. Although the emergence of digital platforms such as Mubi and Netflix raises significant questions about the channels through which Italian films come to be distributed, and how these platforms may influence the kind of Italian cinema with which international audiences become familiar, we should note that this is still a relatively recent phenomenon. Garofalo's piece indicates a shift in power that has undoubtedly been accelerated by the unprecedented rise in online film

5 See Hipkins (2008), Rigoletto (2014), O'Rawe (2008), Schoonover (2012) and O'Leary (2017), respectively.

6 The festivals are: Cannes, Venice, Berlin, Toronto, Locarno, San Sebastian, Sundance, Turin, Rome and London. Garofalo (2018) describes these as "ten of the most important international film festivals," although the criteria for selection are not defined within the piece.

streaming during the COVID-19 pandemic. However, the extent to which this has resulted in films that otherwise would have screened at festivals being distributed through major online platforms is not yet clear (Johnson, 2021). In any case, despite the changes that have taken place over the last ten years, film festivals have been consolidating notions of both art cinema and Italian cinema for almost a century. If film festivals were to disappear tomorrow, their legacy would continue in the notions of artistic value that they have established over a long history of influence.

Over the course of this history, Italy and Italian cinema have been crucial to both the development of the film festival phenomenon and the construction of global art cinema. The first international film festival was an Italian festival: Venice, then known as the *Mostra internazionale d'arte cinematografica*. The earliest of early adopters, Venice's first edition afforded an initial iteration of the international festival template in 1932. The *Mostra* exhibited films from around the world and held an international competition. The competition eventually fell prey to the Fascist state's cultural politics, awarding prizes only to Italian and German films that promoted fascistic ideals, and launching a controversy that would inspire the founding of Cannes soon after. Yet, after the fall of Fascism and the end of World War II, Venice continued to be one of the hegemonic centres of European cinema and the film festival network, constituting one half of the "Venice-Cannes duopoly" and one of the so-called "big three" international film festivals alongside Cannes and the Berlinale.[7]

Together with Cannes, Venice was also one of the first festivals to receive "A" accreditation from FIAPF, and Italian film industry members wielded considerable influence over the federation in its early years. FIAPF was based in Rome between 1950 and 1956 and led by an Italian, Renato Gualino.[8] Meanwhile, the only festival director invited to the federation's first congress in 1950 was Antonio Petrucci of the Venice film festival. Reenforcing its influence over the European festival circuit, Venice also established the first film market in 1950. Cannes quickly emulated, holding its own market in 1951. Historically, Italy and, in particular, Venice, affords the origin of many features that characterise the European A circuit: the existence of an international competition, "A" accreditation by FIAPF, and close links

7 The notion of the "big three" festivals is as ubiquitous in industry and academia as it is reflective of the Eurocentrism discussed above. See, among others, Fehrenbach (1995), Wong (2011), Chan (2011) and Loist (2016).

8 The historical data used here and throughout the rest of this paragraph is taken from Pisu (2018, p. 111).

to international trade prioritised by such festivals and exemplified by the presence of film markets at some of them. This influence continues today, with Venice remaining one of the most prestigious film festivals worldwide.

Venice's global prominence secures a measure of influence for the Italian film industry as well. Historically, this was particularly the case in film festivals' "nationalist" phase, in which each festival's primary aim was to showcase the cinema of its host nation (de Valck, 2007, p. 58). While festivals have moved into a globalised or "post-national" phase, as signalled by their installation of international juries, these events continue to be important tools in the development of national film industries, as evidenced by their continuing state support, justified on precisely such grounds (de Valck, 2007, p. 68; Andrews, 2010, p. 10). The Venice festival is no exception, receiving state funding from the Fascist era to the present as a means of supporting the Italian film industry at large (Wood, 2005, p. 111). Meanwhile, European A festivals still manifest a commitment to national cinema through their selection and recognition of domestic films in the main competition, and their inclusion of programme sections dedicated to domestic films.[9]

It is therefore little coincidence that the three national cinemas historically associated with art cinema often correspond to the three biggest film festivals' countries of origin: Italy (Venice), France (Cannes) and Germany (Berlin). (We might also add Spanish cinema, which the San Sebastián film festival has done much to promote alongside Lusophone cinema more generally.) Besides the importance of Venice to the development of the European A circuit, we can also observe the importance of Italian cinema to the development of concepts of art cinema promoted by film festivals and scholars alike. The notions of art cinema reenforced in both scholarship and at film festivals have traditionally been grounded in a European cinema defined largely in relation to Italian neorealism and the French New Wave. The initial examples of art cinema that Neale (1981) gives are not only European, but Italian—neorealism and the auteur cinema represented by Michelangelo Antonioni and Federico Fellini. Neale then moves on to case studies of three European national cinemas: French, German and Italian. That this Eurocentric conceptualisation of art cinema persists in academic accounts of global art cinema today has been amply shown, and critiqued, by scholars, as discussed above.

Italian neorealism has often been treated as foundational to global art cinema. Historicising the development of art cinema as a concept, Galt and Schoonover (2010, p. 15) argue that "art cinema's cohesion as a category

9 See Chapter 6.

first emerges with the popularity of Italian neorealism, and it retains a close association with the thematic and aesthetic impulses of that postwar tradition." Schoonover (2012, p. 218) continues:

> Neorealism [...] sets the standard for European new wave cinemas, post-colonial cinemas, cinemas of social change and political liberation, the American "new independents" of the 1970s and late twentieth-century explorations of realism by Italian, Danish, Romanian, and Chinese cinemas.

Indeed, we can observe that one of the founding moments of European A festivals also marks the inauguration of Italian neorealism's international success. The first iteration of Cannes in 1946 sparked the development of the European festival phenomenon in the context of postwar reconstruction and anti-fascist sentiment. This edition culminated in the jury awarding Italian neorealist film *Rome, Open City* (*Roma città aperta*, Rossellini, 1945) its highest accolade. De Valck (2007, p. 49) underlines the importance of Rosselini's film to Cannes: "the revelation of the 1946 festival was the anti-fascist *Roma, Città Aperta*." This moment highlights the reciprocal relationship between Italian cinema and film festivals. *Rome, Open City*'s presentation at Cannes helped to generate the mythology surrounding the festival and then the festivals that came to emulate it. Meanwhile, Cannes contributed to the mythology surrounding Italian neorealism and, later, the notions of global art cinema set against such a standard.[10]

This reciprocity characterises festivals' relationship not only with Italian neorealism, but also with Italian auteur cinema (a trope established through 1950s and '60s filmmaking in relation to directors such as Fellini and Antonioni). Reading Mary Wood's (2005) analysis of auteur cinema alongside Cindy Hing-Yuk Wong's (2011) examination of film festivals renders the comparison clear. Wood (2005, p. 135) argues that competing for recognition on the festival circuit has been a crucial strategy for Italian directors from the heyday of auteur cinema to the present. She observes that contemporary auteurs such as Nanni Moretti "follow the regular pattern of authorial stylistic flourishes and serious themes, playing the festival circuits in order to gain recognition, which will lead to international distribution"

10 This mythology has repeatedly been shown to hold influence over institutional accounts of Italian and world cinema alike. See descriptions of neorealism (and the notions of an ethical, humanist realism that accompany it) as the "insidious common sense" of Italian film studies (O'Leary & O'Rawe, 2011, p. 109). I explore the legacy of neorealism and a very European humanism in relation to *Fire at Sea* and migration narratives in Chapter 5.

(Wood, 2005, p. 135). If "playing the festival circuits" in this way is typical of Italian directors' strategies to access recognition and distribution, so nurturing auteurs is part of film festivals' attempts to define themselves and art cinema. Wong (2011) argues that Cannes's cultivation of Antonioni is typical of the way in which film festivals celebrate certain directors to define the kind of cinema they value, and on which they stake their prestige. It is perhaps telling that the case study Wong uses is that of the archetypal Italian auteur I have already mentioned twice in this introduction: Antonioni. In fact, as recent archival research shows, the canonisation of Antonioni—and, we can now add, Fellini—was part of a conscious strategy on the part of the festival director, Robert Favre Le Bret, to build Cannes's reputation through the nurturing of Italian auteurs (Coladonato, 2021).

Film festivals have thus been crucial to the development of a certain kind of exportable Italian cinema, beginning with Italian neorealism and auteur cinema, while neorealism and auteur cinema have been crucial to the creation of a certain "image" for European festivals. Tropes of neorealism and auteur cinema recur in this book's analysis of the ideology of European A festivals. Such an analysis has required me to repeatedly grapple with notions of art associated with the auteur and the political vision associated with neorealism. Both continue to appear in contemporary representations of Italian cinema by European film festivals. Moreover, the development of Italian cinema by festivals also appears to have influenced these institutions' construction of their "image" and that of art cinema in general.

Italian film is a key example of a national cinema that depends upon film festivals for international legitimisation and circulation. Moreover, it is the source of several tropes through which European A festivals construct art cinema more generally. Italian cinema constitutes a significant example of the kind of film valued by European A festivals, through which the circuit both defines itself and the cinema it seeks to construct. While the examples cited above are largely historical (with the exception of Nanni Moretti) this book seeks to demonstrate the reciprocal relationship between European film festivals and Italian cinema in the new millennium, a relationship marked by an enduring attachment to the mythologies of neorealism and auteurism, and the exclusions on which they are based.

Book Outline

This book offers in-depth analyses of five case studies—five Italian films that have won Best Picture or equivalent at a European A festival since the year 2000. I supplement these analyses with a discussion of other Italian award-winners in the conclusion. Since my primary concern is with how festivals construct Italian cinema, I have used festivals' own designations of a film's nationality when selecting Italian films for the corpus. This book initially takes European A festivals' symbolic representation of cinema at its word, yet does so precisely as a means of critiquing them. This approach is, in part, informed by Slavoj Žižek's (2005, p. 71) proposition that the most effective critique of ideology entails "over-identification" with it: taking it at its word as a means of bringing its implicit laws into view.[11] The corpus reproduces the hegemony of the Northern Hemisphere by focusing on European A festivals, and it reproduces the assumptions regarding art cinema by focusing on Italian films that have won top prize at such festivals. It also reproduces, on a basic level, European A festivals' definition of Italian cinema in that it treats films as Italian if they are defined as such by the European A festival that has awarded it top prize. Such a definition is, as I discuss extensively in Chapter 3, a gendered one, too: the films awarded top prize are all directed by cisgender men (though not entirely, albeit mostly, white and heterosexual). This corpus reproduces, in short, the dominant ideas of art cinema and the geopolitical and gendered power structures in which such ideas are embedded. However, I do not take such notions as either fixed or universal: I treat concepts such as the Global North and Europe, art cinema and Italian cinema as inherently unstable and thus open to critique. Initially drawing from these ideological constructions provides the terrain from which we might destabilise such terms at their foundations.

Following a discussion of the study's theoretical framework and methodology in chapter 1, the book proceeds in three sections, with chapters alternating between considerations of overarching ideological structures and their particular expressions. Section 1 analyses European A festivals' claims to an artistic universality predicated on the celebration of the auteur and, moreover, an auteur who is typically gendered male and his artistic vision masculine. I examine these constructions through the hysterically auteurist Nanni Moretti film, *The Son's Room* (*La stanza del figlio*, 2001) and indulgent, Fellini-esque male melodrama, *The Great Beauty* (*La grande bellezza*, Paolo Sorrentino, 2013). Section 2 focuses on political universality, with Chapter 4 identifying European A festivals' preoccupation with figures of the other, as exemplified in Karlovy Vary's representation of queer Holocaust melodrama *Facing Window* (*La finestra di fronte*, Ferzan Özpetek, 2003). Chapter 5 focuses in on a particular figure of the other

11 On ideology critique, film festivals and Žižek, see the next chapter.

integral to European A festivals' geopolitically-inflected humanism, that of the North African migrant, represented in the contentious docu-fiction *Fire at Sea* (*Fuocoammare*, Gianfranco Rosi, 2016).

An investigation of the role of European A festivals' embeddedness in global capitalism guides the book. While I begin this line of reasoning in Chapter 2, examining auteurism's role in disavowing commercial constraint, Section 3 provides a sustained analysis of the relationship between film festivals, ideology and capital. The final case study, *Gomorrah* (*Gomorra*, Matteo Garrone, 2008), highlights European A festivals' displacement of the excesses of capital onto a fantasmatic Global South. Meanwhile, the conclusion outlines the generative function of capital in European A festivals' ideological construction of art cinema, and finishes by calling for a decolonial, anti-capitalist cinephilia.

I have chosen to analyse the films that are most representative of the ideological procedures and effects that I have found when examining the entire corpus. To avoid duplication, I have not included in-depth analyses of films that present similar information. The secondary case studies in the corpus, and discussed in the conclusion, are: *A Children's Story* (*Certi bambini*, Andrea and Antonio Frazzi, 2004), *Private* (Saverio Costanzo, 2004), *Caesar Must Die* (*Cesare deve morire*, Paolo and Vittorio Taviani, 2011, and *Sacro GRA* (Gianfranco Rosi, 2013). For reference, lists of A festivals and the Italian films that have won Best Picture or equivalent at a European A festival since 1946 can be found in the appendices. I include this to help clarify some of the general points I make in the book, including those above. I also hope that this data will facilitate future work on European film festivals and Italian cinema, offering an indication of some of the broad trends in Italian cinema's awarding and representation by European A festivals more generally. (The trends are necessarily superficial but can help to spur for more detailed analyses of the phenomenon.) I also include the synopses of the secondary case studies (Appendix 3) for reference while reading the conclusion.

Bibliography

Ahn, S. (2012). *The Pusan International Film Festival, South Korean cinema and globalization*. Hong Kong University Press.

Andrews, D. (2010). Art cinema as institution, redux: Art houses, film festivals, and film studies. *Scope: An Online Journal of Film and Television Studies*, *18*, 1–21.

Bergfelder, T. (2005). National, transnational or supranational cinema? Rethinking European film studies. *Media, culture & society*, *27*(3), 315–331.

Bhambra, G. K. et al. (2018). *Decolonising the university.* Pluto Press.

Chan, F. (2011). The international film festival and the making of a national cinema. *Screen, 52*(2), 253–260.

Cheung, R. (2016). Ever-changing readjustments: The political economy of the Hong Kong International Film Festival (HKIFF). *New Review of Film and Television Studies, 14*(1), 59–75.

Coladonato, V. (2021). "Mon cher Fédérico": Fellini and the Cannes Film Festival. *Journal of Italian Cinema & Media Studies, 9*(1), 117–132.

Cordoba, C. (2022). The Locarno Film Festival under the influence? Programming Eastern European movies in anti-communist Switzerland (1946–1962). *Contemporary European History: First View, 1*(1), 1–19.

Damiens, A. (2020). *LGBTQ festivals: Curating queerness.* Amsterdam University Press.

De Valck, M. (2007). *Film festivals: From European geopolitics to global cinephilia.* Amsterdam University Press.

De Valck, M. (2013). Migration and film festivals. In I. Ness (Ed.), *The encyclopedia of global human migration* (Vol. 3, pp. 1502–1504). Wiley-Blackwell.

De Valck, M. (2014). Film festivals, Bourdieu, and the economization of culture. *Canadian Journal of Film Studies, 23*(1), 74–89.

Dovey, L. 2015. *Curating Africa in the age of film festivals.* Palgrave Macmillan.

Dovey, L. et al. (2013). "From, by, for" – Nairobi's slum film festival, film festival studies, and the practices of development. *Jump Cut: A Review of Contemporary Media, 55*(1). Available from: http://ejumpcut.org/archive/jc55.2013/DoveySFFNairobi/index.html

FIAPF (International Federation of Film Producers Associations). (2023). *Accredited festivals: Competitive feature film festivals.* [Online]. Available from: https://fiapf.org/festivals/accredited-festivals/competitive-feature-film-festivals

FIAPF (International Federation of Film Producers Associations). (2019). *FIAPF accredited festivals directory: 2016 edition.* [Online]. Available from: https://fiapf.org/festival_file/fiapf-accredited-festivals-directory-2019-edition/

FIAPF (International Federation of Film Producers Associations). (2016). *International film festivals signed FIAPF's mutual trust contract and received accreditation in 2016.* [Online]. Available from: http://www.fiapf.org/intfilmfestivals.asp

Elsaesser, T. (2005). *European cinema: Face to face with Hollywood.* Amsterdam University Press.

Fehrenbach, H. (1995). *Cinema in democratizing Germany: Reconstructing of national identity after Hitler.* University of North Carolina Press.

Galt, R., & Schoonover, K. (2010). Introduction: The impurity of art cinema. In R. Galt & K. Schoonover (Eds.), *Global art cinema: New theories and histories* (pp. 3–27). Oxford University Press.

Garofalo, D. (2018). Italian Cinema in the Shadow of Film Festival Crisis. *International Circulation of Italian Cinema*. [Online]. Accessed 01/04/2019. Available from: https://www.italiancinema.it/italian-cinema-in-the-shadow-of-film-festival-crisis/

Harbord, J. (2002). *Film cultures*. Sage Publications.

Higson, A. (1989). The concept of national cinema. *Screen, 30*(4), 36–47.

Higson, A. (2020). *Soft power and national cinema: James Bond, Great Britain and Brexit*. In R. Dwyer (Ed.), *Cinema and soft power: Configuring the national and transnational in geo-politics* (pp. 210–235). Edinburgh University Press.

Hipkins, D. (2008). Why Italian film studies needs a second take on gender. *Italian Studies, 63*(2), 213–234.

Hipkins, D., & Renga, D. (2016). A new canon? Contemporary Italian cinema and television and the role of quality in the anglophone curriculum. *Comunicazioni sociali, 1*(3), 375–397.

Hjort, M., & MacKenzie, S. (2000). *Cinema and nation*. Routledge.

Iordanova, D. (2009). The festival circuit. In D. Iordanova & R. Rhyne (Eds.), *Film festival yearbook 1: The festival circuit* (pp. 23–39). St Andrews Film Studies and College Gate Press.

Iordanova, D., & Rhyne, R. (2009). Introduction. In D. Iordanova & R. Rhyne (Eds.), *Film festival yearbook 1: The festival circuit* (pp. 1–9). St Andrews Film Studies and College Gate Press.

Jeong, S. (2021). World cinema in a global frame. *Studies in World Cinema, 1*(1), 29–38.

Johnson, R. (2021). Film circulation in times of coronavirus. *Curating and Exhibiting Visual Culture in Times of Coronavirus*. [Online]. Available from: https://ahc.leeds.ac.uk/downloads/download/230/sadler_blog_post_1_film_circulation_in_times_of_coronavirus

King, G. (2022). *Positioning art cinema: Film and cultural value*. Bloomsbury.

Loist, S. (2016). The film festival circuit: Networks, hierarchies and circulation. In M. de Valck, D. B. Kredell, & S. Loist (Eds.), *Film festivals: History, theory, method, practice* (pp. 49–64). Routledge.

Loist, S. (2017–2022). *Film circulation on the international film festival network and the impact on global film culture*. Project website: http://www.filmcirculation.net/

Manzoli, G., & Minuz, A. (Eds.). (2017). *Il cinema di stato: finanziamento pubblico ed economia simbolica nel cinema italiano contemporaneo*. Il Mulino.

Mazdon, L. (2006). The Cannes Film Festival as transnational space. *Post Script, 25*(2), 19–30.

Mezias, S. et al. (2008). Much ado about nothing? Untangling the impact of European premier film festivals. *Creative Encounters Research Paper Series, 14*, 1–31.

Mezias, S. et al. (2011). Transforming film product identities: The status effects of European premier film festivals, 1996–2005. In B. Moeran & J. S. Pedersen (Eds.),

Negotiating values in the creative industries: Fairs, festivals and competitive events (pp. 169–196). Cambridge University Press.
Neale, S. (1981). Art cinema as institution. *Screen*, *22*(1), 11–40.
Nichols, B. (1994). Discovering form, inferring meaning: New cinemas and the film festival circuit. *Film Quarterly*, *47*(3), 16–30.
Nornes, A. M. (2013). Asian film festivals, translation and the international film festival short circuits. In D. Iordanova (Ed.), *The film festival reader* (pp. 245–262). St. Andrews Film Studies.
O'Leary, A. (2017). What is Italian cinema? *California Italian Studies*, *7*(1), 1–26.
O'Rawe, C. (2008). "I padri e i maestri": Genre, auteurs, and absences in Italian film studies. *Italian Studies*, *63*(2), 173–194.
Paz Peirano, M. (2021). Between industry labs and audience formation: Film festivals and the transformation of the field of film production in Chile. *Loisir et Société/ Society and Leisure*, *44*(1), 47–65.
Peranson, M. (2008). First you get the power, then you get the money: Two models of film festivals. *Cineaste*, *33*(3), 37–43.
Pisu, S. (2018). A transnational love-hate relationship: The FIAPF and the Venice and Cannes film festivals (1950–1970). In T. Jenkins (Ed.), *International film festivals. Contemporary cultures and history beyond Venice and Cannes* (pp. 109–131). Bloomsbury.
Rhyne, R. (2009). Film festivals circuits and stakeholders. In D. Iordanova & R. Rhyne (Eds.), *Film festival yearbook 1: The festival circuit* (pp. 9–22). St. Andrews Film Studies & College Gate Press.
Rigoletto, S. (2014). *Masculinity and Italian cinema: Sexual politics, social conflict and male crisis in the 1970s*. Edinburgh University Press.
Robbins, P., & Saglier, V. (2015). Introduction. Other networks: Expanding film festival Perspectives. *Synoptique*, *3*(2), 1–8.
Schoonover, K. (2012). *Brutal vision: The neorealist body in postwar Italian cinema*. University of Minnesota Press.
Sendra, E. (2020). Dak'Art. 30 years of arts curation and reception in postcolonial African societies. *Arts Management Quarterly*, *135*(1), 65–71.
Shambu, G. (2019). For a new cinephilia. *Film Quarterly*, *72*(3), 32–34.
Strandgaard Pedersen, J., & Mazza, C. (2011). International film festivals: For the benefit of whom? *Culture Unbound*, *3*, 139–165.
Stringer, J. (2001). Global cities and the international film festival economy. In T. Shiel & T. Fitzmaurice (Eds.), *Cinema and the city: Film and urban societies in a global context* (pp. 134–144). Blackwell.
Tuck, E., & Wang, K. W. (2012). Decolonization is not a metaphor. *Decolonization: Indigeneity, Education & Society*, *1*(1), 1–40.
Vallejo, A. (2020). Rethinking the canon: The role of film festivals in shaping film history. *Studies in European Cinema*, *17*(2), 155–169.

Wong, C. H-Y. (2011). *Film festivals: Culture, people, and power on the global screen.* Rutgers University Press.
Wood, M. P. (2005). *Italian cinema.* Bloomsbury Academic.
Žižek, S. (2005). *The metastases of enjoyment: Six essays on women and causality.* Verso.

Filmography

A Children's Story (*Certi bambini*) (2004). Frazzi, A., & Frazzi, A. dirs. Italy.
Ceasar Must Die (*Cesare deve morire*) (2012). Taviani, P., & Taviani, V. dirs. Italy.
Facing Window (*La finestra di fronte*) (2003). Özpetek, F. dir. Italy.
Fire at Sea (*Fuocoammare*) (2016). Rosi, G. dir. Italy.
Gomorrah (*Gomorra*) (2008). Garrone, M. dir. Italy.
The Great Beauty (*La grande bellezza*) (2013). Sorrentino, P. dir. Italy.
Private (2004). Costanzo, S. dir. Italy.
The Son's Room (*La stanza del figlio*) (2001). Moretti, N. dir. Italy.
Sacro GRA (2013). Rosi, G. dir. Italy.

1. Film Festivals and Ideology Critique

Abstract: This chapter outlines the book's theoretical framework and methodology. I reframe ideas of quality, taste and aesthetics through ideology—a term long present, yet under-theorised in film festival studies. I argue that rehabilitating the study of ideology is necessary for the development of rigorous, left-wing analyses of contemporary art institutions such as festivals, intervening in both the discursive and economic realities they (re)produce. This chapter adapts theories rooted in Lacanian psychoanalysis, and particularly the work of Slavoj Žižek, to examine the workings of festival apparatuses, paratexts, and cinematic excess. The methodology follows a three-tier critical procedure, bringing into dialogue festivals' operational and material contexts, their representation of themselves and the films they exhibit, and the excessive qualities of such films.

Keywords: art cinema, cinematic excess, cultural value, paratexts, psychoanalysis

Introduction: From Quality to Ideology

In 2012, film curator Roya Rastegar announced that film festivals had entered a state of "curatorial crisis" (p. 310). With the proliferation of digital technologies for making and exhibiting films, the terms used to justify festivals' gatekeeping of an exponentially expanding film culture were beginning to look ever more unstable. In Rastegar's article, festivals' claim to a monopoly on "quality" shows itself as underpinned by "ideologically charged notions of taste and aesthetics" and the exclusion of "cinematic sensibilities that flourish on the margins of film culture and wider society" (p. 310). While later chapters in this book grapple with several questions that Rastegar's polemic raises—questions of exclusion and difference, national identity and the framing of the Global South—I would like to pause on the implications of bringing together these two ideas: quality and ideology. Although ideology

Johnson, R., Film Festivals, *Ideology and Italian Art Cinema: Politics, Histories and Cultural Value.* Taylor & Francis Group, 2024
DOI 10.5117/9789463720366_CH01

plays only a brief (if significant) role in Rastegar's piece and, as I discuss below, remains relatively un-theorised in film festival studies, the article represents something of a culmination of debates around the mobilisation of "quality" as a vague and sometimes obscurantist term used to secure the legitimacy of film festivals in global film culture. By following the short history of polemics against "quality" in film festival studies, we can trace the roots of the crisis Rastegar decries, as well as the importance of apprehending this crisis through the study of ideology.

At an early conference on film festivals, programmer and critic B. Ruby Rich (2003) argued that such institutions operate according to "the worship of taste." Rich observes that any suggestion that film festival programming might follow an agenda is "seen as interfering with the magical and utterly unsubstantiated notion of quality." Taste and quality, therefore, are the subjects of "worship" or "magic," unaffected by earthly concerns such as commerce and beyond question by those mortals outside of the festival covenant. Thomas Elsaesser (2005) takes the argument further, stating that Rich "underestimates the ritual, religious and quasi-magical elements necessary to make a festival into an 'event'" (p. 99). Such elements are written into the very fabric of film festivals as institutions capable of legitimising films: the festival "requires an atmosphere where an almost Eucharistic transubstantiation can take place; a Spirit has to hover that can canonise a masterpiece or consecrate an auteur, which is why the notions of 'quality' or 'talent have to be impervious to rational criteria or secondary elaborations" (Elsaesser, 2005, p. 99).

Andrews (2010) continues Elsaesser's theistic metaphor, but in a more satirical vein: film festivals "have increasingly adopted an air of bogus religiosity" in which the "objects of reverence" that they consecrate appear "absolute" (p. 9). Andrews posits that this "bogus religiosity" is a result of film festivals' need to legitimise not only art cinema, but *themselves*, to position themselves as crucial nodes in the film industry. In this way, the requirement for festivals to claim cultural relevance (and, ultimately, attract funding) appears to result in these events' cultivation of a deific authority regarding the consecration of certain films and, in turn, the construction of art cinema. As we will see below, the constitution of meaning through a series of unwritten yet seemingly absolute rules is the ideological structure *par excellence*: ideology functions not through the explicit representations of its objects, but rather through a set of implicit laws that afford such representations an illusory consistency, that function only to the extent they remain unarticulated, or "unsubstantiated," much in the way that "quality" does above. For now, it suffices to note that, if ideology can broadly be thought of as the attempt to designate a fixed meaning to an unstable object of representation, film festivals' apparent drive to fix art cinema's meaning so firmly that it takes on a quasi-religious absolutism pushes this definition to its extreme.

On the other side of discussions of the "Eucharistic transubstantiation" of films into art cinema lies the study of the practices and influences behind this process. In one of the first international workshops for film festival studies, Dina Iordanova (in Brown, 2009, p. 217) outlined several aspects of film festivals yet to be investigated. Among these was the way in which "the choice of films at a festival reflects a certain ideological standpoint, be that entirely coherent or otherwise." Another concern, which intersects with the first, was the situation of "film festivals as part of an enormous global culture industry" (p. 217). Indeed, one of the most discussed points at the workshop appeared to be film festivals' self-mythologisation,[1] discussed by Saer Maty Ba and David Slocum (cited in Brown, 2009) in relation to ideology and economics: "[f]ilm festivals always (seek to) represent something or someone (consciously or not, they reflect an ideology), and they always serve political (and economic) interests" (pp. 218–219). Several scholars have examined the intersections between the mediation of interests and representation at film festivals—in short, their particular ideological standpoints—for example in relation to the welcoming or exclusion of migrants (Ostrowska, 2019), the geopolitics of the Cold War (de Valck, 2007; Fehrenbach, 1995) and the maintenance of colonial power relations (Dovey, 2015). However, there has not yet been a systematic study of the ideological mechanisms through which film festivals function, particularly on the level of representation or discourse. Nor has there been an attempt to identify common ideological operations and shared values across a specific festival circuit.

To respond to such absences, this book develops a method for studying the relationship between economic and geopolitical factors, shared norms or values, and film festivals' representation of both films and themselves. My emphasis throughout is on representation: the ways in which film festivals' production of texts and other pronouncements on films are at once conditioned by the factors I have just mentioned and, in turn, condition the construction of ideas about cinema, as well as aesthetic value and political expression. As I discuss at length below, this lattice of material

1 A term that builds on Barthes's theory of myth. Theories of ideology and myth have been taken as complementary by Barthes himself, and scholars who interpret and apply his theory (Barthes 2012 [1957]; Lule 1995; Walton 2012).

(e.g., economic) and discursive (i.e., representational) elements can be helpfully conceptualised as ideology, both from a theoretical standpoint and in dialogue with writing on film festivals' *modus operandi*. Building on this conceptualisation, I propose a methodology of ideology critique adapted to, and created through, the study of film festivals.

Due to my focus on representation, the methodology I propose adapts theories of ideology critique with roots in poststructural analysis—in particular, contemporary reformulations of the psychoanalytical theories of Jacques Lacan. Outlining concepts such as the festival apparatus, the festival paratext and the cinematic Real, I trace the coordinates of a three-tier critical procedure that brings into dialogue festivals' operational and material contexts, their representation of themselves and their films, and the unruly or excessive qualities of the films themselves. I use this method to analyse film festivals' production of values around Italian art cinema—that is, their creation of canons, counter-canons and taxonomies, as well as their circulation of ideas about aesthetics and politics. Through ideology critique, the structures of meaning implicit within those notions of "quality" at the centre of film festivals' rhetorical operation (and crisis) can be rendered explicit and thus interrogated, creating a ground from which we might better understand film festivals and, if we wish, advocate for change.

Film Festival Studies and Ideology Critique

Since its brief utterance at the 2009 workshop cited above, the term "ideology" and the methods of studying it have remained relatively absent from film festival scholarship. Film festival studies, as an interdisciplinary field of inquiry, brings together a wide range of theories and methods, largely motivated by the complexity of film festivals themselves. The majority of these methods have been qualitative, ranging from archival research to ethnographic studies, to Marijke de Valck's (2007) and Thomas Elsaesser's (2005) pioneering applications of Bruno Latour's (1996) Actor Network Theory. Film festival studies, too, has repeatedly engaged in methodological self-reflection, with scholars coming together often to "collectively think about how to methodologically study the messy objects that film festivals are in their everyday business" (Loist, 2020, p. 42). Given the diversity of approaches and commitment to self-reflection that characterise the field, the latency of a methodology of ideology critique merits consideration. This method has remained conspicuously absent from qualitative studies of the festival phenomenon, and is often considered antithetical to the quantitative methods becoming more prevalent in film festival studies.[2]

The latter charge is grounded in the anti-empiricist polemics of twentieth-century and particularly 1970s Marxist literature (e.g., Horton, 1972), the arguments of which have been developed in more recent work on ideology and media (e.g., Taylor 2010). Yet, such challenges to empiricism have also inadvertently given rise to the view that studies of ideology may be subject to imprecision, incapable of the kind of systematic rigour to which academic inquiry, quantitative or qualitative, is bound. This view is epitomised in Noël Carroll's (1998, p. 360) claim that

> ideology critique is not usually an investigation into the conditions of possibility of the objects of study [...]. It is criticism, most frequently negative criticism, and not critique, properly so called.

Although writing from a cognitivist and "post-theoretical" position, expressed elsewhere in his and David Bordwell's *Post-Theory* (1996), Carroll presents a common challenge to scholars engaged in studying ideology and film, in the Anglophone academy at least. Carroll was writing of what he perceived as a trend in cultural studies to denigrate all forms of mass art as *a priori* politically and morally regressive, a position that would determine an investigation's conclusions in advance. Following this challenge, Carroll suggests two features of ideology critique "properly so called": it should investigate the "conditions of possibility" of its objects and should not entail negative criticism for negative criticism's sake.

That scholarship conducted in good faith should not conflate critique and negative criticism is, I hope, relatively uncontentious. Studies of certain phenomena may proceed from critique to criticism if necessary, as has been the case in the research into Eurocentric film cultures previously cited, and to which this book contributes. The crucial tenet of Carroll's challenge to ideology critique, then, is that it should entail a study of the "conditions of possibility" of its objects. That which constitutes such conditions of possibility is open to contention, and different theories of ideology have emphasised different factors. For Carroll (1998, p. 360), the "structure of economic arrangements" is the determining condition for the development (and ideology) of film. However, political-economic structures are not the only conditions of possibility for cultural objects, or even social

2 See recent and ongoing data-driven projects by Skadi Loist (2017–2022) and Maximilian Schich et al. (2020–).

formations.[3] Ernesto Laclau (2014) takes an oppositional stance, arguing that the conditions of possibility of political formations are instead rhetorical: "each political institution, each category of political analysis, shows itself today as the locus of undecidable language games" (p. 80). While Laclau's account of ideology favours the rhetorical over the economic, scholars such as Samo Tomšič (2015) posit the need to apprehend a productive intersection between economic *and* discursive conditions of possibility. He calls for scholarship to reinvigorate a "discursive materialist" approach founded on an understanding of the productive reciprocity of both economic and discursive structures (Tomšič, 2015, pp. 61–62). This argument recalls the relationship between film festivals' appearance of "discursive independence" and actual "financial dependence" highlighted by Ragan Rhyne (2009) and discussed in the previous chapter. As I hope this book will demonstrate, a theory and method of ideology critique may therefore be most fruitful when it analyses the relationship between the economic and discursive dimensions of its object, investigating how each might condition the other.

Theorising Ideology

While the economic conditions of possibility of phenomena, including film festivals, are relatively well-theorised, the notion of discursive conditions of possibility requires further elaboration. To do this, we must delve into the poststructuralist and psychoanalytical theories that have come to underpin conceptions of discourse and ideology. Such theories range from the work of Roland Barthes, on whose "mythologisation" Marty Ba and Slocum draw, to that of the "*Screen* theorists" (such as Jean Louis Commoli, Laura Mulvey, Christian Metz and Jean Louis Baudry) at whom Carroll implicitly takes aim. Yet today we find an important update: the recuperation of theories of ideology critique by "New Lacanian" scholars working since the 1990s: Slavoj Žižek, Joan Copjec, Todd McGowan, Sheila Kunkle, Fabio Vighi and others. This recuperation seeks to address the limitations of 1970s poststructuralist philosophy and film theory by re-articulating and re-theorising ideology, often through a re-interpretation of the works of Jacques Lacan.

Copjec (1994, p. 30) situates 1970s film theory in an important historical context: writing before several of Lacan's seminars were published and subsequently translated, scholars were understandably reliant on the

3 For a discussion of the complexities of economic determination "in the last instance," particularly in relation to culture, see Stuart Hall (2018 [1977]).

psychoanalyst's earlier writings on the "mirror stage" (Lacan, 2004 [1949]). Copjec updates these theories with an interpretation of Lacan's later "Gaze" seminars (Lacan, 2004 [1964]). In so doing, she locates the crucial point of difference between Lacanian theories based on his earlier and later work, namely in the latter's mobilisation of the concept of "the Real"—the lack underlying (and generative of) our desire for symbolic meaning. Likewise, Todd McGowan and Sheila Kunkle (2004, p. xiii) discuss the "mistaken use of Lacan" in the work of the *Screen* theorists, which they argue focused solely on the "imaginary" and "symbolic" registers of meaning, resulting in "a near-total exclusion of the Real." To elucidate this difference, and the theoretical framework that underpins this book's deployment of a certain kind of Lacanian theory, I turn to define the three registers, and the conceptualisation of ideology that emerges from them.

Rooted in Lacan's (2004 [1949]) theory of the mirror stage, discussions of the imaginary tend to describe it as the register of experience in which a person identifies with an image of their likeness. The imaginary refers to our relationship with a figure of "imaginary resemblance" such as our mirror image, or a character on screen (Žižek, 2001b, p. 61). This has given rise to notions of films as operating in the register of the imaginary—collections of images that the spectator is ideologically "duped" into believing represent their likeness (McGowan, 2007, pp. 2–3). Here we find the basis of Mulvey's (1975, p. 12) theory that mainstream cinema produces "misrecognition" between spectators and male protagonists, resulting in audiences' idealisation of the male, misogynistic hero (their "ideal ego"), for example.

This identification with the image is facilitated by the symbolic register, which operates on the level of words or language. The symbolic is "the structure supporting our experience, providing not only the words we use to describe ourselves and our world, but also the very identities we take up as our own" (McGowan, 2007, p. 3). The symbolic provides the language through which we make sense of imaginary identification, naming subject positions such as "man" or "woman." It is only through the symbolic that the "male gaze" can be conceptualised as "male," as expressing the subject position of "man."

Together, the registers of the imaginary and symbolic comprise the order of explicit meanings, the "network of signifiers" used to describe our experience (Lacan, 2004 [1964], p. 43). This network of signifiers is not dissimilar to the notion of discourse used by theorists such as Michel Foucault (2012 [1975]) and Edward Said (2003 [1978]). According to such frameworks, our relationship to reality is constructed through a network of explicit meanings with straightforwardly observable effects (Vighi & Feldner, 2007, p. 153).

In this understanding, our reality is constructed by and through explicit discourse, historically specific articulations that determine our senses of ourselves, our practices and the world around us. Conceiving of ideology as discourse would mean that reality, and our interpretation of it, is constituted by these explicit representations of reality.

In contrast, recent Lacanian theories argue that the ideological procedure does not lie in the creation of particular, false representations of reality that "dupe" subjects. Rather, all representation is inherently illusory: the best it can do is stand in for its object, providing terms that offer communicative efficacy, yet are not the object itself. The implication of this understanding of representation is that all discourse is internally and intrinsically undermined by the Real, the "inherent failure of symbolisation," an inherent senselessness (Žižek, 1997, p. 217). We might thus recall scholars such as Rich (2003), Elsaesser (2005) and Andrews (2010) underlining the unsubstantiated and ritualistic deification of films at film festivals. While such descriptions of festivals could sound harsh, through Lacanian theories of ideology it becomes clear that this kind of mystical irrationality—in other words, senselessness—is a feature of discourse, and festival discourse, as such.

While this could be taken to mean simply that discourse is never absolute—it is but "a series of floating signifiers"—ideology functions, rather, *at this point of non-totality* (Žižek, 1989, p. 140). Rather than the production of discourses that fail to represent their objects (that is, all discourses), the ideological procedure is distinguished by the enjoyment and concealment of the Real, the ways in which "ideology takes its own failure into account in advance" (Žižek, 1989, p. 142). Our relationship to reality is in fact organised around an awareness that discourses fall short. We are not duped by discourse; rather, it is at the very moment that we attempt to approach discourse's failure that we find ourselves caught in ideology: "*Les non dupes errant:* the unduped go astray," as Lacan (2011 [1973]) puts it. This is because the Real generates the very search, the desire, for some deeper network of meanings that would compensate for the failure of discourse, and it is this desire that drives the ideological operation.

Ideology entails the negotiation between representation and the Real through "fantasy" (Žižek, 1989, p. 45). Fantasy is an umbrella term for a series of ideological forms that compensate for the inherent failure of representation.[4] It is the hidden "support for our 'reality' [i.e., discourse]

4 The different forms that fantasy can take are described by a sub-set of terms: "superego," "suture," "the sexual relationship," the "institutional unconscious" and, in certain usages, "hegemony." Each term in this sub-set brings with it a different nuance; they are different forms

itself" (Žižek, 1989, p. 45). These ideological formations are best conceived as "unwritten rules that effectively regulate our speech and acts" (Žižek, 2000c, p. 657). Crucially, they occur on the level of the hidden, the unwritten—or the unconscious. In this way, ideology pertains not solely to that which is visible or signifiable (i.e., discourse) but, rather, can be found in the implicit, "generative matrix that regulates the relationship between visible and non-visible" (Žižek, 2012, p. 1). Such rules comprise a matrix of hidden associations that fill terms with meaning. They compensate for the split that undermines explicit discourse, enabling us to conceal the Real, and with it the traumatic knowledge that our reality is ultimately senseless. Fantasy is that which ensures we can act and interact despite meaning being neither transparent nor total. It enables scholars, film critics, audiences and programmers to continue acting as if "art cinema" has a stable meaning, even in light of its constitutive impurity, for example.

Ideology critique is animated by the inquiry into these fantasy structures. At the first level, it is the investigation into the hidden rules that create the conditions of possibility for explicit representations. (The second level entails a return to the Real, which I discuss at the end of this chapter.) Therefore, this book's aim to identify and analyse the ideology that conditions European A festivals' awarding and representation of Italian art cinema can be reformulated thus: it aims to identify and analyse the fantasy structures that condition European A festivals' awarding and representation of Italian art cinema; it considers the means through which such festivals compensate for the inherent inability to represent their objects.

The critique of ideology must centre on identifying and intervening in the implicit level: "not directly changing the explicit text of the law, but, rather, intervening in its obscene virtual supplement" (Žižek, 2008, p. 145). Importantly, however, to do so is not to posit an exit from ideology as such. (Assuming such an exit is possible would return us to the condition of the "unduped," erring ever deeper into ideology.) Rather, it is to provide a position from which certain ideological formations can be refigured. This distinction is summarised by Vighi and Feldner (2007):

> If fully endorsed, in other words, attachment eventually turns into disattachment, producing a rift in the seemingly unbreakable consistency of ideological formations from which the radical rearticulation of the very ideological framework suddenly appears possible. (p. 156)

that the fundamental fantasy structure can take. The forms I identify and analyse throughout this book are those of hegemony, suture, and the sexual relationship.

Moving the implicit laws that support ideology onto an explicit level removes their power: by fully endorsing these laws, one's attachment to ideology turns into disattachment. This provides the possibility of "the radical rearticulation of the [...] ideological framework." Ideology critique aims to provide an (albeit limited) agency over the very structures of meaning-making, intervening in the implicit rules that produce the impression of "full" meaning, or even rejecting the illusion of fullness itself.

Although the associations that regulate representation may initially be implicit (their ideological efficacy depends on it), they can be uncovered and interceded by certain modes of analysis. The one I offer below is, I believe, a relatively holistic method founded on theories of ideology and the Real, tempered by the commitment to material discursive analysis outlined above. This approach is, too, developed through the encounter between Lacanian theory and its application to a particular phenomenon: the film festival phenomenon. As such, I reformulate the theory of ideology into a method that centres on three key aspects of film festivals and the films they represent: festivals' material features, the festival apparatus; their representational practices, festival paratexts; and their objects, the unruly texts of the films they exhibit and rhetorically construct.

The Festival Apparatus

The first stage of the method focuses on the material side of the discursive-material intersection posited by Tomšič and other scholars of ideology (Žižek, 2006). It investigates the organisational features of festivals, which I term the festival apparatus. I follow Wong's (2011) use of the term "apparatus" to refer to the institutional structures and practices that constitute a film festival, including: histories; models of funding; processes of selection; organisation of different programme sections; rituals of prize-giving; cultivation of media attention; the roles of Festival Directors and other stakeholders; and the geopolitics of location. This conception of material and organisational features of film festivals also profits from the association with poststructuralist definitions of apparatus as a configuration of institutions and practices through which ideology functions, although I later complicate these through analyses that foreground representation and the Real.[5]

5 See Althusser (2014 [1971], p. 184): "An ideology always exists in an apparatus and in the practice or practices of that apparatus. This existence is material." On the distinction between ideology *solely* as apparatus and ideology as a function of the Real, see Copjec (1994).

We find a basis for framing the apparatus as ideological in studies of film festivals as "field configuring events" (Rüling, 2009; Lampel & Meyer, 2008; Strandgaard Pederson & Mazza, 2011; Mezias et al., 2011). These studies suggest that an important condition for film festivals' representations of films or construction of film canons is the very "institutional logics" by which they operate (Rüling, 2009, p. 51). Jesper Strandgaard Pederson and Carmelo Mazza (2011) trace the formation of these logics by analysing the development of the international film festival model: the institutionalisation of practices and values first set out by "early adopter" international festivals, most of which today constitute the European A-list (Strandgaard Pederson & Mazza, 2011, p. 145). Expanding Elsaesser's (2005, p. 91) claim that Cannes "set the template for film festivals the world over," Strandgaard Pederson and Mazza conclude that early adopter festivals have "managed to define the field and invent tradition," to "create and institutionalise a model for international film festivals that has become an 'unchallenged given'" (p. 159). The notion of an unchallenged given resounds with conceptions of ideology as a system of common-sense propositions or, as defined above, "implicit rules." These are concepts that have been afforded such salience that they remain broadly unchallenged; challenging them may even appear inconceivable (Žižek, 2004b).

For European A festivals, these "unchallenged givens" constitute many of the features discussed in the previous chapter, some of which are determined by FIAPF regulations while others have emerged more organically. These features include: taking place in a fixed, usually tourist-friendly, metropolitan location; reliance on support from a mix of public (state) and private (commercial) stakeholders; the presence of a main competition arbitrated by an international jury; screening at least fourteen premieres in said competition; and the time-limited hyper-spectacularisation that Janet Harbord (2009) defines as the festival "time-event." Analysing the festival apparatus not only identifies these common features but seeks to situate them within shared economic arrangements as well as historical and geopolitical contexts. Such an exploration constitutes the first level of inquiry into film festivals and ideology, which, as I show later, offers a foundation for the analysis of the norms of representation that festivals might adopt.

Analysing even one festival's apparatus is an ambitious task that can easily fill an entire study. Therefore, this stage of the method, as one part of a multi-faceted analysis of ideology, synthesises insights from existing scholarship and theorises them through the framework of ideology to offer an account of broad institutional logics that characterise a festival circuit.

Generally speaking, rather than an in-depth analysis of a singular film festival, subsequent chapters traverse several European A festivals, sometimes with a focus on the "big three" trend-setters on the circuit (Cannes, Venice and Berlin). In focusing on shared logics and models, the analysis begins to theorise festivals at the structural level, producing a ground from which to analyse particular iterations—a specific festival or singular edition, and its representations of its prize-winners.

Paratexts and the Meaning of Film

One of the implicit rules of film festival studies, as well as research into Italian cinema's institutions, is that the meanings of films are produced in a space that is at once beyond and part of the film text. Such an apprehension of film's meaning is one of the fundamental tenets of this book: that "art cinema" and "Italian cinema" are more than the sum of the films produced under such categories, that their meaning is the product of a continual negotiation that takes place primarily off-screen. This off-screen negotiation can be considered part of the ideological struggle between representation—the discourses that surround individual film texts—and the Real—the impossibility of such discourses fixing such texts' meanings.

To apprehend films in this way, it is necessary to distinguish between three terms: cinema, film and the film text. Cinema, as suggested above, refers primarily to institutionally-produced categories of filmmaking. This idea of cinema as an institution comprised of systems of production, exhibition, distribution and criticism is reasonably commonplace and can be found in works on art cinema cited in the previous chapter, as well as in Pierre Sorlin's (1996) *Italian National Cinema 1896–1996* and numerous studies of, and debates about, world cinema, Third Cinema, and the various other categories used to taxonomise films. In brief, cinema is an abstraction, an idea of a certain kind of filmmaking, produced and reproduced by institutions such as film festivals, film criticism, higher education, cultural policy and sometimes filmmakers themselves.[6]

While this definition of cinema is relatively established within film studies, the distinction between film and film text is less so. To make such a distinction is to suggest that a film may be more than a collection of sounds

6 See, for example, filmmakers' manifestos, perhaps the most famous being Fernando Solanas and Octavio Getino's *Towards a Third Cinema* (1970). For an anthology of such manifestos, see Mackenzie (2014).

and images that appear on screen for a fixed duration. That collection of audiovisual content is the *film text*, but not necessarily the film. Rather, by "film" I refer to the entire constellation of materials and practices that contribute to the production of meaning both within and besides the film text, on and off screen. A number of these off-screen features are suggested in Harbord's (2002) foundational work, *Film Cultures*. Harbord extends the meaning of film to include "production strategies, marketing, film festivals, reviewing, distribution channels and sites of exhibition" (p. 5). Such practices, as Harbord calls them, "engender [...] particular film cultures, embedding film within practices of everyday life" (p. 5). While Harbord's description of the constitutive practices of film cultures is similar to the notion of cinema proposed above—there is a productive overlap between conceptions of "cinemas" and "film cultures"—it can also be applied to the unit of the singular film.

Asking "che cosa è un film?" (what is a film?), Marco Cucco (2014, p. 101) also extends the meaning of film to include its production, distribution and reception. Each can be thought of as procedures by which the meaning of a film is created, whether they occur during a film text's actual production process, thus influencing the creation of the film text itself, or after production, influencing the various practices by which a film's meaning is (re)constructed. Cucco's essay focuses on production, above all the collaborations and funding deals that secured not only *The Great Beauty*'s creation but much of the film's iconography (the giant Martini sign that looms over Jep's Rome, for example). However, Dominic Holdaway's (2014) study of another *cause célèbre* of Italian cinema offers a complementary approach close to the one that underpins this book. Holdaway (2014) analyses the construction of meaning in *Gomorrah*'s promotional materials, specifically the "rhetoric of realism" achieved through the press packs that accompanied the film's premiere at Cannes (Holdaway, 2014, p. 202). Here, *Gomorrah*'s rhetoric extends beyond the film text, being produced through promotional materials that accompanied, and framed, the film's exhibition at a major European film festival.

The extended conception of film that Cucco and Holdaway evoke inadvertently develops the key tenets of Jonathan Gray's (2010) call for "off-screen" studies. Gray's emphasis, much like my own, is on practices of meaning-making that follow a film's production. Promotional materials, such as *Gomorrah*'s press packs, complement film texts to form part of "the massive, extended presence of the filmic and televisual texts across our lived environment"—in other words, their situation within "practices of everyday life" (Gray, 2010, p. 2; Harbord, 2002, p. 5). This extended presence, and thus extended meaning, proliferates across billboards, publications, video sites and social media platforms, from the film poster one might see on the side of a bus to the "promoted" trailer that pops up on a user's Instagram feed.

These materials are paratexts: objects that exist "besides" and "adjacent to" film texts, while also being "intrinsically part of the text" (Gray, 2010, p. 5). Much more than simply marketing materials, to be derided by critics and fans alike, paratexts "create texts, they manage them, and they fill them with many of the meanings that we associate with them [...] a paratext constructs, lives in, and can affect the running of the text" (p. 5). Gray (2010) writes specifically against modes of film criticism that would position the film text as the only significant source of meaning:

> [R]arely if ever can a film or program serve as the only source of information about the text. And rather than simply serve as *extensions* of a text, many of these items are filters through which we must pass on our way to the film or program, our first and formative encounters with the text. (p. 3)

Gray (2010) thus argues that paratexts provide "filters" or "early frames" for a film's meaning, sometimes before the film text itself is viewed (pp. 2–3).

These materials can contribute to the retroactive construction of meaning too. Audiences, and particularly film festival audiences, might encounter paratexts beyond those Gray considers, such as red carpet performances, interviews at press conferences, festival reviews, or even awards speeches, each one re-iterating and re-constituting a film's meaning. Many of these paratexts are produced by and at film festivals. Cindy Hing-Yuk Wong (2011, p. 100) has demonstrated the importance of "extratextual" (or paratextual) materials to film festivals' construction of films, auteurs and global art cinema. She highlights the role of film festivals' "critical discourses" about films: reviews by critics attending festivals, festival catalogues, retrospectives and press conferences (Wong, 2011, pp. 112, 122–125). Each of these, she argues, contributes significantly to the canonisation of films and auteurs, influencing notions of the kind of cinema that film festivals promote. Each film, in its extended sense, is partially constituted by film festivals' textual representations of it as well as the meanings generated within the film text itself.

The cumulative effect of these texts is the construction of meaning for films and, as they are repeated and reiterated over a body of films (such as Italian, award-winning films), the abstract meaning of the "cinema" under which such films are taxonomised. These paratexts are not only crucial for the construction of films', and cinemas', meanings, however. Festivals not only represent films through paratextual materials, they also "represent themselves" (Wong, 2011, p. 122). This is a perspective held by the majority of film festival scholars who have analysed the production of texts at and by film festivals—from Julian Stringer's (2008, p. 53) investigations into the textual construction of a "festival image" to Daniel Dayan's (2000, p. 52) emphasis on a festival's "verbal architecture," which has been recently developed into a multi-modal "visual architecture" by Antoine Damiens (2020, p. 158). Yet such studies tend to understate the importance of these texts to the construction of films' meanings too. In order to better apprehend festivals' role in constructing film canons, we must insist on the reciprocity of meaning between festival and film within the paratext, emphasising how a festival's cultivation of its self-image conditions its representation of films. Bringing Gray's theory into dialogue with studies of festivals' verbal-visual architectures, we can thus posit the "festival paratext," a text that constructs a film exhibited by a festival, and whose representation of that film is mediated by the festival's need to construct an "image" for itself.

While festival paratexts, paratexts produced by and at film festivals, comprise a range of media objects, scholars have previously focused on printed matter. Dayan (2000, p. 52) underscores the relevance of written matter to the study of film festivals, as these institutions annually produce "a Niagara of printed paper [...] spelling out meanings, offering captions, telling and retelling daily events until they reached a stable, paradigmatic form." Stringer (2008, p. 53) argues that this telling and retelling in festival print culminates in a festival's "image," confirming the importance of festival brochures and other printed materials to this complementary relationship of meaning-making for film and festival through the printed paratext. Narrowing our focus to one particular kind of paratext, Rich (1998, pp. 31–32) asserts that "for an instant replay of the festival mind-set, there's no quicker access than the catalogues published to accompany the screenings." Rich suggests that not all festival print is of equal importance, positioning the catalogue, the brochure of films on exhibition each year, as the critical festival paratext.

In the digital age, however, we must extend our focus to include online materials too. Printed brochures are still distributed in print and remain collectable items for the dedicated festival-goer. However, a more common mode of disseminating information about festivals' programmes is online, via film festival websites, social media accounts and sometimes apps. By far the most extensive resource of these is the festival website. They present not only a festival's current edition, as a printed brochure might, but also function as archives of past festival editions, extending the "telling and retelling" of festival events beyond that which was previously possible in print. The curious audience member (or researcher) need only click the year of a past edition to access the plethora of synopses, interviews, press releases and awards lists that constitute a festival's annual paratextual production. These pages, nested within a section of the website explicitly named the "archive," historicise a festival and the films it has shown, creating ever more paradigmatic meanings for each.

While all these effusions of ephemera contribute to the creation of myths surrounding festivals and the films they show, it is the film synopsis that appears at the zenith of the reciprocal relationship between film and festival. These short-form summaries comprise the majority of the text in the catalogues that Rich (1998, pp. 31–32) argues is paramount to a festival's self-representation. These are one of the primary means by which a festival represents, and promotes, its programme. The aim of these texts is not simply to give an objective summary of a film on exhibition; synopses are a crucial part of the marketing that takes place through festival brochures and websites. They provide those "first and formative encounters" with the films that festivals show, helping audiences navigate the films on offer and their prospective meanings (Gray, 2010, p. 3). As suggested above, this is as significant to representing the festival as it is to representing the film. It is well known that festivals are in part defined by their film selections, carefully curated expressions of a "brand identity" or "curatorial profile" (Bosma, 2015, pp. 71–72). As the written representation of these film selections, synopses must frame films in a manner that aligns with the festival image.

This is not a matter of misrepresenting films but rather foregrounding aspects that match a festival's profile. While the features of European A festivals' "identities" will emerge throughout this book, I would like to offer an illustrative example from the world of migration film festivals. The London Migration Film Festival aims to expand definitions of migration beyond the dominant tropes found in mainstream British media, which depicts suffering, racialised refugees travelling to the UK by boat (Parrot & Stahnke, 2021). To achieve this, the programmers select films that might not fit into obvious categories of "migration film," such as experimental movies about movement or documentaries of displacement within nations rather than between them. These aspects of the festival's aims and programming (its apparatus) are articulated through its textual representations of films: LMFF uses its synopses to re-frame films, constructing their meaning in relation to the theme of migration.

The London Migration Film Festival has considerable control over the paratexts they produce, with synopses written by the programmers in dialogue with filmmakers and distributors. This is not always the case, particularly in larger organisations such as A-list film festivals. With their greater scale comes increasing complexity, and it is not always clear how, or by whom, a synopsis might be produced. However, regardless of whether the text is provided by a filmmaker, distributor, festival programmer or marketing team—or through negotiation between several of these agents—the conditions of possibility and purpose of the synopsis remain the same. As text produced with the express aim of representing a film within the context of that festival, the synopsis is very likely to be conditioned by a festival's institutional identity. To write a synopsis that does not align with a festival's image is to risk a film appearing out of place or, worse, being completely overlooked. Moreover, where synopses are not written in-house by festival staff, they are often the product of a negotiation between the original writer and festival, with communications teams requesting proofs and returning edits before the material is published.

Vitally important, moreover, is the *effect* of the synopsis: these texts, however they are produced, become constitutive of a film and festival's image. Appearing in print and archived online, they contribute to the creation of films' meanings, the cumulative effect of which is the creation of cinemas within the festival framework. Analysing a body of synopses, such as synopses of Italian award-winning films, can indicate how certain cinemas have been constructed within such frameworks. This becomes yet clearer as tropes associated with that cinema recur across the corpus, such as Fellini-esque auteurs or humanist (neo)realism. Such repetitions demonstrate how festivals' paratextual representations of films are at once conditioned by, and constitutive of, certain ideas of cinema.

It is worth heeding Loist's (2020) caution against relying solely on festival paratexts, including synopses, when studying film festivals. As Loist (2020, p. 43) argues, studying only "publicly available material such as program booklets provide only very limited insight into the world of a film festival." While these materials do not necessarily provide insights into the decision-making process behind the programming and awarding of films (*pace* Rich), they are of vital importance when analysing how precisely the outward-facing (or "publicly available") materials of film festivals participate in and reproduce dominant ideas about art cinema and its attendant concerns—concerns that include, but are not limited to, cultural value, aesthetics, geopolitics and identities. Furthermore, Loist is correct in her assessment that paratexts fall short of representing the festivals and films they take as their objects. Yet we can transform this failure into a mode of analysis. Much less than a shortcoming of festival research, the "gap" between a festival paratext and the experience of attending a festival or watching the films it exhibits offers a productive point of fissure that can be exploited in ideology critiques of these institutions.

The Cinematic Real

To focus on this point of failure within the context of film festivals requires us to redefine the theories of the Real discussed above. The third and final stage of the method I propose below builds a concept of the "cinematic Real": the failure of meaning that at once motivates and limits a film's meaning. I locate this Real between the film text and paratext: it is expressed in points of contradiction between the meanings we find a in a film text and those we find in its institutional representation. My approach to analysing the films that festivals screen is deliberately atypical. It aims to emphasise the points at which the representation of the film in the synopsis fails— irruptions of the Real that highlight the constitutive impossibility of paratextual representation. This stage further demonstrates the ideological procedure of the synopsis as such: the attempt to conceal its intrinsic misrepresentation of its object. Moreover, by foregrounding the precise moments in which this failure becomes clear, my analysis offers further accuracy in interpreting the "implicit rules" that govern a festival's representation of the films it exhibits.

My treatment of films as objects that can highlight the Real is grounded in studies that emphasise films' potential to make manifest the inherent failure of ideology. As McGowan (2007, p. 171) argues, "rather than seducing us into accepting our symbolic prison, film tends to show us the [R]eal openings within that prison" (McGowan, 2007, p. 171). In contrast with Mulveyan notions of films as constructing totalising "symbolic prisons," such as rigid structures of gender identity, films also register moments in which a symbolic order might falter. These irruptions of the Real in film at once constitute and challenge ideology. Their duality is summarised well by McGowan and Kunkle (2004):

> [T]he ideological dimension of film lies in its ability to offer a fantasy scenario that delivers us from a traumatic Real. At the same time, film's radicality lies in its ability to involve us in an encounter with this Real. Thus, the ideological and radical dimensions of film overlap; both involve a relationship to the traumatic Real. (p. xviii)

These scholars define film in relation to the Real, highlighting its potential to either reinforce ideology through a compensatory "fantasy scenario" or radically challenge it by "involving us in an encounter with this Real." To conceptualise films in this way is to define them in relation to a fundamental ambiguity: registering moments of symbolic failure, films can alternately reinforce or challenge an ideological formation.

The Real dimension of film at once generates and challenges its inscription within institutions of cinema. For example, debates about neorealist cinema, even when they define neorealism through lists of stylistic features (see Hayward, 2002), find continual frustration in the texts of so-called neorealist films. As early as the 1948 edition of Venice, Luchino Visconti himself stated that "neorealism" constituted no more than "un assurda etichetta" (an absurd label) for his film *La terra trema* (1948), a film that has since been treated as the "formula of cinematic neorealism" by critics and scholars alike (Leavitt, 2020, p. 15). In fact, Charles Leavitt IV highlights the textual impurity of films such as *La terra* and, another neorealist archetype, *Obsession* (*Ossessione*, Visconti, 1943), underscoring the latter's status as "as much *noir* as neorealist" (2020, p. 28), since it is based on James M. Cain's novel *The Postman Always Rings Twice* (1934). Meanwhile, studies of neorealist film texts have highlighted their melodramatic, comedic and even camp dimensions—for example, the use of slapstick humour in *Rome, Open City* (Forgacs, 2004). Just as abstract notions of art cinema are challenged by the heterogeneous "marks of enunciation" within individual films (Neale, 1981, p. 15), so those of one of its founding pillars, neorealism, are undone by elements of each film text. Such marks can be considered stains of the Real, traumatic openings that underscore the ultimate failure of a particular notion of a "cinema" to capture its object, those fundamentally ambivalent films that appear under such terms. This is applicable to notions of cinema in general but, above all, their construction through the paratexts produced within "art cinema's central institution," film festivals (Andrews, 2010, p. 7).

Thus, while McGowan and Kunkle's theorisations of the cinematic Real remain within the domain of the film text (the "symbolic prison" is created within this text, even as it registers its own failure), we can extend their framework to the constellation of film texts and paratexts discussed above. Several parts of a film, in its extended sense, can register dominant norms and moments of representational failure, as well as the fantasy scenarios and traumatic encounters that emerge from this failure. Within the numerous paratexts that constitute a film, we can narrow our analysis to an ideological critique of a specific institution and, moreover, the institution proper to films' ideological construction, film festivals. If film festivals ideologically construct films, the difference between the film text and its representation can make manifest the Real, the point at which the festival's symbolisation of the film fails. In the context of my analysis, the encounter with the Real that film affords is, therefore, the encounter with the Real of European A festivals' representations of films. By highlighting the specific differences between the film text and a festival's representation of it, I identify the points at which the ideological fantasy is likely to emerge, and the forms it might take.

Film Festivals and Ideology Critique: A Method

Based on the concepts just discussed, this book offers a three-tiered method for analysing the ideology conditioning European A festivals' awarding and construction of Italian cinema in the new millennium. Each chapter begins with an analysis of the European A festival apparatus, attempting to identify the explicit rules through which they claim to function. This analysis proceeds through the synthesis of previous insights into European A festivals' organisational features and practices. As such, it is greatly indebted to the work of other film festival scholars. This debt is, I hope, repaid by bringing such studies not only into dialogue with each other, offering a more holistic picture of the European A circuit, but into dialogue with key concepts in ideology critique, offering an indication of the circuit's common ideological structures or fantasies. I seek to reframe understandings of the festival phenomenon using a Lacanian theory of ideology that draws predominantly on the work of Slavoj Žižek. Of the New Lacanian scholars on whom I draw, Žižek's theoretical oeuvre constitutes the most sustained attempt to conceptualise ideology through the Real and, crucially, the economic-discursive conditions of possibility for numerous social, political and cultural formations. While contentious, Žižek's writings offer key coordinates for psychoanalytical, and Marxist, analyses of cultural phenomena in late capitalism. This book seeks to take the best of these theoretical concepts, reappropriating them for the study of film festivals, and calling for anti-capitalist, decolonial film futures.

This syncretic approach to studying the film festival apparatus offers initial hypotheses concerning how a festival's explicit operation might be underpinned by a hidden, fantasmatic supplement. I treat the apparatus as one aspect of ideology, one part of the material-discursive lattice that constitutes film festivals and their construction of cinemas. I do so as a means of conjecturing about the fantasmatic structures that underpin European A festivals, offering grounding for the interpretations of paratexts and film texts that follow. Each chapter tests these hypotheses through an examination of a specific case study.

To examine each case study—an Italian film awarded top prize by a European A festival—I first concentrate on the synopsis through which the awarding festival represents the film. This constitutes the second tier of the book's method. I begin this analysis with a review of scholarly interpretations of the film in question, which I treat not only as a means of gathering information about the film, but as another institutional discourse symptomatic of the ideology conditioning the construction of a certain kind of Italian cinema internationally. (I do so based on Italian film studies' treatment of itself as ideological, discussed in the previous chapter.) Having identified common tropes and contradictions associated with the film in question, I then undertake a psychoanalytically-inflected discourse analysis of the synopsis presented by the European A festival that awarded the film. This is informed by Ian Parker's (2005, pp. 167–178) model of discourse analysis, focusing on the elements that he identifies as central to a text's construction of meaning: rhetorical constructions, rhetorical conclusions, repeated words that anchor representation, the implicit norms or "rules" that the text refers to and points of contradiction. In a procedure complementary to its analysis of the European A festival apparatus, each chapter's interpretation of synopses identifies the explicit ways in which such festivals represent Italian art cinema. Meanwhile, employing Parker's focus on the points of contradiction in the text, I identify how such representations may fall short. I do so initially by using the findings gathered from my readings of film festival scholarship and critical interpretations of the film. Such a move begins our approach towards the Real, continued further as I turn to analyse the text of the film under examination.

The third tier of this book's methodology is therefore an analysis of the ways in which films can make manifest the Real points of failure in festivals' representations of them. To demonstrate and clarify the ideological procedures that regulate European A festivals' representation of Italian cinema, I mobilise a reading of film texts that emphasises how they escape the meanings ascribed to them. If film festivals ideologically construct films, the difference between the film text and its representation can make manifest the Real, the point at which the festival's symbolisation of the film fails.

Each chapter culminates in an analysis that uses the film text as a means of "looking awry" at the festival apparatus and the synopsis, attempting to identify the hidden laws structuring festivals' paratextual representation of films by analysing their "hidden inconsistencies" (Žižek, 1992, p. 3). This is an entirely heuristic approach, which locates compensatory structures (fantasy) in the paratext and the Real in the film, and does so as a means of better interpreting the ideological procedure of the former. While this reading highlights the functioning of ideology, as well as the specific values that an ideological formation might attempt to highlight or repress, it does not aim at an interpretation of the truth of a film. It does not imply that a synopsis or even critical interpretation that could totally represent the film being studied exists. Rather, I offer a deliberately partial interpretation that acknowledges the film's status as an ambivalent text, and use that status as a means of critiquing the film's ideological representation by European A festivals. Yet in staging an encounter with the Real, the method I propose finishes on a moment of undecidability: the analysis opens a utopic space, one at the precipice between the infinite possibilities of meanings for art cinema and the closure of those meanings through European A festivals' ideological operation.

Bibliography

Althusser, L. (2001 [1971]). Ideology and ideological state apparatuses (notes towards an investigation). In L. Althusser, *Lenin and philosophy and other essays* (pp. 85–126). New York University Press.

Andrews, D. (2010). Art cinema as institution, redux: Art houses, film festivals, and film studies. *Scope: An Online Journal of Film and Television Studies, 18*, 1–21.

Barthes, R. (2012 [1957]). *Mythologies*. Hill and Wang.

Bordwell, D., & Carroll, N. (1996). *Post-theory: Reconstructing film studies*. University of Wisconsin Press.

Bosma, P. (2015). *Film programming: Curating for cinemas, festivals, archives*. Columbia University Press.

Brown, W. (2009). The festival syndrome: Report on the International Film Festival Workshop, University of St Andrews, 4 April 2009. In D. Iordanova & R. Rhyne (Eds.), *Film Festival Yearbook 1: The Festival Circuit* (pp. 216–225). St. Andrews Film Studies & College Gate Press.

Carroll, N. (1998). *A philosophy of mass art*. Oxford University Press.

Copjec, J. (1994). *Read my desire: Lacan against the historicists*. Verso Books.

Cucco, M. (2014). Che cosa è un film? *La grande bellezza* in una prospettiva di economia e politica di media. In M. Cucco (Ed.), *La trama dei media. Stato, imprese, pubblico nella societa dell'informazione* (pp. 101–119). Carocci editore.

Damiens, A. (2020). *LGBTQ festivals: Curating queerness*. Amsterdam University Press.

Dayan, D. (2000). Looking for Sundance: The social construction of a film festival. In I. Bondebjerg (Ed.), *Moving images, culture and the mind* (pp. 43–52). University of Luton Press.

De Valck, M. (2007). *Film festivals: From European geopolitics to global cinephilia*. Amsterdam University Press.

Dovey, L. (2015). *Curating Africa in the age of film festivals*. Palgrave Macmillan.

Elsaesser, T. (2005). *European cinema: Face to face with Hollywood*. Amsterdam University Press.

Forgacs, D. (2004). Space, rhetoric, and the divided city in *Roma città aperta*. In S. Gottlieb (Ed.), *Roberto Rossellini's* Rome Open City (pp. 106–130). Cambridge University Press.

Fehrenbach, H. (1995). *Cinema in democratizing Germany: Reconstructing of national identity after Hitler*. University of North Carolina Press.

Foucault, M. (2012 [1975]). *Discipline and punish: The birth of the prison*. Vintage.

Gray, J. (2010). *Show sold separately: Promos, spoilers, and other media paratexts*. NYU Press.

Hall, S. (2018 [1977]). Re-thinking the "base-and-superstructure" metaphor. In D. Morely (Ed.), *Essential essays, volume 1: Foundations of cultural studies* (pp. 143–171). Duke University Press.

Harbord, J. (2002). *Film Cultures*. Sage.

Harbord, J. (2009). Film festivals as time-event. In D. Iordanova & R. Rhyne (Eds.), *Film festival yearbook 1: The festival circuit* (pp. 40–46). St Andrews Film Studies & College Gate Press.

Hayward, S. (2013). *Cinema studies: The key concepts* (4th ed.). Routledge.

Higson, A. (1989). The concept of national cinema. *Screen, 30*(4), 36–47.

Holdaway, D. (2014). Osservazioni sulla retorica di *Gomorra*. In W. Hope, S. Serra, & L. D'Arcangeli (Eds.), *Un nuovo cinema politico italiano? Il passato sociopolitica o, il potere istituzionale, la marginalizzazione* (pp. 198–210). Troubador.

Horton, J. (1972). Combatting empiricism: Toward a practical understanding of Marxist methodology. *Insurgent Sociologist, 3*(1), 24–34.

Lacan, J. (2004 [1949]). The mirror stage as formative of the *I* function as revealed in psychoanalytic experience. In J. Lacan (Ed.), *Écrits: A selection* (pp. 3–9). Norton & Co.

Lacan, J. (2004 [1964]). *The four fundamental concepts of psychoanalysis*. Norton.

Lacan, J. (2011 [1973]). Seminar XXI: Les non-dupes errant. In C. Gallagher (Ed.), *Lacan in Ireland*. Available from: http://www.lacaninireland.com/web/translations/seminars/

Laclau, E. (2014). *The rhetorical foundations of society*. Verso.

Lampel, J., & Meyer, A. (2008). Field-configuring events as structuring mechanisms: How conferences, ceremonies, and trade shows constitute new technologies, industries, and markets. *Journal of Management Studies, 45*(6), 1025–1035.

Latour, B. (1996). On actor-network theory: A few clarifications. *Soziale Welt, 47*(4), 369–381.

Leavitt, C. (2020). *Italian neorealism: A cultural history*. University of Toronto Press.

Loist, S. 2020. Film festival research workshops: Debates on methodology. In A. Vallejo & E. Winton (Eds.), *Documentary film festivals Vol. 1* (pp. 41–52). Palgrave MacMillan.

Lule, J. (1995). Enduring image of war: Myth and ideology in a *Newsweek* cover. *Journal of Popular Culture*, *29*(1), 199–211.

MacKenzie, S. (2014). *Film manifestos and global cinema cultures: A critical anthology*. University of California Press.

McGowan, T. (2007). *The real gaze: Film theory after Lacan*. State University of New York Press.

McGowan, T., & Kunkle, S. (2004). Introduction: Lacanian psychoanalysis in film theory. In T. McGowan, S. Kunkle, & F. L. Restuccia (Eds.), *Lacan and contemporary film*. Other Press.

Mezias, S. et al. (2011). Transforming film product identities: The status effects of European premier film festivals, 1996–2005. In B. Moeran & J. S. Pedersen (Eds.), *Negotiating values in the creative industries: Fairs, festivals and competitive events* (pp. 169–196). Cambridge University Press.

Mulvey, L. (1975). Visual pleasure and narrative cinema. *Screen*, *16*(3), 6–18.

Neale, S. (1981). Art cinema as institution. *Screen*, *22*(1), 11–40.

Ostrowska, D. (2019). "The migrant gaze" and "the migrant festive chronotope" – Programming the refugee crisis at the European human rights and documentary film festivals. The case of the One World International Human Rights Documentary Film Festival. *Studies in European Cinema*, *16*(3), 266–281.

Parker, I. (2005). Lacanian discourse analysis in psychology: Seven theoretical elements. *Theory & Psychology*, *15*(2), 163–182.

Parrot, L., & Stahnke, L. (2021). *Curation as research: A masterclass with the London Migration Film Festival*, 1 July, University of Leeds.

Rastegar, R. (2012). Difference, aesthetics and the curatorial crisis of film festivals. *Screen*, *53*(3), 310–317.

Rich, B. R. (1998). *Chick flicks: Theories and memories of the feminist film movement*. Duke University Press.

Rich, B. R. (2003). Abstract from "Taste, fashion, and service: The ideology of film curating." In *Terms of address: The pedagogy and politics of film and video programming and curating, 7–8 March 2003, Centre for Media and Culture in Education (CMCE), Ontario Institute for Studies in Education, Toronto*. Available from: http://fcis.oise.utoronto.ca/~cmce/terms%20of%20address%20symposium.htm

Rüling, C. C. (2009). Festivals as field-configuring events: The Annecy International Animated Film Festival and Market. In D. Iordanova & R. Rhyne (Eds.), *Film festival yearbook 1: The festival circuit* (pp. 49–66). St Andrews Film Studies and College Gate Press.

Said, E. (2003 [1978]). *Orientalism: Western conceptions of the Orient*. Penguin
Schich, M. et al. (2020–). *Cultural Data Analytics* (CUDAN). Project website: https://cudan.tlu.ee/
Solanas, F., & Getino, O. (1970). Toward a third cinema. *Cinéaste, 4*(3), 1–10.
Sorlin, P. (1996). *Italian national cinema: 1896–1996*. Routledge.
Strandgaard Pedersen, J., & Mazza, C. (2011). International film festivals: For the benefit of whom? *Culture Unbound, 3*, 139–165.
Stringer, J. (2008). Genre films and festival communities: Lessons from Nottingham, 1991–2000. *Film International, 6*(4), 53–60.
Taylor, P. (2010). *Žižek and the media*. Polity.
Tomšič, S. (2015). Materialism between critique and speculation. In A. Hamza (Ed.), *Repeating Žižek* (pp. 58–71). Duke University Press.
Vighi, F., & Feldner, H. (2007). Ideology critique or discourse analysis? Žižek against Foucault. *European Journal of Political Theory, 6*(2), 141–159.
Walton, D. (2012). *Doing cultural theory*. Sage.
Wong, C. H-Y. (2011). *Film festivals: Culture, people, and power on the global screen*. Rutgers University Press.
Žižek, S. (1989). *The sublime object of ideology*. Verso.
Žižek, S. (1992). *Looking awry: An introduction to Jacques Lacan through popular culture*. MIT Press.
Žižek, S. (1997). *The plague of fantasies*. Verso.
Žižek, S. (2001b). *The fright of real tears: Krzysztof Kieślowski between theory and post-theory*. British Film Institute.
Žižek, S. (2004b). *The reality of the virtual* [lecture]. Recorded 11 December 2003. Ben Wright Film Productions.
Žižek, S. (2006). *The parallax view*. MIT Press.
Žižek, S. (2008). *Violence: Six sideways reflections*. Profile Books.
Žižek, S. (2012). *Mapping ideology*. Verso Books.

Filmography

Obsession (Ossessione) (1943). Visconti, L. dir. Italy.
The Postman Always Rings Twice (1934). McCain, J. United States.
Rome, Open City (Roma, città aperta) (1945). Rossellini, R. dir. Italy.
La terra trema (1948). Visconti, L. dir. Italy.

Section I

Artistic Universality

2. Enjoy Your Auteurism! *The Son's Room* at Cannes

Abstract: Through the case study of Cannes award-winner, *The Son's Room* (Nanni Moretti, 2001), this chapter interrogates film festivals' self-presentation as institutions that "take nothing into account other than the art of film" (Gilles Jacob cited in Elsaesser, 2005, p. 98). I argue that European A festivals mobilise the auteur as a figure of artistic universality and anti-commercial purity—a means of disavowing their statuses as enterprises engaged in a struggle for the very definition of art. I use Nanni Moretti's ambivalent authorial persona in *The Son's Room* to "speak back" to such disavowal, showing how Moertti's self-conscious performance of auteurism highlights the contradictions of the auteur as at once a symbol of artistic freedom and product of commercial constraint.

Keywords: auteur theory, art cinema, Nanni Moretti, film festivals, Italian cinema, film authorship

A close family in a small northern Italian city. The father, Giovanni, the mother, Paola and their two teenage children: Irene the elder and Andrea, the younger. Giovanni is a psychoanalyst. In his consulting-room next to his flat, his patients confide their neurosis to him, which contrasts strongly with his own quiet existence.
One Sunday morning, Giovanni is called by a patient for an emergency. He is not able to go jogging with his son, like he had told him. Andrea leaves to go scuba diving with friends and he never comes back from it...
– *Synopsis of* The Son's Room *in the Cannes 2001 print and online programme*

Introduction

It has been well documented that European A festivals differentiate themselves from other cinematic institutions through their "professed

Johnson, R., Film Festivals, *Ideology and Italian Art Cinema: Politics, Histories and Cultural Value.* Taylor & Francis Group, 2024
DOI 10.5117/9789463720366_CH02

commitment to artistic excellence and nothing else" (Elsaesser, 2005, p. 95). This was demonstrated recently in a contradictory and politicised edition of Cannes. The 2018 edition took place in the context of the #MeToo and "Time's Up" movements, both of which called for an end to discrimination against women in the film industry. That year, Cannes's main competition was judged by a female-majority jury led by Cate Blanchett, and the festival was marked by several protests for gender equality. Some appeared orchestrated, such as the women's march on the red carpet before the premiere of *Girls of the Sun* (Eva Hussan, 2018), and others spontaneous, such as juror Kristen Stewart refusing to wear high heels on the same red carpet. (It has been a controversial unwritten rule that women must wear heels on this strip of fabric.)[1] These performances contributed to a sense that this edition of the festival was to be a politicised one, raising the possibility that other aspects of the Cannes 2018 edition might respond to recent, high-profile calls for gender equality. However, when asked if these issues would influence the jury's awarding of prizes, both the festival director Thierry Frémaux and Blanchett insisted that films would be selected and judged on the basis of artistic merit alone (Mumford, 2018).

Such statements enact a familiar demarcation between art and politics and place one of European A festivals' central rituals (prize-giving) firmly on the side of "art." Yet this obscures the political nature of the very construction of "art" as an evaluative notion, and "art cinema" as a contested term. As discussed in the introduction to this book, ideas of art cinema and the concepts of artistic value that underpin them are by no means pure: they are produced and reproduced by institutions that exist in contingent historic, economic, geographic and cultural contexts, and that operate according to political and commercial interests. As Liz Czach (2004, p. 84) puts it, "politics is never removed from the question of taste." This chapter explores how film festivals obscure the contested, and thus political, dimension of their selection and awarding of films through their appeals to artistic purity and celebration of the figure of the auteur. I do so through not only an analysis and theorisation of film festivals' common practices in relation to art and the auteur, but through the case study of Cannes awarding the Palme d'Or to *The Son's Room*, a film that highlights the contradictory nature of auteurism as a sign of artistic autonomy and quality.

1 The controversies surrounding Cannes's unofficial policing of women's footwear, including at the 2018 edition, have been reported in trade publications such as *Screen Daily* and *Variety*. See Wiseman (2015, 2016) and Saperstein (2018).

Constructing Universals: "The Art of Film"

Film festivals, particularly A festivals, occupy a paradoxical position. They are at once differentiated from and closely related to highly commercialised sections of the film industry: for example, Hollywood, a commercial film producer whose films circulate at major film festivals, and film theatres, commercial exhibition sites that draw on festivals as part of their supply chain (de Valck, 2007, p. 58; Burgess & Kredell, 2016, p. 165). On the one hand, film festivals tend to privilege the exhibition and awarding of films that would not otherwise succeed at the box office: "festival screenings typically serve a *cultural* purpose, not an economic one" (de Valck 2016, p. 104, italics in the original). In this sense, film festivals are driven by cultural—and within this, artistic—concerns above financial ones. On the other hand, A-list festivals are required, by definition, to serve the interests of the film industry. They are "expected to implement quality and reliability standards that meet industry expectations" (FIAPF, 2016). Scholars such as Mezias et al. (2008), Peranson (2009), de Valck (2007, 2014), Ostrowska (2016) and Loist (2016) have repeatedly highlighted the commercial aspect of these events, from their role in facilitating the modest commercial success of cinema produced outside Hollywood, to the impact of commercialisation on the processes of film selection and awarding.

As Dina Iordanova (2009, pp. 23–24) has argued, while film festivals are, on the surface, sites of exceptional cultural celebration, when we look closer, "seemingly secondary concerns like the rank of celebrities on the red carpet and the numbers of accredited journalists take over the art of cinema." This chapter seeks to examine the effects of this contradiction between A festivals as cultural, political and commercial events. What interests me is not necessarily whether European A festivals are primarily cultural or commercial; such binary opposition would do injustice to the complexity of the festivals in question. Rather, I am concerned with how European A festivals represent themselves and the films they award, given their need to negotiate this contradictory opposition. What do such festivals foreground, and what do they disavow? What does this mean for the notions of art cinema that they reproduce?

Fremaux and Blanchett's comments about the 2018 edition of Cannes suggest one possible answer to these questions: festivals claim to dedicate themselves to the promotion of artistic merit at the exclusion of all else. This claim was a prevalent feature of Cannes before 2018, for example. Fremaux's predecessor, Gilles Jacobs, claimed that

> [o]ur aim is always to place film at the centre of our acts. Generally, to take nothing into account other than the art of film and the pre-eminence of artistic talent. (Jacob in Elsaesser, 2005, p. 98)

The claim to "take nothing into account other than the art of the film" implies purity—no concern but that of "the art of film" should influence the organisation of the festival and, above all, its selection and awarding practices. Film festivals depend upon this sense of their extraordinary significance to the cultivation of the cinematic art for their legitimacy. Film festivals are given "faith" on the basis of their "adamant insistence that the sole criterion applied is that of quality and artistic excellence" (Elsaesser, 2005, p. 98). Much more than an idealistic statement, the image and success of festivals such as Cannes are intimately bound up with their claim to be influenced solely by notions of artistic merit. Film festivals are legitimated, and legitimate films, through the idea of a sanctified commitment to "art." Yet, paradoxically, film festivals are themselves involved in the continual redefinition of what counts as art. The "art of film" that festival directors such as Jacob claim to privilege is not a fixed concept that straightforwardly guides the selection and awarding of films, but a changeable and contested one.

Film festivals' self-definition in relation to "the art of film" obscures the highly contingent and complex nature of these organisations and their selection, awarding and representation of art cinema. We might therefore theorise "the art of film" as the *universal signifier* of A-list film festivals. A universal signifier is a concept or phrase that does not have any specific content in itself—it is "empty"—but has enough of a semblance of meaning that it can function as the ideal under which an institution might operate.[2] For example, we might say that a government operates under the universal of "democracy." This functions as an ideal, even though the particular expression of democracy might change depending on the historical moment or the governing party. Similarly, "the art of film" can be considered to operate as the empty signifier of film festival ideology. It is posited as pristine, a "pure" idea through which film festivals define themselves.

As the example of democracy shows, however, universals are subject to an inherent tension between their empty ideality and the particular meaning

2 See the theories of Ernesto Laclau, Judith Butler and Slavoj Žižek. All three theorists' work has been brought into dialogue in the collection of essays and responses *Contingency, Hegemony, Universality* (2000). The notion of universal as empty signifier is the basic agreed concept for the interventions made by all (though the arguments they make from this starting point differ). I emphasise Žižek's theory of the universal predominantly for its compatibility with the overarching theoretical framework of this book.

they are given at a certain time (Žižek, 1999, p. 176). A universal is never truly universal, never "pure": its actual meaning is always circumscribed by some particular content. In the West, at our present historical juncture, democracy often refers to a specific system of parliamentary, representative democracy. Likewise, "the art of film" refers to the canons of filmmaking that institutions such as film festivals have promoted and cultivated over the last century. The particular meaning ascribed to a universal is secured through a process of contestation, the struggle between different actors or stakeholders. This is the struggle of ideology, the "level on which [...] ideological battles are won or lost" (Žižek, 1999, p. 175). It is this process of contestation that drives A-list film festivals; the struggle between programmers, jurors and a whole range of stakeholders for the meaning of "art," and, with it, the meaning of art cinema.

However, in order for ideology to function effectively, this contingency must be disavowed: "a minimum of 'naturalisation' is a condition of effectiveness of the hegemonic [or ideological] operation" (Žižek, 2004a, p. 96). This is the ultimate function of the universal. Although film festivals advertise some aspects of this process of contestation—the debates and disagreements between jurors even constituting part of the festival spectacle—such processes are ultimately subsumed back into a discourse that operates under the sign of "art." As we have seen, even moments in which contestation and contingency manifest themselves (as in the 2018 edition of Cannes) are ultimately presented under the sign of a universal. They either serve or are secondary to the commitment to "the art of film and nothing else." The product of such contestation—the selection and awarding of certain films at each festival edition—is not presented as contingent, the eccentric quirk of a particular festival or year. Such films are defined through, and come to define, "the art of film." As discussed above, the faith stakeholders afford A-list film festivals depends upon this operation. In short, the efficacy of film festival ideology depends upon the naturalisation of festival actors' decisions, their contingency veiled under the universal of "the art of film."

From Universal to *Sinthome*: The Enjoyment of Auteurism

So far, I have outlined two levels of the ideological construction of the universal: (1) the universal as an empty signifier, an ideal notion without content; (2) the ideological universal, the universal given a particular content, even if this particularity is disavowed. Thus, we find that the universal of European A festivals is "the art of film," while its ideological expression, the ideological universal, is the actual canon of art cinema that such festivals produce. To fully understand film festivals' ideological mobilisation of "art," however, we must add a third level: the *sinthome*. The *sinthome* is a particular example, often a figure, in which the meaning of the ideological universal is crystallised. This figure is presented as the "typical case," the perfect expression of the universal notion (Žižek, 1999, p. 175). The efficacy of the universal in ideology depends on its meaning being condensed in "some particular content" which stands in as the universal's representative. This particular content is known as the *sinthome*, the typical case of a universal notion. The *sinthome* is not just any representation of the universal idea, but the crucial representation, the "point at which all the lines of the predominant ideological argumentation meet" (Žižek, 1999, p. 176). In other words, all the assumptions and values implicit in an ideological universal are condensed into this singular figure.

The *sinthome* is therefore a contradictory signifier: it is both highly particular while representing the universal. We might think of the *sinthome* as internally split, divided between its particularity and the claim to universality it effects. The contingency of the *sinthome* must, too, be disavowed. In its contingency, the *sinthome* is an ultimately senseless signifier, yet its presentation as typical (rather than nonsensical) secures the effective functioning of ideology. Treating a senseless signifier as though it were meaningful is described in Lacanian theory as *jouissance* or enjoyment. We "enjoy" the *sinthome*, affording it significance while disavowing its highly contingent nature.[3] The *sinthome* is, in this sense, "the kernel of idiotic enjoyment" that secures the efficacy of an ideology (Žižek, 1992, p. 128). It represents the ideological universal in the form of a highly contingent, senseless signifier that we nonetheless enjoy as though it were universal.

"The art of film" is the universal under which A-list film festivals operate, and the particular canon of art cinema that such festivals construct is the ideological universal. What might be the *sinthome* of this ideological formation? Surely the notion of film as "art" finds no more common figuration than that of the auteur. The auteur is the *sinthome*, a "kernel of idiotic enjoyment" that stands in for "the art of film." This was summarised by one film critic's description of Cannes's motto as "Live by the Auteur, Die by the Auteur," a phrase that exemplifies the senseless subjection of *jouissance* (McCarthy, 1999).

3 In fact, it is the senselessness that the subject "enjoys," since it is experienced as the "secret," the greater knowledge of the big Other, of ideology, to which one quite literally subjects oneself. This is the same procedure as the move from the Real to fantasy described in the previous chapter.

One of the reasons that the auteur can represent film festivals' claim to a single-minded commitment to artistic purity is that the concept has been associated with artistic autonomy since its inception. First appearing in *Cahiers du Cinéma*'s provocative *politique des auteurs*, the auteur is, as the journal's editor, André Bazin, argued, "always subject to himself [*sic*]," producing artworks that transcend their industrial "conditions of existence" (Bazin, 2008 [1957], p. 25). In this line of reasoning, the auteur may work within an industrial context, but the films they create are not constrained by it. While Bazin's account is relatively balanced, still accounting for technological and industrial factors, it is in Andrew Sarris's (1962) transformation of the *politique des auteurs* into so-called "Auteur Theory" that the figure of the auteur, and their films, assumes the burden of artistic purity. Sarris's account of the auteur rejects the historicisation of a director's work, advocating readings that consider only their aesthetic dimension and, crucially, their artistic virtuosity: "the third and ultimate premise of the *auteur* theory is concerned with interior meaning, *the ultimate glory of cinema as an art*" (Sarris, 1962, p. 7; italics added). This idea of the director's powerful artistic vision takes on an evaluative function, securing some films' legitimation as "art," while those films that are not perceived to bear such a vision are dismissed as less-than-worthy reflections of historical influences, usually bound up with the commercial demands of the Hollywood film industry (Buscombe, 2008 [1973], p. 80). While scholars have repeatedly and persuasively challenged this mode of auteurism, it remains a stubborn assumption underpinning the evaluation of films. As Dana Polan (2001, para. 21) puts it, even when "we admit that directors take up their place in larger structures of meaning-production, [...] in the long run, we want to imagine that auteurs are of interest independent of all that context." The auteur endures as a figure that ultimately disavows the contingent nature of filmmaking, positing the transcendence of contextual factors as a marker of a film's artistic value.

The figure of the auteur is not only exemplary for its value-laden signification of artistic freedom. The auteur *sinthomatically* bears the contradictions between the universal and the particular. It does so on a structural level and on the level of its actual expression. On a structural level, although the auteur signifies art in its ideal sense, this process of signification also requires the restriction of that ideality. The universal of "the art of film" cannot be expressed without the figure of the auteur, thus restricting the meaning of art cinema to auteurist cinema, a process well documented in accounts of art cinema from Neale (1981) to Bordwell (1979) to Galt and Schoonover (2010). Meanwhile, on the level of the individual film, meaning is also restricted through its relation to the auteur. Rather than a "pure" artwork, a film's meaning is delimited by its auteurist interpretation. As Paul Sellors (2010, p. 43) argues via Roland Barthes, the auteur conditions the meaning of a film via the "fiction" of their presence within the text—in most cases, the dominance of their "artistic vision." Therefore, paradoxically, the evaluation of film via the concept of the auteur actually restricts a film's meaning in the name of artistic purity. This replicates the structural contradiction between the universal as a pure, or empty, notion, and the *sinthome* as a contingent, particular expression of the universal.

The fiction and contradictions of the auteur are as much a product of commercial necessity as an expression of the theoretical permutations of auteurism outlined above. Central to the tension between the auteur as a signifier of artistic freedom and its effective restriction of a film's meaning lies another contradiction: the presentation of films under the sign of the auteur delimits their meaning for commercial purposes. This tension is characteristic of the notion of the auteur, its function having been, historically, to delimit the meaning of art cinema in such a way as to make it saleable. Neale (1981) discusses the importance of the figure of the auteur to the institutional construction of art cinema, identifying film festivals as an important example of the institutions engaged in such a process. Although raising the possibility of art cinema being subject to contested and fluid definitions, Neale (1981) argues that the institutional nature of the mode means that this possibility is foreclosed as it is subject to auteurism, or "an ideology of art as individual expression" (p. 36). This grounds his description of the way in which the institutionalisation of art cinema entails its homogenisation for commercial purposes: the institution "mobilises [art cinema's] meaning in accordance with commodity-based practices of production, distribution and exhibition" (p. 15). Paradoxically, while signifying transcendence from commercial constraints, the auteur is also "used as a kind of brand name, to mark and to sell the filmic product" (p. 15). The endurance of auteurism is a product of the same structures of capitalism and commodity exchange that it, as *sinthome*, serves to disavow.

These processes of delimiting art cinema's meaning via the figure of the auteur, and doing so in such a way as to secure some measure of commercial success for films, are particularly clear when we examine the operation of A-list film festivals. As these festivals moved to a "post-national" system in 1972, international selection committees became prevalent, and a greater variety of films were selected for exhibition and competition.[4] With this

4 See also de Valck (2007) and Ostrowska (2016).

greater diversity came the need for a sign under which festivals could organise themselves as both gatekeepers of art cinema and nodes in the film industry. This sign became the auteur: "by stressing 'the auteur' and other signs of universalism, film festivals could better facilitate the international flow of cultural and economic capital on which they depended" (Andrews, 2010, p. 10). The construction of the auteur as a "sign of universalism" may have originated at Cannes: Elsaesser (2005, p. 91) states that "the gold standard of the European festivals under the rule of Cannes became the auteur director." The auteur has since become the central figure used to define and promote both films and film festivals worldwide. Film festival directors and programmers are well aware of the marketing value of the auteur: the auteur is a "reified [...] marketing category" (Ma, 2010, p. 346) that film festivals mobilise to secure "value-added prestige" for each edition (Falicov, 2016, p. 214).

The value—symbolic and, ultimately, economic—that an auteur's presence at a festival might add can even override the importance of a film's quality in programming decisions. Tamara Falicov (2016, p. 214) has argued that a particular film's shortcomings may be overlooked for a festival to maintain the continuity of the auteur "brand." Further expressing the paradoxes of film festivals' deployment of the universal of "art," the auteur's very mobilisation is an expression of these events' contingency. Film festivals' selection of a director's films, and thus legitimisation of such films as "art," is conditioned by that festival's need to secure prestige and brand continuity.

Thus, the auteur has become a central figure in film festivals' organisation under the sign of "art," the universal through which they attempt to define both themselves and the films they exhibit and award. This *sinthome* at once delimits the meaning of art cinema and disavows festivals' status as sites of contestation conditioned by commercial interests: it is the paradoxical signifier of festivals' "anti-commercial purity" (Andrews, 2010, p. 9). The auteur assists the disavowal of the contingent relationship between the actual films presented at festivals (the ideological universal) and the ideal of "the art of film" (the empty universal). However, the auteur also instantiates the contradictions of this ideological operation. The auteur is, paradoxically, a signifier of artistic freedom that delimits films' meanings for commercial purposes. The auteur condenses the same paradox I have described in relation to film festivals above: the economic viability of festivals and the films they exhibit is dependent upon their semblance of anti-commerciality, their organisation around the notion of artistic purity. We can therefore observe an overlap between commerciality and contingency that cuts through ideological construction of "the art of film," and art cinema. The auteur is symptomatic, or rather *sinthomatic*, of the contradictory relationship between universality and contingency, artistic purity and commercial constraint that characterises European A festivals.

Performative Contradiction: Untying the Knot of Auteurism

This paradox becomes clearer when we examine the auteur's status as a representative of artistic autonomy who is nonetheless constrained by their relationship to film festivals. Although promoted as the signifier of artistic freedom rather than commercial constraint, auteurs depend on film festivals for their consecration, just as film festivals depend on auteurs for their legitimation as tastemakers (Elsaesser, 2005, p. 97). As argued above, film festivals construct the very notions of "art" that they present as universal in order to, paradoxically, market themselves, and the films they award, on the basis of their anti-commerciality. Likewise, by cultivating relationships with directors and repeatedly selecting their films, festivals construct the category of the auteur, determining who belongs to it as a means of securing both symbolic and financial capital. In so doing, they delimit the meanings of the films they reward, constraining their universality as "art" through the particularity of auteurism.

As directors are ascribed the role of auteur, they are required to perform the role of an autonomous artist. Another contradiction emerges: the director-as-auteur is required by film festivals to perform the role of one whose works are not subject to institutional or commercial limitations. As Elsaesser (2016) has observed,

> a dynamic of reciprocal dependencies is implicit in this relationship between auteur and festival, chief among these being that the festival, in order to fulfil its mission, has to encourage and even *constrain* the filmmaker to behave as if he/she [/they] was [were] indeed a *free agent and an autonomous artist*, dedicated solely to expressing a uniquely personal vision, and thus to *disavow* the very pressures the festival has to impose. (p. 25; italics added)

Another paradox is condensed in the figure of the auteur that film festivals mobilise, since these filmmakers are "constrained" to behave as though they were "autonomous artist[s]." The circulation of symbolic and financial capital through film festivals depends upon their (contradictory) requirement for the auteur to act as a free agent. While Elsaesser theorises this relationship neither in terms of ideology nor psychoanalysis, his use of the term "disavowal" alludes to the ideological procedure at work in this "dynamic of reciprocal tendencies" that structures film festivals' relation to the auteur. The very category of the auteur is contingent upon film festivals' consecrating function, which necessitates auteurs' performance of freedom from contingency.

It is through this paradox that we can approach the *sinthome* of the auteur as a contradictory signifier of artistic freedom and universality that disavows commercial constraint and contingency. The auteur must act as though their films are free expressions, universal artworks, but, in doing so, their freedom is limited by: (1) the director's identity being delimited by their construction as an auteur (a role they must perform); and (2) their films' meanings being delimited by their construction in relation to the auteur (we could say that the film, too, is made to "perform" a contingent, auteurist meaning).

The paradoxes that the figure of the auteur represents—particular and universal, free and contingent—can be made manifest through performative contradiction. This procedure will be central to the rest of this chapter, which aims to untie the knot of the auteur as *sinthome*, simultaneously demonstrating and interpreting film festivals' disavowal of contingency. Žižek (2000a, p. 102) uses the notion of performative contradiction to theorise a model for ideology critique:

> [T] he proper critique of "false universality" does not call it into question from the standpoint of pre-universal particularism, it mobilises the tension inherent to universality itself [...] if the ruling ideology performatively "cheats" by undermining—in its actual discursive practice and the set of exclusions on which this practice relies—its own officially asserted universality, progressive politics should precisely openly practice performative contradiction, asserting on behalf of a given universality the very content this universality (in its hegemonic form) excludes.

If film festivals performatively "cheat" by undermining the officially asserted universality of art through their construction of and dependence on the exclusive categories of art cinema and auteur, the director-as-auteur can disrupt claims to universality through performative contradiction. For example, directors can assert on behalf of "art" that which the concept disavows, the constraint on which it depends—for example, the constraint of a director's identity as that of auteur.

Continuing his analysis of auteurism, Elsaesser (2016, p. 25) has considered the means by which the auteur may perform self-contradiction, assisting an understanding of how the auteur as *sinthome* can demonstrate the contradictory universality mobilised by film festivals. Elsaesser (2016, p. 37) gives the example of Lars von Trier attending the Berlinale while wearing a T-shirt bearing the words "persona non grata" and the Cannes logo, a response to having been banned from the French festival.[5] Elsaesser defines this as a case of "performative contradiction" in which the claim (von Trier's autonomy, i.e., his freedom to wear polemical T-shirts) is contradicted by the means used to make it (his appearance at a film festival, and thus dependence on it to make such a claim publicly). This example demonstrates one way in which directors can simultaneously perform and resist the "auteur" label applied to them by film festivals. Although having cultivated a "personal genre identity" and "brand name" for strategic gain (that is, an auteur persona or brand), von Trier's appearance at the Berlinale performed the contradiction of this identity: his dependence on festivals such as Cannes and Berlin enabled him to, paradoxically, assert his autonomy (Elsaesser, 2016, pp. 36–37). Von Trier's performance dramatises the contradictions in the construction of the auteur as a signifier of artistic freedom.

The Son's Room: A Hysterical Auteurism

The case of *The Son's Room*'s presentation and awarding at Cannes in 2001 clarifies the process of performative contradiction yet further. As I show below, Cannes's representation of *The Son's Room* as an artwork, its evaluation as a product of free creative expression, is contradicted by the means used to make it: the festival's ascription of legitimacy to the film is dependent upon Moretti's status as an auteur. This contradiction is not performed, but rather *appears hidden* in Cannes's synopsis of the film. While on an explicit level

5 Lars von Trier was banned from Cannes in 2011 for making antisemitic remarks, claiming to sympathise with Adolf Hitler. He returned to the French Riviera in 2018, when his film *The House that Jack Built* (2018) was selected for Cannes's main competition. (The film was disparaged by critics for its patent sexism.) The inclusion of von Trier in this book, even if via Elsaesser, is not intended to excuse or celebrate this director. Indeed, while this example is useful in a purely theoretical sense, outlining the model of performative contradiction that I expand on, we cannot ignore the other aspects of the contradiction that von Trier performs: his very ability to appear at the Berlinale, and later Cannes, is enabled by the auteurist structure of film festivals and film criticism more generally, permitting him to make antisemitic comments and still be afforded attention and prestige on the basis of his status as auteur. There is not the space to elaborate on the role that the media system, film festivals and the politics of provocation play in such cases here. However, my analysis of Nanni Moretti provides, I hope, a useful counterexample of a director who can perform the contradictions of auteurism without recourse to "provocation."

the text seems to present *The Son's Room* as an artwork unconstrained by Moretti's authorial persona, it can only do so on the basis of the unwritten law of auteurism, thanks to the strength of Moretti's authorial persona, in this case. Reading the synopsis against the film, and vice versa, I analyse some of the ways in which the film highlights this contradiction. In so doing, I further demonstrate the paradox around which film festival ideology is, in part, structured: the universal of "the art of film" being delimited by the very *sinthome* that supposedly represents it.

Nanni Moretti's career and authorial persona have been cultivated by Cannes since the late 1970s, finding most recent expression in the festival's selection of *A Brighter Tomorrow* (*Il sol dell'avvenire*, Moretti, 2023) for the main competition in 2023. Although awarded his first major festival prize at the Berlinale, Moretti has been a regular presence at Cannes for over forty years: first as an actor in Palme d'Or winner *Father and Master* (*Padre Padrone*, Taviani & Taviani, 1977) and then as director, screenwriter and lead actor of *Ecce bombo* (Moretti, 1978), which also premiered in the main competition. At the time of writing, the Italian filmmaker is credited in sixteen films screened at Cannes and has won two of the festival's most prestigious awards: Best Director for *Dear Diary* (*Caro diario*, Moretti, 1994) and the Palme d'Or for *The Son's Room*. He has also sat on the festival jury twice.[6] This confirms the well-established notion that film festivals are "in the business of making new authors," capitalising on such discoveries to secure their own prestige (Elsaesser, 2005, p. 99). The evidence so far suggests that *The Son's Room*'s selection at the festival, and its winning the Palme d'Or, were at least partially influenced by Moretti's status as one of Cannes's privileged auteurs.

Both Moretti and the film that won top prize highlight the contradictions of the *sinthome*. Moretti's extremely successful cultivation of an authorial persona through his role not only as director but also (among other things) as lead actor and often protagonist in his films has resulted in a scenario in which every film he directs is marked by his "overwhelming authorial presence" (Vighi, 2005, p. 80). Scholars' interpretations of *The Son's Room* indicate that Moretti both performs and undermines his status as auteur, highlighting its constructed dimension. This, in turn, underlines the contradiction that he

6 This information appears in the biography of Moretti on Cannes's website (Festival de Cannes, 2019b). This paratext flaunts Moretti's auteurist credentials, as well as the festival's long-standing relationship with him. The festival's production of biographies for the auteurs they promote (a common feature of European A festivals' websites) attests to the centrality of the figure of the auteur to its apparatus.

should be constrained to play the role of the auteur—that he should "behave as if he was indeed a free agent and an autonomous artist, dedicated solely to expressing a uniquely personal vision" (Elsaesser, 2016, p. 25). While a departure from Moretti's previous autobiographical filmmaking, *The Son's Room* remains marked by the indelible stain of Moretti's "authorial presence," producing a tension between the film's diegetic and metacinematic levels—its status as a film as such, and as a "Moretti film." As we will see later, the film represents a refusal to perform its status as a free artwork, with Moretti appearing on screen to highlight the inescapable, auteurist constraint of its meaning.

Alongside his cultivation by Cannes, Moretti has developed a particularly strong authorial persona through his extensive involvement in filmmaking, often playing the roles of director, screenwriter, producer, lead actor and, through his films' use of the autobiographical mode, lead protagonist. Ewa Mazierska and Laura Rascaroli (2004, p. 44) argue that Moretti's greatest achievement is to have created a fictional persona whose autobiography runs across his films. Playing protagonists such as Michele Apicella (whose surname is Moretti's mother's maiden name), Don Giulio, Nanni and Giovanni (permutations of Moretti's given names), the director has managed to consistently "put himself at the forefront of his cinematic discourse" (Mazierska & Rascaroli, 2004, p. 8).

However, *The Son's Room* was commonly received as a departure from Moretti's autobiographical oeuvre, a film in which his authorial persona recedes. Reviewing the film in *Variety*, for example, David Rooney (2001, para. 1) describes the film as a "refined, uncharacteristic work" that transcends "Moretti's customary narcissism." The film is conceived as more mature, a refinement of Moretti's previous works, due to its perceived distance from the Moretti persona. Mazierska and Rascaroli (2004, p. 112) respond to those who see Giovanni as "the first 'real' and non-autobiographical protagonist that the film-maker has created." Beyond the continuity afforded by Giovanni taking Moretti's birth name, Mazierska and Rascaroli also identify the common thread of irony running through *The Son's Room* and Moretti's other films. This irony develops from negative irony in films such as *Aprile* and *Caro diario* into a positive irony that allows Giovanni and his wife Paola to learn to laugh at the absurdity of life (p. 113). They conclude that Giovanni is "best seen as the mature and more successful version of the old character [Apicella]" (p. 112).

Their analysis points to one of the ways in which *The Son's Room* both is and is not a typical Moretti film. Mazierska and Rascaroli locate the film within Moretti's oeuvre in such a way that places Moretti's persona at the centre. Whether considered a break from or development of the Moretti figure, the meanings ascribed to *The Son's Room* depend upon its relation to Moretti's body of work, taken as the yardstick against which to compare and contrast the film. Crucially, however, Mazierska and Rascaroli's reading foregrounds the constructed nature of Moretti's persona, elucidating the performance of a cinematic ego that conditions, even forms a fundamental part of, his films' representational strategies.

Other scholars have interpreted *The Son's Room* in relation to Moretti's persona and the trope of irony or, in some cases, the questioning of identities that runs across his body of work. Fabio Vighi (2005) also positions *The Son's Room* as different from, yet related to, Moretti's oeuvre in important ways. Vighi interrogates the claim that *The Son's Room* can be considered a departure from Moretti's other films. Vighi (2005) concludes that the film inaugurates a "new" Moretti (but a Moretti, nonetheless) as it "radicalises the implicit achievement of his previous filmography" (p. 105). Specifically, Vighi (2005) argues that, until *The Son's Room*, the ironic self-questioning common to Moretti's films was that of the "Beautiful Soul": "the subject who laments the shortcomings of the world around him and, at the same time, keeps at a safe distance from it through an ironic relativistic gaze" (p. 84). Yet in *The Son's Room*, this ironic safe distance breaks down. Upon the death of his son, Giovanni must confront not only the immediate, mortal loss, but also a much deeper, intrinsic loss: the fundamental impossibility of ever having a full relationship with, of ever fully knowing, his son. In doing so, Giovanni takes on the position of the radical hysteric: he begins to confront the lack intrinsic to his identity as a father (Vighi, 2005, p. 92). The son's death sets Giovanni on a course of radical questioning that touches the lack inherent to identity as such, the impossibility of ever fully being that which we are supposed to be.

Vighi's reading of hysteria in *The Son's Room* relates well to the project of untying the *sinthome*, highlighting the contingency of the relation between the *sinthome* and the universal. We, as subjects, must negotiate the abyss between our individual, particular experience and our participation in abstract identities, such as father, woman or even human. We are also split between particularity and universality. Likewise, "auteur" can refer to a symbolic identity, a *sinthome*, and an individual director. When one shifts focus from Giovanni-as-hysterical-subject in *The Son's Room*'s narrative to Moretti-as-authorial-presence in the film, we can start to consider whether this radical questioning might also entail the performance of a contradiction inherent to the very notion of *The Son's Room* as a Morettian film. We might interpret *The Son's Room* as performing a confrontation with the fundamental lack *inherent to itself* as an Italian, auteurist film valorised by a European A festival. In this way, the Palme d'Or winner has the potential to effect a "full hystericisation" of not only the subject (Vighi, 2005, p. 92), but the auteurist festival film.

While writing primarily about hysterical masculinity in *Aprile*, Paul Sutton (2004) also raises the question of undermining identity in *The Son's Room*, and relates this to Moretti's constructed or "public" persona. Sutton's analysis of both films shows how they simultaneously perform and undermine Moretti's identity as a masculine figure and an auteur.[7] Sutton (2004) argues that Moretti's status as a father is a central part of his public persona: he appears as both a "cinematic father" and, since the release of *Aprile*, a father in the everyday sense of the term (p. 151). Sutton (2004) argues that the model of fatherhood in both cases is "represented as fragmented and open," while *Aprile* can be read as a film marked by "the splintering of Moretti's already precarious identity" (p. 152). This interpretation leads him to reinforce the notion of Moretti's authorial power, however, concluding that "[t]he plural, problematic and cinematic Nanni Moretti is offered in place of the singular and dangerously alluring Silvio Berlusconi" (p. 153). Sutton thus takes the representation of a fragmented identity to be an authorial signature and political statement that culminates in Moretti's opposition to the masculinity represented by Italy's former Prime Minister. Read with Vighi's analysis, we might note that such an interpretation characterises Moretti's persona, and *The Son's Room*, as splitting "Moretti" into a multiplicity of identities. Sutton's discussion of the relationship between Moretti's status as cinematic father (auteur) and his characters' statuses as on-screen fathers provides an important frame through which to interpret *The Son's Room* as a film simultaneously about paternal grief and Moretti's authorial persona. However, we should contrast this with the film's potential to perform the split inherent to identity as such—that is, its capacity to make manifest the contradictions internal to each identity it presents, rather than the tensions between different identities.

De Gaetano's (1999, p. 116) interpretation of Moretti's satirical and exaggerated acting style suggests how this splitting might manifest on screen. His theory highlights the centrality of Moretti's performance of a multiplicity of identities, which makes apparent a rupture between them. De Gaetano's interpretation of Moretti's performance also has the potential to be reformulated to account for both the splitting *between identities* and the split, or lack, *fundamental to each identity*. De Gaetano (1999) demonstrates

7 On masculinity and the auteur, see the next chapter.

how Moretti's performance style constructs a "gap in the mask" that destabilises the identities that appear on screen (p. 116). When Moretti plays a character such as Michele Apicella, he never fully mimics his character but reveals their face as a mask. De Gaetano shows how this operates on both a diegetic and a metacinematic level. On the diegetic level, Moretti's grotesque, over-exaggerated acting style effects an over-identification between the character and their identity, like with Apicella as the over-zealous Communist (pp. 115–116). Through exaggeration, this identity is ridiculed, revealed in its constructed dimension.

Meanwhile, on a metacinematic level, Moretti allows his mask as actor to slip, usually by momentarily breaking character (De Gaetano, 1999, p. 117). In this case, Moretti's sudden appearance *as Moretti*, his "presence as actor" (*presenza d'attore*), constructs a distance between the character and the actor (De Gaetano, 1999, p. 117).[8] In this way, Moretti's acting style contributes to the destabilisation of identity that Sutton argued is central to both Moretti's persona and *The Son's Room*. When we add to this the dimension of Moretti as not only actor and character, but *auteur*, we can perceive a third level of destabilisation. Moretti's identity as both actor and character is, as we have seen, overdetermined by his status as auteur; his acting and autobiography contribute, ultimately, to the construction of his authorial persona. When Moretti appears on screen, all three identities appear; however, they are overdetermined by his persona as auteur. De Gaetano's concept of the construction of gaps in the actor's mask, to which I add the actor-auteur's mask, highlights how Moretti's on-screen performance might reveal the constructed dimension of his authorial status. In other words, Moretti's films, including *The Son's Room*, have the potential to make manifest Moretti's presence as *auteur* (or *presenza d'autore*), constructing a distance between the character, actor and the auteur, eventually revealing a tension inherent to the latter.

Taking these interpretations of *The Son's Room* together, the pertinence of the film as a case study for interrogating the *sinthome* of the auteur is clear. Moretti's auteur status has been repeatedly consecrated by Cannes, and his films are characterised by the construction and performance of an unmistakeable authorial persona. While Moretti initially appears to play the role of auteur designated by European A festivals, he does so in a way that highlights its performative dimension, suggesting the contradiction that this entails. Bringing this into relation with the status of auteur as *sinthome* raises the possibility of interpreting *The Son's Room* as a film that

8 All translations from Italian to English in this book are my own, unless otherwise stated.

performs the contradiction of film festivals' ideological construction of both the auteur and the universal "the art of film." Rather than an impossibly "free" artistic expression, *The Son's Room* is constrained by the necessity that it be a "Moretti film"—that it bear the traces of its auteur. However, reading Moretti's performative questioning of this aspect of the film can make manifest such a contradiction. This understanding of the film provides a basis from which to analyse Cannes's construction of it. To what extent is *The Son's Room* represented in its ideality as artwork, while in fact being constrained by its status as a "Moretti film"? To answer this question, let us turn to the festival's synopsis of *The Son's Room* and clarify the extent to which the film's construction is mediated by, and instantiates, European A festivals' auteurist apparatus and the ideological structures that underpin it.

Synopsis Analysis

The synopsis of *The Son's Room* that represents the film in Cannes's 2001 programme appears to omit any detail that would indicate Moretti's presence in the film, whether as auteur, lead actor or protagonist. The synopsis precludes explicit reference to Moretti as well as features that might imply the director's authorial presence, such as thematic or stylistic tropes associated with his filmmaking. The paratext presents *The Son's Room* as a narrative film in its own right: the film, as well as Cannes's celebration of it, is shown as untouched by Moretti's authorial presence.

Although not the focus of this chapter, Cannes's synopsis of one of Moretti's earlier films, *Dear Diary*, the film which won him Best Director at the festival, brings into relief Cannes's omission of any indication of Moretti's persona in the synopsis of *The Son's Room*. The earlier text presents *Dear Diary* as autobiographical and inward-gazing, expressing the author's "most hidden thoughts and ideas." Moreover, the synopsis expresses a playfulness around auteur theory, eliding director and protagonist in ambiguous references to "the author" of this "visual diary." Such playfulness alludes to auteurism, even invites us to enjoy it. While space does not permit a more detailed comparison of the two synopses here, these details indicate that Cannes's presentation of *The Son's Room* may build on the festival's establishment of Moretti as an auteur and his films as expressions of his authorial vision. However, the differences between the two synopses also suggest that the latter downplays the auteurism that characterised Cannes's representation of *Dear Diary*, highlighting omissions in the festival's textual framing of *The Son's Room*.

Yet, in both cases, the auteurist dimension of Moretti's filmmaking and Cannes's repeated selection of his films cannot be approached directly. It takes on an indirect, even ironic, character in the synopsis of *Dear Diary*, and is rendered absent in that of *The Son's Room*. It is as though Moretti's "overwhelming authorial presence" and, to a greater extent, his hysterical questioning of his status as auteur or "cinematic father" disrupt the smooth functioning of film festivals' elision of "the art of film" and the auteur (Vighi, 2005, p. 80; Sutton, 2004, p. 151). As such, it must be redirected in the festival's textual representations of his films. From this perspective, it may be unsurprising that it was *The Son's Room*, a film celebrated as a departure from Moretti's narcissistically auteurist style, that won the Palme d'Or. This impression of the film permitted a modicum of distance between *The Son's Room* and its director, side-stepping the contradictory constraint of a film's meaning and value via the figure of the auteur, as a signifier of the opposite of constraint: free, idealised artistic expression.

Cannes's synopsis of *The Son's Room* emphasises aspects of the film that run counter to an interpretation of it as a Moretti film (even an a-Morettian Moretti film). In doing so, it participates in the celebration of *The Son's Room* as a departure from Moretti's previous works, a film free of the Moretti persona. (As discussed above, this interpretation is not only partial, but paradoxical: such a claim depends upon Moretti being the film's director.) As such, the synopsis suggests that the prize-winning film has been selected for its purity as "art," unconstrained even by the auteur's presence (or rather, over-presence). The opening sentence of the text places us in "a small, northern Italian city." The first thing to note is the description of film's setting: we are initially confronted with a setting other than the well-known one of Moretti's home city, Rome. We can see the significance of this when we recall that Clodagh Brook (2005) identifies a setting based on the director's home city as a key feature of autobiographical cinema, and Eleanor Andrews (2014) defines this setting as Rome in Moretti's films. The synopsis initially posits a geographical distance between Giovanni and Moretti.

The paratext also opens on a "close family" rather than the image of the individual, narcissistic father that constitutes another trope of Moretti's films (or at least the auteurist progression from *Aprile* to *The Son's Room* highlighted in Sutton [2004] and MacDonald Carolan [2013]). Foregrounding the family unit at the expense of the protagonist sets the scene for a description of *The Son's Room* that disperses our attention across the characters rather than towards Moretti's persona. Although highlighting the protagonist's identity as a father, the following sentence presents this identity alongside a list of others: "The father, Giovanni, the mother, Paola and their two teenage children: Irene the elder and Andrea, the younger." In this context, the opening of the synopsis frames *The Son's Room* less as about Moretti and fatherhood and more about a fictional family unit.

The text eventually settles on Giovanni as protagonist but elides aspects that would indicate that he may be another Morettian alter-ego. Rather than a hysterical questioning of Moretti's identity as both diegetic and cinematic father (a key trope associated with Moretti's filmmaking) in the synopsis, hysteria is transformed into "neurosis," and dispersed among Giovanni's patients.[9] The patients "confide their neuroses" to Giovanni, while he (for a time, at least) has a "quiet existence." Moreover, rather than the radical questioning of identity (hysteria) that Vighi (2005) argues constitutes *The Son's Room*'s status as a development of Moretti's previous work, we have the impression of a generic mental condition (neurosis). While scholars have interpreted *The Son's Room* as a film in which Giovanni and Moretti's identities might be radically questioned, the synopsis frames the film through another reading. *The Son's Room* appears here as a film untouched by any kind of radical hysteria, much less one that permeates the metacinematic dimension of its status as a Moretti film.

The only interruption to Giovanni's "quiet existence" is presented as originating from outside his psyche. The synopsis presents Giovanni's trauma as being caused by a singular event (the disappearance of Andrea) rather than as a foundational lack confronted through hysteria. This is effected through the text's continuing, albeit subtle, focus on events external to the protagonist's subjectivity, in contrast with the subjective, even "narcissistic" gaze associated with Moretti's autarkic and autobiographical style. A series of external events cause the only conflict that the synopsis depicts. First, "Giovanni is called by a patient." The use of the passive tense ("is called") places the focus on the patient—the bearer of neurosis, as we saw before—rather than Giovanni. Then, when Giovanni "is not able to go jogging with is son," the son "goes scuba diving" and climactically "never comes back from it." Taken together, these sentences create the impression of external events culminating in tragedy.

How this might contrast with *The Son's Room*, as well as tropes associated with Moretti's persona, becomes clearest in relation to Vighi's (2005) analysis of the film and Moretti's hysterical discourse. As we have seen, Vighi argues that *The Son's Room* can be interpreted as a continuation and

9 Along with the work of Mazierska & Rascaroli (2004), Sutton (2004) and Vighi (2005, 2003), see also Antonello & Barotsi (2009) and Bonsaver (2001).

radicalisation of Moretti's authorial signature of self-questioning (Vighi, 2005, p. 105). While hysteria is triggered by the death of Andrea, its radicality depends upon recognition that the symbolic loss of Andrea pre-existed his death; it involves a confrontation with a lack foundational and internal to Giovanni's paternal subjectivity (Vighi, 2005, p. 92). As such, and in contrast with the synopsis, conflict is shown to begin within Giovanni's psyche and then is made manifest through external events in the narrative. The reversal of causality should be clear: in the synopsis, an external event causes conflict; in Vighi's reading of the film, the conflict pre-exists the external event. The Cannes synopsis, then, elides the hysterical aspect of *The Son's Room*, re-instituting the idea of the lack as external rather than internal, foundational to the subject. This directs our focus away from Giovanni/ Moretti's hysterically split subjectivity, be it that of the character or the auteur. Overall, we can observe an intriguing effect: the synopsis presents *The Son's Room* as existing in a sort of vacuum, free even of the authorial signatures that would constrain it to the definition of a "Moretti film." This disavows the contingency of *The Son's Room*'s presentation at Cannes—the centrality of Moretti's authorial status to the significance that the festival ascribes to the film.

One could argue that this is simply because Cannes synopses tend to contain less detail about films than synopses at other festivals. They are often shorter and more narrative-focused (this will become clear throughout the book, as we encounter synopses from a range of European A festivals). However, this testifies to the nature of Cannes as a festival aimed at those already initiated into the order of European A festivals and art cinema. It is the only festival in this study that is not wholly open to the public, with the majority of screenings being accessible only to industry figures. As such, Cannes is considered a particularly influential "field-configuring event" for the film industry, an event that reproduces and reinforces dominant norms among professionals (Mezias et al., 2008; Rüling, 2009, p. 51).

Such norms make up the symbolic order of film that festivals reproduce; they are the implicit "rules of the game" or "symbolic laws" to which festivals subscribe (Žižek, 2000c, p. 669). Therefore, each edition of Cannes, and its representations of films, is directed first towards those who already know "the rules of the game." The festival presents itself and its films in a way that assumes knowledge of certain symbolic laws, chief among these being auteurism. Given the festival's long-standing relationship with Moretti, we can assume that one of the laws governing Cannes's representation of *The Son's Room* is that it is a worthy film precisely because it was directed by a man whom the festival has cultivated and consecrated from his first appearance in the 1970s to his Best Director award in 1991. Moretti's status as an auteur, and the worth conferred on *The Son's Room* by this status, constitute the unwritten symbolic order of Cannes's selection, presentation and awarding of the film.

The guarantee afforded by Moretti being the film's auteur constitutes the "obscene unwritten law" that does not appear in the text itself but structures it nonetheless (Žižek, 2005, p. 54). The Cannes synopsis can therefore be read as framing *The Son's Room* as an a-Morettian film, supporting the claim that the film is a neutral artwork, unconstrained by Moretti's authorial presence, all the while depending on the hidden law of auteurism for the legitimation of that artwork. Omitting *The Son's Room*'s (and the festival's) auteurist dimension, the Cannes synopsis therefore produces the effect of supporting the *sinthome* and the ideology it represents. Hiding the *sinthome* of the auteur hides the contradictions that constitute and can be made manifest by it.

The Cannes synopsis can thus be read as a text that frames *The Son's Room* not as a text that performs the contingency of Moretti's many identities, nor as an a-Morettian Moretti film. Rather, it appears as an artwork in its own right, untouched by Moretti's status as auteur. The synopsis instantiates the ideological procedure of presenting film as unconstrained art—in line with the universal notion of the art of film—all the while being underwritten by a contingent, particular law, that of auteurism. In this way, the synopsis makes manifest a crucial tension at work in European A festivals' selection, awarding and representation of films: the tension between the ideal of evaluating a film on the basis of some pure criterion of artistic merit, and the impact of contingent factors (including a festival's relationship with a particular director) that condition not only the evaluation of films, but the very formulation of artistic merit.

Film Analysis

To investigate the relationship between the synopsis of *The Son's Room* and the context in which the film was shown and awarded—that is, the context of an auteurism characteristic of both the film festival circuit and the persona cultivated by Moretti—I now turn to the film text. I have described above how European A festivals ideologically represent films such as *The Son's Room* as though they are free, idealised artworks while simultaneously constraining their meaning through the *sinthome* of the auteur. While my analysis of *The Son's Room* aims to interpret this contradiction, it is, in a sense, marked by a similar one. Since it is a fundamental assumption of this book that film texts are unstable, with no fixed meaning, it is necessary to acknowledge that any interpretation I give of a film text is also partial—contingent and constrained. I argue that this is a productive constraint, however, since it is grounded in the aims of my analysis. The reading of *The Son's Room* that I give below are contingent upon the findings of my work above, and delimited by my aim to further investigate and interpret the *sinthome* and, with it, the ideology at work at European A festivals. Below I offer an interpretation of the ways in which *The Son's Room* performs the contradiction of its status as an a-Morettian Moretti film and its presentation at Cannes according to the same paradoxical logic. In this way, I use the aspects of *The Son's Room* that could be read as performing contradiction to aim at the "truth" of its ideological construction by Cannes, rather than the truth of the film itself.

The Body of the Auteur, the Name of the Character

One of the most inescapable, and contradictory, aspects of Moretti's films is the actor-auteur's physical embodiment on screen. Furthermore, the auteur's effigy represents the authorial signature *par excellence*, the indelible stain of the auteur on his work. The first shot of *The Son's Room* is marked by precisely such a stain, as the film opens on the figure of Moretti jogging along a port.

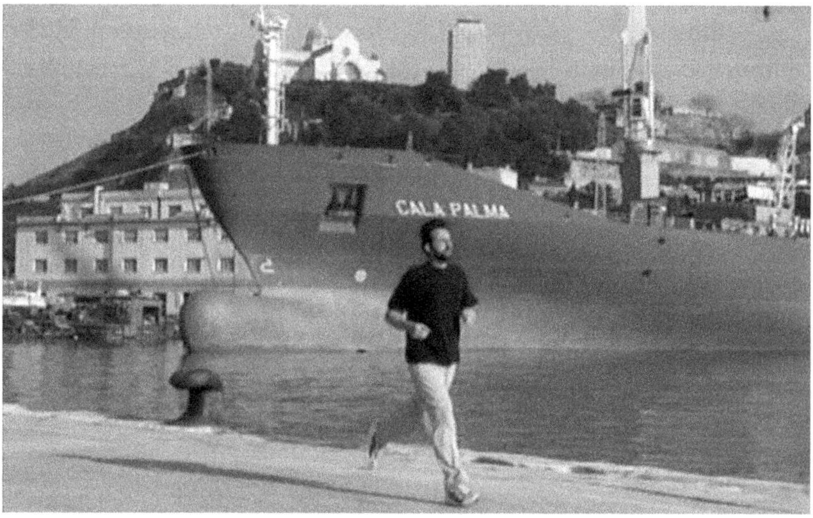

Figure 1: Moretti jogging in the opening scenes of *The Son's Room* (Moretti, 2001). Miramax Pictures.

We are presented with no contextual information (with the exception of the setting, which I will discuss shortly). The only signifier we are given is the body, a body that can signify a character or an actor but that is, due to Moretti's extra-diegetic authorial persona and the autobiographical style of his previous films, overdetermined by its association with the auteur. With no context to establish these other identities, it appears that Moretti the auteur has run out of the past—perhaps his previous film, *April*—and into the first frame of *The Son's Room*. This sense of the auteur's appearance on screen is reinforced as the figure finishes jogging and begins enacting two tropes associated with Moretti's films and persona: singing and dancing.[10] In this instance, he dances with *hare krishnas* and sings to himself in the hallway as he returns home. The opening of the film establishes the presence of the auteur through the appearance of his body and tropes that characterise him as Nanni Moretti. In contrast with the opening of the Cannes synopsis, which places a "close family" at the centre, here the film opens on the image of the director, framing *The Son's Room* as a Moretti film before establishing its other diegetic features such as the characterisation of Giovanni and the exposition of the plot. From the very beginning, *The Son's Room* performs the auteurism that the Cannes synopsis obscures.

The opening scene is, however, ambiguous due to its setting, the port of Ancona, which, as we know, differs from the autobiographical setting of Rome common to Moretti's oeuvre. The film's setting highlights a split in the film text: the port suggests that the figure on screen is a character and that *The Son's Room* may eschew the usual autobiographical representation of the auteur that marked Moretti's previous works. This is in tension with the effect produced by Moretti's appearance on screen. This tension, perhaps, is also conferred onto the figure; the setting implies that he is a character, while the image of the figure himself implies that he is the auteur, Moretti. The contradiction between the body and its context in this shot thus reinforces and externalises the internal contradiction of Moretti's body representing both the character and the auteur. In this way, the film seems to allude to the radical instability of identity, this figure appearing internally split between identities, even from its first appearance on screen. The unfamiliar setting might direct the viewer to perceive this figure as a character, while the brute fact of the body, as well as the lack of a name that confers any specific identity onto this body, encourages a perception of this figure as Moretti the actor-auteur.

We can see how this also makes manifest a split in the film text when we analyse the composition of the establishing shot. Most of the frame is

10 On Moretti's dancing and singing, see De Gaetano (1999, pp. 118–120).

taken up by an enormous red ship which signals the port setting and, in its size and brightness, draws the eye away from Moretti. While Moretti's figure stands out against the background, the diegetic space dwarfs him. Signifying the film's setting as Ancona rather than Rome, the ship further alludes to the film's narrative dimension, and thus its status as "a-Morettian." This enacts the explicit law governing the Cannes synopsis's representation of the film: the idea of the film as an artwork in its own right. Meanwhile, Moretti's body indicates the hidden law of the film's structural constraint as a "Moretti film." In this shot, the auteur appears as a small but immovable stain: the grain of sand highlighting a split in the large diegetic space of the film, and its status as both "free" artwork and constrained auteur film.

Scenes of jogging recur at key narrative junctures throughout the film. In contrast with the first one, later scenes can be interpreted as re-articulating Moretti's body, re-signifying its meaning within the diegetic space of the film. Subsequently, the body is ascribed another signifier, a name: Giovanni Sermonti. In Lacanian theory, naming marks the subject's entry into the symbolic (Lacan 2004 [1949]). It is, in a sense, one of the explicit laws of the symbolic order—that subjects should have names. However, this process is also constitutive of the alienated subjectivity that Lacan (2004 [1964], p. 205) argues defines all humans: the split in identity which, as discussed above, hysteria forces the subject to confront. This is because the symbolic signifier, the name, does not totally correspond with the being it designates.[11] The name, as a particular signifier of identity, produces the same split between ideality (here, a person's transcendental being) and signification (the name). Moretti's transformation into Giovanni via naming effects his entry into the explicit symbolic order of the film, and this requires the alienation of his embodied being as auteur. Subsequent repetitions of the first jogging scene can be seen to function on an explicit symbolic level in which the figure becomes re-articulated as character. This depends upon, to an extent, a repression of the figure's identity as auteur. Moretti as auteur is thus repressed as the fictional narrative and characterisation of Giovanni takes precedence.

11 Lacan pursues this line of reasoning in several of his seminars. The one I refer to in this paragraph is "The Subject and the Other: Alienation," from *Book XI: The Four Fundamental Concepts of Psychoanalysis* (Lacan, 2004 [1964]). In this seminar, Lacan refers to two lacks that define the subject, one primary and one secondary. The primary one is "the real, earlier lack, to be situated at the advent of the living being" (Lacan, 2004 [1964], p. 205). The subject loses this lack upon entry into the symbolic through being named. This produces, however, a second lack—that which we might understand as a symbolic lack, the lack which defines the (split) subject ($), most commonly referred to in Lacanian theory.

Breaking the Fourth Wall of the Clinic: Metacinematic Hysteria

Lacan designated the clinic the space proper to hysteria; the psychoanalyst's role is to hystericise the analysand in this controlled setting (Fink, 1995, p. 135). It should therefore be unsurprising that we find much of *The Son's Room*'s representation of hysteria actually taking place in Giovanni's practice, and that scholars such as Sergio Benvenuto (2001) and Mignon Nixon (2005) have discussed the film's representation of psychoanalysis at length. However, the representation of the patients' treatment shows them not as fully hysterical, but in a state of transference, a stage of psychoanalysis in which "the subject is still looking for his [*sic*] certainty" in the analyst and is continually frustrated in this search (Lacan, 2004 [1964], p. 129). In this stage, the patient has not yet confronted the reality that the analyst (as an authority figure) does not "know" and so cannot provide certainty Lacan, 2004 [1964], pp. 129–130). This frustration, in the case of negative transference, results in suspicion (Lacan, 2004 [1964], p. 124).

The Son's Room's representation of Giovanni's patients can be understood through this notion of negative transference rather than radical hysteria. They appear to be caught in a cycle of questioning but also to still, ultimately, believe in the authority of the analyst. The film depicts the majority of Giovanni's patients complaining about the ineffectiveness of his treatment but returning to him nonetheless. The first patient is shown saying that she does not think Giovanni understands her and implies that the only real therapy she receives is her trip to buy a new dress after every session. The film also shows a patient who threatens to leave Giovanni's practice during every appointment, since she thinks the treatment is little more than a means of extorting money from her. That the patients repeatedly return and address their questions to Giovanni implies a continuing belief in the analyst's authority. This cycle of questioning and return recalls, and complicates, another Morettian trope: Moretti's distrust of the medical profession, which rose to prominence in the "Medici" section of *Dear Diary*. Through Moretti's character, *Dear Diary* seems to comment on the ineffectiveness of medical treatment, and yet, like the patients in *The Son's Room*, Moretti continues to undergo a variety of therapies. In this way, the characterisation of the patients in the latter film effects a displacement of one of the tropes of Moretti's persona onto a series of characters. The film is, again, split. On the one hand, it can be read as a Moretti film since it contains the trope of cynical questioning and, more specifically, the mistrust of the medical profession that was a key theme in the film that won Moretti the Best Director award at Cannes. On the other hand, the displacement of this mistrust from Moretti's character onto a series of other characters signifies the film's difference from Moretti's oeuvre, echoing the synopsis's presentation of it as an a-Morettian film.

This sense is initially reinforced through the position of Giovanni, no longer the mistrustful patient, but the clinician being questioned. Within this context, the film also characterises Giovanni in a way that distinguishes him from Moretti's previous alter-egos, appearing to privilege the film's fictional narrative over its metacinematic, auteurist dimension. During the analytical sessions, the camera frequently rests on Giovanni's tranquil expression, and sometimes slowly zooms in to emphasise and reinforce the advice he gives his clients. This aspect of the film echoes the synopsis's description of Giovanni's "quiet existence" in contrast with his patients' neuroses.

However, Giovanni goes on to exhibit a distinctly Morettian distrust of the medical profession following the death of Andrea. Giovanni becomes unable to perform as a psychoanalyst due to his grief, and both his authority as analyst and tranquillity are undermined. At the climax of this, Giovanni rants at Oscar, a patient who has been diagnosed with cancer (again recalling Moretti's own situation in *Dear Diary*). This can be read as part of the narrative's overall hysterical quality. Depicting the lack in an authority figure, such as a psychoanalyst, appears as a reference to the trope of cynical questioning associated with Moretti's oeuvre. However, in previous films such as *Dear Diary*, and in the initial stages of *The Son's Room*, the questioning character(s) and authority figure were presented as separate: rather than addressing the subject's inherent lack, this lack is repeatedly displaced onto a separate authority figure. In contrast, Giovanni/Moretti's questioning of his own authority (as psychoanalyst) creates an overlap between the lack in the authority figure (indexical of medical authority as such) and the lack in the subject (questioning character). This scene therefore breaks down the distance required for the cynicism of cynical questioning. In occupying both positions as hysteric and authority figure, Giovanni/Moretti is shown to confront the lack in himself.

The hystericisation afforded by the clinical setting also takes the form of metacinematic hysteria in an unusual scene during one of Giovanni's sessions with a client. Giovanni is agitated and bored while his client speaks to him of her neurosis, a form of obsessive-compulsive disorder. Foreshadowing the undermining of Giovanni's authority as analyst that the film shows later, the camera cuts to the familiar sight of Moretti playing a frustrated, self-critical and impatient character that echoes his previous alter-egos. As Moretti/Giovanni gets up from his chair, he appears to step out of the diegetic reality into what we discover afterwards is a daydream. In this dream, Moretti/

Giovanni occupies his previous persona, expressing exasperation with the patient, insulting her and himself at the same time ("I'm just as boring as you"). He also shows the patient and audience his collection of sports shoes, alluding to another Morettian trope—an obsession with footwear.[12]

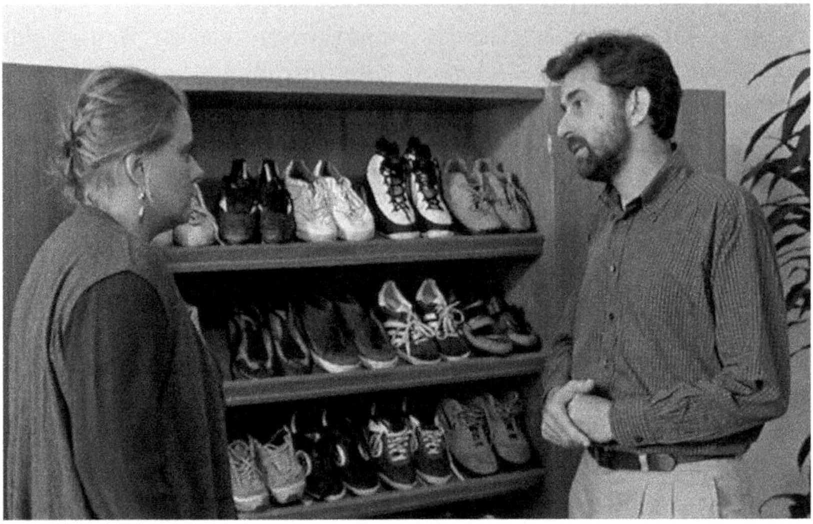

Figure 2: Moretti/Giovanni steps out of his role as analyst and out of the diegesis. *The Son's Room* (Moretti, 2001). Miramax Pictures.

The figure who steps out of the film's immediate narrative to address the patient is, it seems, Moretti rather than Giovanni. The figure leaves the film's diegetic space and enters an interstitial space, a space between the narrative world Giovanni inhabits and the metacinematic world Moretti inhabits. As such, we glimpse a gap in Moretti's mask (the gap between actor-auteur and character) which, in turn, opens up a gap between the metacinematic (auteurist) and diegetic (narrative) dimensions of the film. This image of Giovanni daydreaming that he is Moretti recalls Zhuang Zhi's dream that he is a butterfly, which Lacan (2004 [1964], p. 76) describes as exemplary of the split subject's predicament. The problem can be articulated as such: "now I do not know whether I am a man dreaming he is a butterfly or if I am a butterfly dreaming he is a man." In *The Son's Room*, the formulation becomes: "now I do not know whether I am a character dreaming he is an auteur or an auteur dreaming he is a character." In this moment, it becomes unclear what is the dream: Giovanni's daydream or the diegesis of the film.

12 Marcus (1996, p. 239) lists Moretti's "fascination with shoes" among his "usual obsessions," catalogued in *Dear Diary* and elsewhere. See also Sutton (2004, p. 150) on the resurfacing of this trope in *Aprile*.

From an auteurist perspective, the diegesis is in fact the dream—a dream that covers over the traumatic reality of the film's contingency on Moretti's auteur persona. This reality can be thought of as the film's ultimate, repressed meaning being a senseless manifestation of the same *sinthomatic* auteurism that conditions European A festivals' construction of art cinema. As such, this scene pushes the contradiction of *The Son's Room* as an a-Morettian Moretti film to its hysterical limit. *The Son's Room* does not resolve the contradictions in its meaning, but performs them. In this reading, it highlights the inherent tension between the notion of the "art of film" and the *sinthomatic* auteurism through which this notion is constituted. It at once gestures towards the instability of meaning proper to art as a universal notion (its emptiness) and highlights the constraint of this meaning through the very signifier of art's universality, the auteur as a metacinematic stain on the text.

Conclusion

Film festivals are in the business of constructing universals. Their core ideological operation is to define themselves and the films they exhibit in relation to a universal notion, thus disavowing the contingency of their selection, awarding and representation of certain films. Yet this procedure is marked by a fundamental tension: film festivals in fact *constrain* the meaning of films—and eventually art cinema—through the very claim to universality. As I show above, European A festivals delimit the meaning of the films they award through the notion of "the art of film" and its *sinthomatic* expression via the auteur. These ideas are, while representative of artistic autonomy, also crucial to both the marketing of art cinema and A film festivals' legitimacy as events vital to the film industry. Such constraint entails the subtle expectation that directors should perform the role of auteur, a "free" artist subject to themselves alone. In turn, the films directed by those consecrated as auteurs are evaluated in relation to a perceived authorial vision, simultaneously securing and restricting their meaning as "art."

We have seen a peculiar case of this: Cannes's presentation of *The Son's Room* in a way that disavows the auteurism likely to underpin the film's selection and eventual winning of the festival's top prize. The Cannes festival programme presents *The Son's Room* as an artwork unconstrained even by the structures of auteurism that secure its legitimacy. On the one hand, this may be due to the longevity of the relationship between Moretti and Cannes: that *The Son's Room* is a Moretti film and is therefore "worthy" simply does not need to be said. Auteurism remains the hidden law that underwrites the festival's presentation of the film. On the other hand, the suppression of Moretti's presence in the festival synopsis participates in the critical evaluation of *The Son's Room* as a departure from Moretti's autarkic style, a more "mature" film, unfettered by Moretti's overwhelming authorial presence. The strength of Moretti's persona brings to the fore many of the tensions of a universalised notion of "art" and its auteurist expression. *The Son's Room* is no exception: here, as in the director's other works, Moretti can be seen to perform the role of auteur (or rather, actor-auteur-protagonist), leaving an indelible authorial mark on the text. Moretti's over-presence pushes auteurism to its extreme, and *The Son's Room* can be interpreted as a film that highlights the fundamental constraint of a film's meaning by the very *sinthome* that secures its expression as an autonomous artwork.

The constraint I discuss above is not solely theoretical, however; it is a product of commercial necessity. European A festivals not only reproduce but instantiate the same symbolic structure and the same tensions as the very notion of "art cinema." Such festivals' ability to secure both symbolic and financial capital rests on their self-definition in line with a purified notion of "the art of film," a notion that, in itself, disavows the economic constraints under which film festivals select and award films. This finds expression in European A festivals' construction of ideas of the auteur as a symbol artistic autonomy, obscuring both the auteurs' and the festivals' actual subjection to commercial constraints.

So begins a crucial line of reasoning that this book undertakes. The disavowal of economic contingency suggests a fundamental ideological procedure structuring European A festivals: the repression of their dependence on and reproduction of capital. From such a grounding we can begin to apprehend the effects of this structure: the various fantasies and dislocations, the production of further taxonomies of value, and the construction of other *sinthomatic* figures.

Bibliography

Andrews, D. (2010). Art cinema as institution, redux: Art houses, film festivals, and film studies. *Scope: An Online Journal of Film and Television Studies*, *18*, 1–21.

Andrews, E. (2014). *Place, setting, perspective: Narrative space in the films of Nanni Moretti*. Fairleigh Dickinson University Press.

Antonello, P., & Barotsi, R. (2009). The personal and the political: The cinema of Nanni Moretti. In P. Antonello & F. Mussgnug (Eds.), *Postmodern impegno: Ethics and commitment in contemporary Italian culture* (pp. 189–212). Peter Lang.

Bazin, A. (2008 [1957]). De la politique des auteurs. In B. K. Grant (Ed.), *Auteurs and authorship: A film reader* (pp. 19–28). Blackwell.

Benvenuto, S. (2001). *The Son's Room*, or: The analysis is over. *Journal of European Psychoanalysis, 12*. [Online]. Available from: http://www.psychomedia.it/jep/number12-13/benvenuto.htm

Bonsaver, G. (2001). The egocentric Cassandra of the left: Representations of politics in the films of Nanni Moretti. *The Italianist 21*(1), 158–183.

Bordwell, D. (1979). The art cinema as a mode of film practice. *Film Criticism, 4*(1), 56–64.

Brook, C. (2005.) Screening the autobiographical. In W. Hope (Ed.), *Italian Cinema: New Directions* (pp. 27–52). Peter Lang.

Burgess, D., & Kredell, B. (2016). Positionality and film festival research: A conversation. In M. de Valck, B. Kredell, & S. Loist (Eds.), *Film festivals: History, theory, method, practice* (pp. 159–176). Routledge.

Buscombe, E. (2008 [1973]). Ideas of authorship. In B. K. Grant (Ed.), *Auteurs and authorship: A film reader* (pp. 76–83). Blackwell.

Butler, J., Laclau, E., & Žižek, S. (Eds.). (2000). *Contingency, hegemony, universality: Contemporary dialogues on the left.* Verso.

Czach, L. (2004). Film festivals, programming, and the building of a national cinema. *The Moving Image, 4*(1), 76–88.

De Gaetano, R. (1999). *Il corpo e la maschera: Il grottesco nel cinema italiano.* Bulzoni.

De Valck, M. (2007). *Film festivals: From European geopolitics to global cinephilia.* Amsterdam University Press.

De Valck, M. (2014). Film festivals, Bourdieu, and the economization of culture. *Canadian Journal of Film Studies, 23*(1), 74–89.

De Valck, M. (2016). Fostering art, adding value, cultivating taste: Film festivals as sites of cultural legitimisation. In M. de Valck, D. B. Kredell, & S. Loist (Eds.), *Film festivals: History, theory, method, practice* (pp. 100–116). Routledge.

Elsaesser, T. (2005). *European cinema: Face to face with Hollywood.* Amsterdam University Press.

Elsaesser, T. (2016). The global author: Control, creative constraints, and performative self-contradiction. In S. Jeong & J. Szaniawski (Eds.), *The global auteur: The politics of authorship in 21st century cinema* (pp. 21–41). Bloomsbury.

Falicov, T. (2016). The "festival film." In M. de Valck, B. D. Kredell, & S. Loist (Eds.), *Film festivals: History, theory, method, practice* (pp. 209–229). Routledge.

Festival de Cannes. (2001). *La Stanza del Figlio* (*The Son's Room*). [Online]. Available from: http://www.festival-cannes.com/en/films/la-stanza-del-figlio

Festival de Cannes. (2019b). *Nanni Moretti.* [Online]. Available from: https://www.festival-cannes.com/en/artist/nanni-moretti-3

FIAPF (International Federation of Film Producers Associations). (2016). *International film festivals signed FIAPF's mutual trust contract and received accreditation in 2016.* [Online]. Available from: http://www.fiapf.org/intfilmfestivals.asp

Fink, B. (1995). *The Lacanian subject: Between language and jouissance.* Princeton University Press.

Galt, R., & Schoonover, K. (2010). Introduction: The impurity of art cinema. In R. Galt & K. Schoonover (Eds.). *Global art cinema: New theories and histories* (pp. 3–27). Oxford University Press.

Iordanova, D. (2009). The festival circuit. In D. Iordanova & R. Rhyne (Eds.), *Film festival yearbook 1: The festival circuit* (pp. 23–39). St Andrews Film Studies and College Gate Press.

Lacan, J. (2004 [1949]). The mirror stage as formative of the *I* function as revealed in psychoanalytic experience. In J. Lacan (Ed.), *Écrits: A selection* (pp. 3–9). Norton & Co.

Lacan, J. (2004 [1964]). *The four fundamental concepts of psychoanalysis.* Norton.

Loist, S. (2016). The film festival circuit: Networks, hierarchies and circulation. In M. de Valck, D. B. Kredell, & S. Loist (Eds.), *Film festivals: History, theory, method, practice* (pp. 49–64). Routledge.

Ma, J. (2010). Tsai Ming-Liang's haunted movie theater. In R. Galt & K. Schoonover (Eds.), *Global art cinema: New theories and histories*, pp. 334–350. Oxford University Press.

MacDonald Carolan, M. A. (2013). Moretti's children: The next generation? *Quaderni d'italianistica, 34*(2), 113–132.

Marcus, M. (1996). *Caro Diario* and the cinematic body of Nanni Moretti. *Italica, 73*(2), 233–247.

Mazierska, E., & Rascaroli, L. (2004). *The cinema of Nanni Moretti: Dreams and diaries.* Wallflower.

McCarthy, T. (1999). High art pays low dividends for Cannes auds. *Variety.* [Online]. Available from: https://variety.com/1999/voices/columns/high-art-pays-low-dividends-for-cannes-auds-1117502356/

Mezias, S. et al. (2008). Much ado about nothing? Untangling the impact of European premier film festivals. *Creative Encounters Research Paper Series, 14*, 1–31.

Mumford, G. (2018). Cannes 2018: Cate Blanchett defends festival's failure to select more female directors. *The Guardian.* [Online]. Available from: https://www.theguardian.com/film/2018/may/08/cannes-2018-cate-blanchett-defends-festivals-failure-to-select-more-women-directors

Neale, S. (1981). Art cinema as institution. *Screen, 22*(1), 11–40.

Nixon, M. (2005). On the couch. *October, 113*, 39–76.

Ostrowska, D. (2016). Making film history at the Cannes film festival. In M. de Valck, B. D. Kredell, & S. Loist (Eds.), *Film festivals: History, theory, method, practice* (pp. 18–33). Routledge.

Peranson, M. (2008). First you get the power, then you get the money: Two models of film festivals. *Cineaste, 33*(3), 37–43.

Polan, D. (2001). Auteur desire. *Screening the Past.* [Online]. Available from: http://www.screeningthepast.com/issue-12-first-release/auteur-desire/

Rooney, D. (2001). Review: *The Son's Room. Variety.* [Online]. Available from: https://variety.com/2001/film/reviews/the-son-s-room-1200467299/

Rüling, C. C. (2009). Festivals as field-configuring events: The Annecy International Animated Film Festival and Market. In D. Iordanova & R. Rhyne (Eds.), *Film festival yearbook 1: The festival circuit* (pp. 49–66). St Andrews Film Studies and College Gate Press.

Saperstein, P. (2018). Kristen Stewart climbs Cannes red carpet stairs barefoot. *Variety.* [Online]. Available from: https://variety.com/2018/film/news/kristen-stewart-cannes-red-carpet-barefoot-1202810872/

Sarris, A. (1962). Notes on the *auteur* theory in 1962. *Film Culture, 27*(1), 1–8.

Sellors, C. P. (2010). *Film authorship: Auteurs and other myths.* Columbia University Press.

Sutton, P. (2004). "Can the man panic?": Masculinity and fatherhood in Nanni Moretti's *Aprile.* In P. Powrie, A. Davies, & B. Babington (Eds.), *The trouble with men: Masculinities in European and Hollywood cinema* (pp. 144–154). Wallflower Press.

Vighi, F. (2005). Nanni Moretti: Trauma, hysteria, and freedom. In W. Hope (Ed.), *Italian cinema: new directions* (pp. 79–106). Peter Lang.

Wiseman, A. (2015). Cannes: Women denied Palais entry for wearing flats. *Screen Daily.* [Online]. Available from: https://www.screendaily.com/festivals/cannes/cannes-women-denied-palais-entry-for-wearing-flats/5088395.article

Wiseman, A. (2016). Kristen Stewart, Julia Roberts kick off their heels in Cannes. *Screen Daily.* [Online]. Available from: https://www.screendaily.com/cannes/kristen-stewart-julia-roberts-kick-off-their-heels-in-cannes/5103878.article

Žižek, S. (1992). *Looking awry: An introduction to Jacques Lacan through popular culture.* MIT Press.

Žižek, S. (1999). *The ticklish subject: The absent centre of political ontology.* Verso.

Žižek, S. (2000a). Class struggle or postmodernism? Yes, please! In J. Butler, E. Laclau, & S. Žižek (Eds.), *Contingency, hegemony, universality: Contemporary dialogues on the left* (pp. 91–135). Verso.

Žižek, S. (2000c). Melancholy and the act. *Critical Inquiry, 26*(4), 657–681.

Žižek, S. (2004a). *Iraq: The borrowed kettle.* Verso.

Žižek, S. (2005). *The metastases of enjoyment: Six essays on women and causality.* Verso.

Filmography

Aprile (2007). Moretti, N. dir. Italy.
Dear Diary (*Caro diario*) (1993). Moretti, N. dir. Italy.
Father and Master (*Padre Padrone*) (1977). Taviani, P., & Taviani, V. dirs. Italy.
Ecce bombo (1978). Moretti, N. dir. Italy.
Girls of the Sun (*Les filles du soleil*) (2018). Hussan, E. dir. France/USA.
The Son's Room (*La stanza del figlio*) (2001). Moretti, N. dir. Italy.
A Brighter Tomorrow (*Il sol dell'avvenire*) (2023). Moretti, N. dir. Italy.

3. Gendering Art: *The Great Beauty* at Cannes and Tallinn

Abstract: This chapter examines the universal of "art" and the figure of the auteur in relation to gender. Presenting new data regarding the history of European A festivals' prize-giving, I respond to the fact that no Italian film directed by a woman has won top prize since and including the first edition of Cannes in 1946. Through an analysis of the book's most celebrated case study, *The Great Beauty*, I show that Italian women directors' exclusion is accompanied by film festivals' implicit gendering of the notions of art that they promote. This chapter responds to recent challenges to cinematic institutions' gender discrimination (e.g., the #MeToo movement), countering notions of artistic universality with theories of male gaze and sexual difference.

Keywords: male gaze, art cinema, Italian cinema, film festivals, Paolo Sorrentino, feminism

In a giant loft apartment in central Rome, a wild party rages on all night long—it's Jep Gambardella's (Toni Servillo) 65th birthday. Jep is the symbol of Roman decadence. In the foot-steps of the Jesuits and the Medicis, he knows more about people's lives than he should and enjoys his influence in the marble gardens of the capital like some autocrat of old. Yet this birthday constitutes a symbolic confrontation with mortality that sends Jep (and us, along with him) on a dream-like tour of Rome's past and present through Jep's memories, passions and crumbled dreams.
"Great Beauty" is too aristocratic to deign to adhere to any kind of narrative structure. Instead it offers us a whirlwind adventure that cuts through time and space gallantly, as if through a fine Parma ham. Anyone familiar with Fellini knows how sometimes one must simply surrender to the filmmaker's whims. Whereas Fellini wrote love letters to Rome, Paolo Sorrentino is preoccupied with the decay of the ages that have been deposited under the gilded superficies. This film is at once an ode and an elegy to Rome. Paolo Sorrentino turned 43 this year and he has now given us his finest film. Is he also gripped by thought of mortality, like Jep? Perhaps it is a

Johnson, R., Film Festivals, *Ideology and Italian Art Cinema: Politics, Histories and Cultural Value*. Taylor & Francis Group, 2024
DOI 10.5117/9789463720366_CH03

> valuable thing for anyone of us to be reminded of our time and place by the rustle of the reaper?
> – *Synopsis of* The Great Beauty *in the Tallinn 2013 print and online programme*

> Aristocratic ladies, social climbers, politicians, high-flying criminals, journalists, actors, decadent nobles, prelates, artists and intellectuals—whether authentic or presumed—form the tissue of these flaky relationships, all engulfed in a desperate Babylon which plays out in the antique palaces, immense villas and most beautiful terraces in the city. They are all there, and they are not seen in a good light. Jep Gambardella, 65, indolent and disenchanted, his eyes permanently imbued with gin and tonic, watches this parade of hollow, doomed, powerful yet depressed humanity. A moral lifelessness enough to make one's head spin. And in the background, Rome in summer. Splendid and indifferent, like a dead diva.
> – *Synopsis of* The Great Beauty *in the Cannes 2013 print and online programme*

Introduction

In the previous chapter, I identified a contradiction that emerged from Cannes 2018 appearing to promote a politics based on gender (via its selection of several films directed by women and a female-majority jury), while claiming nonetheless to judge films solely on the basis of their artistic merit. The deference to "merit" subtly provided the justification for the jury's decision to award the Palme d'Or to *Shoplifters* (*Manbiki kazoku*, Koreeda, 2018), a Japanese film directed by a consecrated male auteur. Meanwhile, films directed by women, whose selection contributed to the image of Cannes as politically engaged, either did not win prizes or won lesser prizes. Thus, it was an ambivalent moment when, for example, an Italian film directed by Alice Rohrwacher, *Happy as Lazzaro* (*Lazzaro felice*, 2018), won the Grand Prix for Best Screenplay. That film festivals, and the media industries in general, reflect and reproduce unequal gender relations is common knowledge, a knowledge that finally penetrated festivals and mainstream media with the rise of the #MeToo movement in 2018. Along with the (equally valid) anecdotal evidence offered by women in the industry, a recent data-driven study has explicitly broached the question of inequality in film exhibition. Although analysing film theatre screenings, Deb Verhoeven et al. (2019) demonstrate the gender inequality that characterises global film exhibition. They found that, between 2012 and 2015, 15% of films released were directed by women. These films, already a small percentage of global releases, accounted for an even smaller share of screenings in cinemas across the globe: 3%.

Reflecting on media industries' responses to #MeToo and other calls for gender equality, Skadi Loist and Deb Verhoeven (2019, p. 69) point to "emerging standards of accountability"—for example the BFI Diversity standards and, most pertinent to this study, all major film festivals' subscription to a 50/50 pledge to achieve gender parity in their recruitment of programmers and the selection of films. Loist and Verhoeven rightly underline that the formal presence of such standards does not guarantee equality, particularly given "patriarchy's notable capacity for perseverance" (p. 69). Indeed, a year after Thierry Frémaux promised Cannes would achieve "5050x2020," the festival had made mixed progress. On the one hand, only four of the films in competition in 2019 were directed by women (the highest number since 2011, but low nonetheless). On the other hand, half the selection committee were women, challenging the "male-dominated gatekeeping" that Verhoeven et al. (2019, p. 137) identify as a major factor in the exclusion of films directed by women from exhibition circuits. As with the strange contradiction of the 2018 edition of Cannes boasting a woman-majority jury and awarding the Palm D'Or once again to a film directed by a man, the presence of a greater number of woman film programmers had a minimal impact on the festival's legitimation of films in the 2019 main competition. This may be changing: in 2021 Julia Ducornau's *Titane* (2021) won top prize, as did Justine Triet's *Anatomy of a Fall* (*Anatomie d'une chute*, 2023) in 2023. (Respectively, these are the second and third films directed by women ever to do so; the first was Jane Campion's *The Piano* [1993].) The last few years have seen European A festivals, in particular the "big three," award top prizes to films directed by women, from the Berlinale's awarding of the Golden Bear to *Touch Me Not* (Adina Pintilie, 2018) and *Alcarràs* (Carla Simón, 2022) to Venice awarding the Golden Lion to *Happening* (*L'Événement*, Audrey Diwan, 2021).

European A Festivals may thus be shifting in their exhibition and awarding of films directed by women, although, as I demonstrate below, the effects of this shift have yet to touch Italian cinema and its canons. At this juncture, it feels ever more necessary to consider the values on which female-directed films' canonisation is predicated, and the potential presence of a *male-dominated paradigm* in the legitimation of films. I refer to the paradigm of auteurism outlined in Chapter 2 of this book. Several feminist scholars have interrogated auteurism as a system of evaluation that repeatedly, if not intrinsically, excludes women filmmakers and/or feminist filmmaking. Carie

Tarr (1999), writing of the French context in which the *politique des auteurs* emerged, argues that "the concept of the *auteur*, if ostensibly ungendered, remains resolutely masculine" (p. 3). Both Angela Martin (2003) and Priya Jaikumar (2015) suggest that this exclusion is intertwined with auteurism as a masculinist paradigm, with Martin (2003, p. 29) stating that the framework of authorship "actually contributes to the omission of women's films from circulation and film theory." Jaikumar (2015), addressing the intersections of gender and race, shows that "the most admired in auteur theory [...] were, without exception, white men working in European and American film industries" (p. 205). Jaikumar outlines the trend of Western feminist film scholarship's interrogation of authorship (which she identifies in White [2015] and Silverman [2003]) to result in "feminist investments in *female* authorship" much as postcolonial interrogations are characterised by an "investment in *non-Western* authorship" (p. 205–206). Such criticism, she suggests, maintains a structure of authorship that renders women and non-Western filmmakers "perennial outsiders who can at best look in" on a paradigm invisibly qualified patriarchal and Western (Jaikumar, 2015, p. 206).

Providing counterexamples of Global Southern films co-directed by women, Jaikumar challenges the very notion of a singular auteur as creator and guarantor of a work. Such examples "reveal that the singular and normatively male director is central to the dominant paradigm of most film industries [and] draws attention to the limitations and exclusions of the category of authorship in cinema" (Jaikumar, 2015, p. 211). Martin and Jaikumar ultimately call for different approaches, each of which underscore what is at stake in the legitimation of films by auteurist means. Martin (2003, pp. 35–36) proposes the replacement of authorship with a new framework, one that might begin with Agnès Varda's *cinécriture*. Jaikumar, meanwhile, argues for a dispersal of the category that ultimately results in a dismantling of the idealisation of a singular, unconstrained creative agent, and thus the paradigm of auteurism we have seen so far.

Whether advocating for female auteurism or challenging the paradigm itself, feminist film scholars have repeatedly demonstrated the dominance of the figure of the male author in the legitimation of films. Bringing their considerations into dialogue with the continuing centrality of the figure of the auteur to European A festivals, we can begin to see a further development of the ideological procedure I outlined in the previous chapter. It thus appears that a useful way of approaching the question of European A festivals' gendered construction of art cinema is through an examination of their structural dependence on the figure of the auteur as *sinthome*, as the representative of such festivals' promotion of the ideological universal "the art of film." One of the paradoxes of the auteur is that they are at once a figure and a real human—a symbol of artistic freedom and a film professional who depends on the festival apparatus for their income, as Elsaesser (2016, p. 29) notes. The auteur, as a human figure, is caught in the symbolic network of identities that constitute all subjects. The auteur is ascribed signifiers such as a name, a race (usually white), a sexuality (usually straight) and a gender (usually male), in part by the festival apparatus.[1]

Given their status as *sinthome*, gendering the auteur may also, in turn, influence the notion of art that this figure represents, and thus the evaluation of films by creators of any gender. This is especially the case given the focus on the subjectivity of the director in auteurist constructions of cinema—the common notion of a film as being the product of the auteur's artistic vision. In other words, through the historical dominance of the *sinthome* of the male auteur, "the art of film" may be constructed as an expression of a masculine creative vision: art made by men and from their perspective or, furthermore, expressing certain stylistic tropes found in canonical male-directed films.[2] The universality of art is not only partial on a purely structural level, as shown in the previous chapter, but may also be partial in a specific way: "art" as masculine. I build on the notion of auteur as *sinthome* and the contradictions it raises to suggest that the particularity of European A festivals' ideological universal, "the art of film," not only disavows the contingency of European A festivals' construction of art cinema, but also colours the notion of "art" with a particular, gendered content. In this chapter, I aim to analyse European A festivals' consecration of solely male Italian auteurs, suggesting the reproduction of a masculine Italian film canon and implicitly setting an aesthetic standard against which Italian art cinema may come to be measured.

1 This is apparent in the case of Ferzan Özpetek being perceived as a queer, migrant auteur; see Chapter 4.

2 The question of the relationship between a director's gender and the gender perspective of a film is a contentious one, and not one I seek to resolve here. For a basic summary of the debates regarding women's cinema on the levels of production, distribution, textual practices and reception, see the entry "Feminist Film Criticism" in Hayward (2002, pp. 137–148). See also B. Ruby Rich's (1998) contention that the women's film movement must concern itself with all the aspects of cinema just listed. Rich's implication that there is not an intrinsic relationship between the gender of the director and a film's strategies of representation works both ways, and contributes to the ongoing debate around paradigms of authorship in feminist film theory.

European A festivals' construction of films (and of themselves) in relation to a canon of "greats" such as Federico Fellini is retroactively validated by their continuing representation of the films they award in relation to this canon. The case study I analyse below, *The Great Beauty*, epitomises this dynamic. *The Great Beauty* is also one of the most successful cases that I analyse in this book as one of highest grossing films and the only Academy Award winner. Furthermore, it was directed by an Italian auteur whose renown extends beyond Europe: Paolo Sorrentino. (See, for example, Sorrentino's television series *The Young Pope* (2016), which premiered in the US on Sky Atlantic.) Having premiered in competition at Cannes in May 2013, the film proceeded to win a series of prestigious awards, including top prize at another European A festival, Tallinn; the Golden Globe, Academy Award and BAFTA for Best Foreign Language Film; and European Film Awards for Best Film, Best Director, Best Actor (Toni Servillo) and Best Editor (Cristiano Travaglioli). The film grossed $24.6 million worldwide between 2013 and 2014 (Box Office Mojo, 2018b). In this respect, it might be seen as the pinnacle of new millennium Italian cinema, and a prime example of how the festival circuit interacts with other institutions, such as the Oscars, to construct Italian cinema in a particular way. The following analysis of *The Great Beauty* and its representation in film festival programmes has clear implications for any consideration of the success of a certain kind of Italian cinema more broadly.[3]

The Great Beauty has been repeatedly evaluated in relation to Italian auteur cinema, most notably in comparisons to *La Dolce Vita* (*La dolce vita*, Fellini, 1960).[4] Reinforcing the construction of Italian cinema through the figure of the (male) auteur, Sorrentino, along with two other auteurs present in this book's main corpus, has become one of the main representatives of Italian cinema on the European A circuit. He, along with Nanni Moretti and Matteo Garrone, has had films repeatedly exhibited in the main competition at Cannes, such as Special Jury Prize-winner *Il Divo* (*Il divo: La vita spettacolare di Giulio Andreotti*, 2008) and, more recently, *Youth* (2015). The latter film premiered alongside Moretti's *Mia madre* (2015) and Garrone's

3 I refer to only "a certain kind of Italian cinema," not all Italian cinema, to avoid collapsing the distinction between a film like *The Great Beauty* and its far more commercially (if not critically) successful counterpart *Quo Vado?* (Checco Zalone, 2016). *Quo Vado?* was released in the same year and earned over two-and-a-half times as much in box offices worldwide—a taking of $65.3 million that made it the highest grossing Italian film of all time. On the implications of *Quo Vado?*'s success for the taxonomy of Italian cinema, see O'Leary (2017) and Cucco (2014).

4 See Donadio (2013), Martini (2015) and Mori (2016). Also see critical discussions of evaluations of *The Great Beauty* in Balicco (2013), Gordon (2015), Minuz (2013) and La Porta (2013).

Tale of Tales (*Il racconto dei racconti*, 2015), cementing them as the three faces of Italian cinema in the new millennium (De Marco, 2015).

As I review both scholarship on the gendered canon of Italian cinema and analyses of the gender politics of *The Great Beauty*, it will become clear that the film's success may have been influenced by interpretations of it that place it within a gendered film canon, reinforcing the notion of "the art of film" within a framework of a masculine artistic universality. Meanwhile, what will emerge from this chapter's analysis of both the synopsis and the film text is that the notions of "the art of film"—in particular, the artistic worth ascribed to a certain canon of cinema—is represented in relation to the figure of the *male* artist or auteur, and constructed as expressing a dominant masculine look. I conclude that this manner of representing Italian cinema is underpinned by a fantasy of sexual difference and thus disavows the inherent non-totality both of masculinity and of the notions of art that European A festivals reproduce.

Gendering the Artist, Gendering Art

While important work has been done regarding women's festivals, as well as the gender politics of film festivals and the film industry more generally, there has not been, to my knowledge, a systematic analysis of gender and the European A circuit's construction of art cinema.[5] While an investigation of these issues may take many forms—from an empirical analysis of the numbers of films directed by women exhibited and/or awarded at European A festivals (which I do, in part, utilise here), to analyses of festivals' representation of women in other sections, such as director retrospectives—I employ a method based on the framework of psychoanalytical theories of film and ideology, and on the findings of previous chapters. Given the scarcity of research into gender and European A festivals, my review of film festival scholarship will be necessarily limited. Instead, I put forward some preliminary data regarding European A festivals' awarding of Italian films since 1946, highlighting the festivals' continuous privileging of films directed by men and exclusion of those directed by women, as enacted by their awarding of top prizes only to the former. I demonstrate the prevalence of this gendering of Italian cinema by highlighting the total exclusion of Italian films directed by women from the ranks of top prize-winners. I suggest that this trend is too consistent to be coincidental, although there

5 See Rich (1998) and Maule (2014).

are some signs of change, with festivals awarding non-Italian films and awarding lower-order prizes to a few Italian films directed by women. I return to the observations made at the beginning of Chapter 2 to highlight a tension between the concepts of art and gender mobilised at European A festivals; the notion of a "universal" artistic merit that festivals claim to promote has been, and continues to be, constructed in line with a masculine canon.

As I have shown, the notion of "art" against which festivals claim to measure films is contested, the product of an antagonistic struggle in which European A festivals themselves are engaged through their central ritual of prize-giving. In fact, European A festivals' disavowal of the politics of their construction of art can be contrasted with other festivals' insistence on it. These festivals' explicit politicisation of their criteria for selecting and awarding films often highlights that which is excluded from the supposedly neutral construction of art cinema by the A circuit. A key example is women's festivals, which explicitly promote a feminist politics through programming and, where applicable, prize-giving. Such festivals are decidedly separate from, and even opposed to, the "mainstream" of the A circuit. Rosanna Maule (2014, p. 368) describes women's festivals as having "consolidat[ed] a niche position in film culture, separate from mainstream or traditional channels of film promotion and distribution, as well as from the big film festivals' circuit." She takes this as being at once their weakness and their strength. On the one hand, they benefit from "a discrete profile" (p. 368). On the other, this distinctiveness may relate to the fact that "mainstream media and even specialised publications (including contributions within the emerging area of film festival studies) tend to disregard women's film festivals" (p. 369). Such comments perhaps highlight the positioning of women and women's cinema as other, excluded from the hegemonic universality of European A festivals' construction of the cinematic art. Maule's passing reference to film festival studies also suggests the reproduction of this in academia, which may explain the lacuna I mention above.

Historically, there has been an undeniable trend for European A festivals' top prizes to exclude films by female directors, and Italian cinema offers a particularly instructive case. Although far more modest than Verhoeven et al.'s (2019) data-driven study of global film exhibition, I offer some preliminary indications of such festivals' consistent exclusion of female directors from the canon of Italian films constructed through prize-giving. As a basis for this book, I collected information regarding the top prizes awarded to Italian films by European A festivals since the first festival edition after World War II—Cannes 1946, hailed as a foundational moment for cinema artistically, politically and institutionally.[6] This long view highlights the precedents set by the historical awarding, and thus construction, of Italian cinema on the European A festival circuit as it has developed over the past seven decades. Between the years 1946 and 2022, no Italian film directed by a woman has won top prize at any European A festival. The films being awarded, the canon and, with it, the international conception of Italian cinema constructed by European A festivals from the postwar period to the present, remain largely founded on a series of films directed by male auteurs.

A study of the Italian woman directors who have had films exhibited at European A festivals further indicates the presence of a "glass ceiling" that inhibits access to the top prizes and, until recently, the most significant festivals (in particular Cannes). Responding to the exclusion of Italian woman directors from the canon, Áine O'Healy (2000) and, later, Danielle Hipkins (2008) have proposed a list of neglected Italian female directors, with the latter considering their legitimation (or not) by institutions such as festivals and the academy. Hipkins (2008) contrasts O'Healy's observation that there is a record number of female directors in Italy today with the number of such directors receiving international recognition. Hipkins (2008, p. 217) records two: Liliana Cavani and Lina Wertmüller. Films directed by Wertmüller were screened in competition at Cannes and the Berlinale on several occasions, while those by Cavani have been screened in competition at Cannes and Venice. In contrast with films directed by Sorrentino and the other male directors in this book, neither have won the festivals' top prizes, although we might note that Wertmüller won an honorary Oscar in 2019, two years before her death in 2021. Along with Wertmüller and Cavani, most of the female directors that O'Healy and Hipkins list have competed in European A festivals, but none have won Best Picture or equivalent: Francesca Archibugi competed in Venice with *Shooting the Moon* (*L'albero delle pere*, 1998); Cristina Comencini competed at Venice twice with *Don't Tell* (*La bestia nel cuore*, 2005) and *When the Night* (*Quando la notte*, 2011); Giovanna Gagliardo competed at the Berlinale with *Via degli specchi* (1983); Antonietta de Lillo competed at Locarno and Venice with *Non è giusto* (2001) and her segment of *The Vesuvians* (*I vesuviani*, 1997), respectively; Roberta Torre competed at Locarno with *The Dark Sea* (*Mare nero*, 2006). None have competed at Cannes.

Since the publication of Hipkins's and O'Healy's studies, an increasing number of films directed by Italian women are being screened in competition

6 The full list of prize-winners can be found in the Appendix. I discuss the legacy of Cannes 1946 in Chapter 5.

at European A festivals. This is, I think, complemented by an increase in awards, although Best Picture and Best Director still remain inaccessible to these films and filmmakers. Alice Rohrwacher's *The Wonders* (*Le meraviglie*, 2014) was awarded the Grand Prix at Cannes, while Valeria Golino's *Honey* (*Miele*, 2013) featured in the Un Certain Regard programme and received a "Mention of the Ecumenical Jury" award. Films by both directors were also exhibited in the 2018 edition of the same festival, and, as mentioned above, Rohrwacher's *Happy as Lazzaro* won Best Screenplay. Meanwhile, Laura Bispurri's *Daughter of Mine* (*Figlia mia*, 2018) featured in the main competition at the Berlinale to critical acclaim, although it did not win a prize.[7] While festivals' gendered practices of prize-giving appear to be changing in general, it remains to be seen if this will result in an Italian woman director winning the elusive Best Picture award. One also needs to consider what such films and their directors must do to gain recognition. For example, critics' praise for *Happy as Lazzaro* placed it in relation to a canon of great male directors, in particular the works of Fellini and Pier Paolo Pasolini (Bianchi, 2018; Romney, 2018). This may suggest that European A festivals and film critics may continue to construct film through the *sinthome* of the male auteur, applying this notion as an implicit evaluative criterion for films directed by women.

While blunt information on the number of prizes Italian woman directors have (or have not) won is indicative, in order to theorise European A festivals' ideological, and gendered, construction of Italian cinema, we must revisit the notions of auteurism and the cycle of symbolic capital outlined in Chapter 2. The auteur is the *sinthome* of the supposedly universal notion of "the art of film" mobilised by European A festivals. The empty universal "the art of film" is filled with a specific content, becoming the ideological universal—the actual canon of art cinema constructed by European A festivals. However, this specificity and ideological character of the universal—in short, its actual particularity—is disavowed through a "typical case": the auteur (as *sinthome*). The auteur is paradoxical: one who is extremely particular while, at the same time, mobilised to signify universality. As *sinthome*, the auteur is particular on a structural level: a

7 As noted previously, a film directed by a woman did in fact win the Golden Bear that year: the Romanian movie *Touch Me Not*. This leads one to wonder if notions of Italian cinema constructed by festivals are even more conditioned by a masculinist film canon, making it more difficult for Italian films directed by women to receive this accolade. My review of scholarship on masculinity and the canon of Italian cinema below adds further credence to this claim, although it is one which requires further investigation involving, most likely, a transnational, comparative analysis of festival cinema.

signifier cannot but be particular, cannot truly be universal. Likewise, the notion of "the art of film" is structurally particular: it is, as I have argued previously, a specific construct created through antagonistic struggle. In the case of European A festivals, this entails the struggle not only between the juries tasked with deciding which films will win Best Picture, and thus become representative of "the art of film," but also between the festivals' various stakeholders, many of which are commercial.

Moreover, the auteur as *sinthome* of "art" bears the traces of the contradiction between the claim to universality and the necessary particularity of its articulation. This takes on a new dimension when we consider the fact that the *sinthome* can be gendered. If the *sinthome* is "the point at which all the lines of the predominant ideological argumentation meet" (Žižek, 1999, p. 176) *and* is masculine, then we can suppose that at least one of these lines of ideological argumentation is that artistically worthy film is masculine in some way—at the very least, directed by a man. If such films are presented as the products of the auteur's artistic vision, and this vision is that of a man, we should question how far award-winning films are represented in relation to a masculine vision—or, more specifically, a "male gaze" that designates the masculine as subject and the feminine as other (Mulvey, 1975).[8] Reflecting on this information, we might ask at what point the claim to consider only artistic merit conceals a gender bias; at what point is "artistic merit" a signifier whose meaning slips towards "masculinity"? Below I demonstrate the presence of such a slippage between the notion of art mobilised at European A festivals and the masculinity of both the auteur and his "vision" (more accurately, the film's vision) in relation to which it is defined.

The Great Beauty and the Masculine Canon

Masculinity and Canonicity in Italian Cinema

Scholars who have taken a similarly critical approach to art, and Italian, cinema's institutions have identified several tropes that characterise the gendered construction of an Italian film canon. One study that considers

8 I use the word "gaze" (lower-case) to refer to its meaning in the Mulveyan sense—a dominant look or perspective over a scene (and, often a feminised object). I discuss the relationship between this theory of the gaze and more recent Lacanian notions of the "Gaze" (upper-case, as in the appearance of the Real in the field of vision) in the film analysis later.

this explicitly is O'Rawe's (2008) "'I padri e i maestri': Genre, Auteurs, and Absences in Italian Film Studies." Throughout, O'Rawe argues that both public discourses (such as film criticism in newspapers) and scholarship on Italian cinema are founded on the tropes of "permanent crisis," "the relation of cinema to national history," "an obsession with great auteurs," "authorial art cinema" and "a nostalgia for neorealism, seen as the founding moment of Italian cinema" (pp. 174–175). Of particular interest here are O'Rawe's comments on the Italian film canon's construction in relation to "authorial art cinema" and the "obsession with great auteurs," since she highlights the gendered implications of this circumstance. Discussing Gian Piero Brunetta's (2007) and then Millicent Marcus's (2002) scholarship on Italian film history, O'Rawe demonstrates that both focus on Fellini's death, taken as a symbolic event for Italian authorial art cinema. She concludes: "For both Marcus and Brunetta it is the traumatised body of the male auteur which is read as universal, and which speaks of and for the nation and national cinema" (pp. 175–176).[9] The status of the male auteur as a universal subject has significant implications for the canon of Italian cinema: the "traumatised body of the male auteur," in this case Fellini, is positioned as a "universal subject" (perhaps *sinthome*) of both Italy and Italian cinema. Although O'Rawe focuses on journalistic and academic writing, we might also question how far other institutional representations, such as those of European A festivals, reproduce a similar structure. To what extent might Fellini and/or the male auteur more generally stand in as the *sinthome* of Italian film?[10]

Hipkins (2008) also analyses the relationship between canonicity, auteur cinema and exclusion of the feminine, adding consideration of the structures of heterosexual desire and Mulvey's gaze theory. This study suggests a connection between the celebration of the male auteur and the notion of cinema as expressing a masculine vision. Arguing that Italian film studies "needs a second take on gender," Hipkins (2008, p. 213) draws a connection

9 Marcus (1996) also suggests that Moretti, both as auteur and on-screen persona, embodies the Italian nation, highlighting the prevalence of this trope within the ideological construction of Italian films and auteurs treated in this book.

10 A tangential consideration may also centre on the ideas of death and trauma that O'Rawe highlights—might we consider institutional representations as haunted by the death of Fellini symbolic of the death of Italian auteur cinema? Although not vital to this chapter's inquiry into masculinity and auteurism in general, these ideas will resurface in its analysis of the specific case of *The Great Beauty* and its representation at Cannes and Tallinn, suggesting that the death of this auteur (and with it Italian auteur cinema) results rather in an extension of his symbolic authority via a the consecration of a new Fellini-esque auteur, Sorrentino. The response of festivals (particularly Tallinn) to the death of Fellini could thus be read as extending such power. "The auteur is dead! Long live the auteur!"

between the canonisation of male auteurs and the prevalence of films that tend to narrate straight male desire in such a canon:

> I would point to the dominance of popular Italian contemporary films that insistently continue to suture Italian history and the male gaze, whilst female protagonists (often contested by two men in a classical Oedipal structure) remain firmly entrenched within the private sphere, and the critical acceptance of this tendency. (p. 213)

These films' "dominance" and the "critical acceptance" of those which "suture Italian history and the male gaze" further underscore the relationship between patriarchal structures and canonicity, a relationship we can productively analyse in relation to European A festivals. Such films thus appear constitutive of, and constituted by, an "auteurist canon" that neglects both female directors and films about female desire (heterosexual or otherwise).

Relating this to the question of film texts themselves, Hipkins (2008, pp. 214–215) distinguishes between "images of women" and "images for women." She posits the latter as a remedy to the former, the former being caught up in patriarchal structures that consider women only in relation to the ways they are looked at (their "looked-at-ness," to continue Hipkins's citation of Mulvey [1975, p. 11]). Films that make it into the canon are, generally speaking, preoccupied with images *of* women. As I suggest above, this indicates that a canon of Italian cinema founded on films directed by male auteurs may also reproduce a notion of artistically worthy film in relation to a masculine vision, characterised by male figures gazing at "images of women" and addressed to a male viewer—"images for men" instead of "images for women," perhaps. Below I consider this in relation to the Tallinn synopsis and its foregrounding of Jep's and Sorrentino's perspectives, as well as the Cannes synopsis making use of the image of a "dead diva" displayed for the film and the viewers. As Hipkins challenges the commitment to an auteurist canon made up of images of women in Italian film scholarship, we can add that European A festivals may be subject to something similar.

In a subsequent study on Italian cinema and masculinity, O'Rawe (2014) underscores the relationship between male filmmakers and masculine representations privileged in the construction of Italian cinema, including in the new millennium:

> The male dominance of Italian cinema is not just restricted to its personnel, but also encompasses a representational economy dominated by the

> concerns of masculinity. In fact, Italian cinema since the new millennium has been marked by strong performances by charismatic male stars, often working together, and by representations of troubled masculinity across a surprisingly wide range of genres. (p. 1)

The confluence of auteur and star is relevant to both the cases of *The Son's Room*, in which the auteur is also the star, and *The Great Beauty*, which is part of a series of celebrated collaborations between Sorrentino and actor Toni Servillo. In relating O'Rawe's comments to those of Hipkins, and my own regarding the logic of European A festivals, we might investigate the extent to which Italian cinema's awarding and representation is conditioned by an evaluation of films based on the triad of consecrated male auteur, charismatic male star, and representation of troubled masculinity.[11] Although O'Rawe considers this trend across Italian films in general, it appears pertinent to consider whether the notion of "art" that conditions European A festivals' awarding and representation of Italian cinema between 2000 and 2017 might be defined by films by men about masculinity. To what extent does the universal "the art of film" mean not only films directed by men, but "film as masculine"?

Along with her overall argument that the canon of Italian cinema is constructed around a masculine logic, O'Rawe (2014) discusses several issues that we might trace through the relationship between *The Great Beauty* and European A festivals' representation of it, such as: the degradation of society represented via ideas of feminisation (pp. 5–6); the (constructed) difference between "serious" actors such as Servillo and "teen heartthrobs" such as Scamarcio (p. 154); and "male melancholy" as the overarching structure of (canonical) Italian cinema (p. 164). Notions of "seriousness" and "male melancholy" are somewhat co-dependent. Male melancholy, O'Rawe seems to suggest, often becomes a signifier for seriousness, a conflation that also attests to the positioning of male subject as universal in various representations of Italian cinema. We can read this through O'Rawe's brief analysis of *The Great Beauty*. She states that while the film's success is often articulated in terms of its engagement with the "big, serious themes of existence," a closer examination reveals that *The Great Beauty* is "primarily a male melodrama" structured around Jep's "quest to remember his great youthful love," Elisa, who functions only as "a structuring absence or loss"

11 For example, the trope of the male star is absent in Cannes's and Tallinn's construction of *The Great Beauty* but appears in Karlovy Vary's exaltation of Massimo Girotti in its synopsis of *Facing Window*.

(O'Rawe, 2014, p. 163). The claim to universal appeal—engaging with "big, serious themes of existence"—covers over the particularity of the film's narrative, the gendered dimension of these themes. Rather than tackling existence per se, we might read *The Great Beauty* as a film about a specifically heterosexual masculine trauma that centres on the loss of the feminine. It will be important to examine the extent to which Tallinn's and Cannes's representations of the film articulate *The Great Beauty*, and thus "the art of film," through a structure of male melancholy, or attempt to represent it as a film that deals with "big, serious themes," omitting the gendered particularity of such themes' articulation.

The Great Beauty and Gender

Despite O'Rawe's (2014) identification of *The Great Beauty* as a case study for the analysis of Italian cinema and masculinity, the film has only been interpreted in relation to gender twice in depth, to my knowledge. This lack of material indicates a need for further investigation, particularly since the two in-depth studies reach contrasting conclusions about the film. Moreover, each depends on an analysis of the film text without considering the implications that a gendered institutional and ideological context might have for *The Great Beauty* and its success or canonisation. Annachiara Mariani (2017, pp. 171–172) advances the proposition that "in Sorrentino's films, the female becomes 'the other,' an object whose existence is defined and legitimised by men who clearly hold the dominant gaze in his cinematic creation." Mariani bases this on Mulvey's (1975) theory that women are fetishised, defined by their to-be-looked-at-ness, in order to neutralise the threat they present to male subjectivity. Across Sorrentino's oeuvre, Mariani argues, the threat that the feminine might subvert masculinity and its dominant position is overcome through female characters' lack of psychological development.

Characters such as Ramona, Elisa and Suor Maria either die, remain fixed in a nostalgic dream-memory space or are depicted as asexual or hermaphrodite (Mariani, 2017, p. 175). Mariani reads *The Great Beauty* as a film centred on Jep's struggle towards an epiphany, a revelation of "great beauty" that will release him from his writer's block. She shows the various ways in which female characters are used as touchpoints on the journey to this epiphany, either blocking or facilitating the male protagonist's progress but never fundamentally challenging the quest itself. While Mariani acknowledges the threatening nature of the feminine, even when fetishised, she demonstrates how *The Great Beauty* contains this threat by locating the feminine in a "heterotopic non-space" (p. 177). That is, the potential for a female character to throw both Jep and the film's diegesis off course is limited by the various ways in which female figures are represented, culminating in Jep's epiphanic memory of Elisa, his first love:

> Ultimately, the great beauty is an indefinite oneiric trace that woman, or women, may leave in the man's conscious reminiscence where she continues to live and to inspire the author, while she is still trapped in a heterotopic, Platonic and metaphysical dimension. (Mariani, 2017, p. 179)

There is one aspect of Mariani's reading of Sorrentino's films, including *The Great Beauty*, of particular interest to us here. Mariani brings together (some might say conflates) Sorrentino's perspective and that of his films' characters. She concludes that misogyny is a kind of authorial signature that runs across Sorrentino's oeuvre. Leaving Mariani's own implicit investment in the category of the auteur aside, her study highlights useful questions regarding the way in which *The Great Beauty* has been constructed by European A festivals as an auteur film, and the implications this has for the gender politics of such a construction. Do festivals present *The Great Beauty* as the product of a genius male auteur, and how is the feminine represented in relation to this? Is the film shown to be the product of, and to contain, a powerful masculine look that fetishises the feminine? Are Sorrentino's and Jep's perspectives conflated in the festival synopses as well? How does the film confirm or undermine this representation? And, finally, what does this mean for the notion of "art" as defined through the figure of a male auteur's gaze over the feminine?

The second study that focuses on gender in *The Great Beauty* draws an opposing conclusion, arguing that it is a film about masculine weakness in relation to women, and thus free from the patriarchal structures that other scholars identify in it. Eszter Simor and David Sorfa (2017) criticise scholars for neglecting the comic element of Sorrentino's films. They argue that films such as *The Great Beauty* parody male desire by representing it as excessive and absurd: Sorrentino's "accentuated style creates room for an ironic interpretation and this permits them to undermine their own representation of sexism" (Simor & Sorfa, 2017, p. 212). The authors take the ending of *The Great Beauty* as a key example of this procedure, although they appear to interpret it in a diametrically opposite way to Mariani. In their interpretation, this scene is so over-stylised as to render Jep's obsession with Elisa ridiculous. They conclude that "[t]he cause of the protagonist's writing block is revealed as being overwhelmed by the physical attractiveness of an idealised woman. It becomes a parody of men's obsession with female beauty" (p. 210).

While there is room for debate about the relationship between style and content in this scene, the authors fail to recognise that this representation maintains the same structure of desire that Mariani (2017) and other scholars have critiqued: the female figure is still positioned in relation to the male protagonist's quest, only this time as an obstacle. *The Great Beauty* may ironise male desire, but it remains entrenched within the structures of sexual difference—the opposition of the masculine and feminine. Psychoanalytically-inflected feminist film theory already highlights the necessity of remaining attentive to reproduction of such binaries in films. For example, Teresa De Lauretis (1984) argues that as long as the categories of masculine and feminine continue to be ideologically invested in (whether they are shown as weak or powerful), the tyranny of sexual difference will continue.[12] This also explains the contradiction between the two interpretations of *The Great Beauty* above: since both appear still to invest in the gender binary, even though both may aim to critique it (or rather one half of it, masculine dominance), they leave its overall structure intact. It might therefore be more productive to analyse the ways in which Jep's perspective itself may be undercut, rather than focusing solely on this perspective's relation to the feminine. I refer to an analysis that identifies manifestations of the Real that destabilise the illusion of internal consistency within the masculine viewpoint and thus may destabilise institutions' investment in the categories of masculine/feminine as such.

Synopsis Analyses

It should be clear that in order to extricate ourselves from the impasse produced by the conflicting readings of *The Great Beauty* above, it is necessary to take a different approach. Its relationship to gender, film canons, and its potential to disrupt these, need to be grounded in the context of its place within certain institutions. If European A festivals are central to the construction of Italian cinema internationally, then it is important to consider how *The Great Beauty*'s relation to gender functions in this context. In what follows, I investigate how the patriarchal aspects of the festival apparatus may be manifest in its ideological construction of Italian cinema in its programmes and paratexts: the vision of art expressed in Cannes's

12 See, in particular, "Snow on the Oedipal Stage," pp. 70–83.

and Tallinn's representations of *The Great Beauty*. I analyse the paratextual construction of the film in the programmes of two European A festivals: Cannes, at which the film premiered, and Tallinn, which awarded the film its top prize. Although *The Great Beauty* only won top prize at Tallinn, analysing the two synopses together provides more information regarding the way in which the film and, in turn, Italian cinema, is constructed across the European A circuit. Therefore, my analysis, while remaining attentive to the differences that might emerge between the two, highlights an important continuity: both synopses represent the *Great Beauty* as a film that expresses a masculine vision through which its status as "art" is secured in one way or another.

The synopsis analysis below takes a form more common to the methodology that this book employs. When interpreting Cannes' representation of *The Son's Room*, we were faced with the unique challenge of interpreting an absence: the preclusion of Nanni Moretti's presence from the film. The synopses of *The Great Beauty* present the opportunity to analyse paratexts in their positive forms: their presentation of signifiers that more or less explicitly construct the film in a certain way. Each synopsis presents *The Great Beauty* as a film whose protagonist, Jep Gambardella, offers us a privileged view of contemporary Rome. In the case of Tallinn, this perspective merges with that of the film's director, and the text invites us to "surrender to the [...] whims" of a genius auteur. This auteur is constructed in relation to a masculine canon of Italian cinema, as the synopsis represents Sorrentino as a new Fellini. Meanwhile, the Cannes synopsis describes Jep as one who "watches" a "parade of [...] depressed humanity" in the "desperate Babylon" that is Rome. I argue that Jep is positioned as the "bearer of the look" (Mulvey, 1975, p. 11) in both synopses, as each attempts to represent the film's meaning in relation to the masculine figure and his perspective.

Cannes: A Male Gaze Over a Feminised Rome

As discussed in the previous chapter, Cannes synopses tend to be more condensed than those of other film festivals. They rarely contain information regarding a film's style, although such information may be inferred from the style of the text. They do not often mention the auteur, who is treated as an implicit symbolic figure around which synopses are structured. The festival's representation of *The Great Beauty* is no exception, being a short and stylised summary of the film's content. Nonetheless, the paratext does give the impression of the film presenting a male look towards a degraded, feminised, and traumatised Rome. This is most apparent in the paratext's slippage between a seemingly neutral perspective and the subjective viewpoint of the film's protagonist, Jep. Initially, the Cannes synopsis does not ascribe a particular point of view to *The Great Beauty.* At first, the perspective it presents is a neutral one that is best understood as representing both that of the synopsis and of the film. The synopsis, in its seemingly direct description of the characters and images that appear in the film, assumes the perspective of the film, as though it were screening these same images for our look. It achieves this at first by not referring to a perspective at all—that is, simply presenting a series of figures: "[a]ristocratic ladies, social climbers, politicians, high-flying criminals, journalists, actors, decadent nobles, prelates, artists and intellectuals…" When the synopsis indicates a relation of looking towards these character-types, it first uses a passive construction, implying an objective viewpoint, for example that of the film: these frivolous character-types "are not seen in a good light." In addition, the text's sole focus on the film's content—its lack of any meta-description, such as we will find in the Tallinn synopsis—contributes to the sense of a neutral perspective both in and over the film.

However, the text reaches a turning point when it describes Jep. Significantly, he is the only character that the synopsis depicts as having the power of vision; he bears the look of the film. The text focuses on his "eyes, permanently imbued with gin and tonic," through which he "watches the parade of […] depressed humanity." This parade is, in fact, the one just described—the long list of character types with which the text opens. This produces an intriguing slippage between what had initially seemed to be a neutral depiction of the film's perspective and its articulation through the viewpoint of the protagonist. Therefore, the point of view we were presented with initially is not objective, but rather that of *The Great Beauty*'s male protagonist. Here, the perspectives of the synopsis and the film are retroactively refigured as Jep's. As reader (and viewer or viewer-to-be), we are encouraged to align our point of view with this character. The text thus could even be said to address the reader-cum-viewer as male: it represents the film and its content from a masculine perspective, thus reinforcing the notion of art as being constituted by "images for men" identified by Hipkins (2008, p. 214).

Once the synopsis presents Jep's as the primary perspective in both the film and the text, the text that follows can be read as reflecting his point of view. It is ambiguous whether "[a] moral lifelessness to make one's head spin" is the view of the synopsis or the protagonist, though, given the above, I would argue that they can be interpreted as Jep's. This leads to the synopsis reproducing a gender binary as the male perspective encounters a feminine figure: "Rome, splendid and indifferent, like a dead diva." This image offers at once the feminised image of social degradation that O'Rawe (2014) identifies as a common trope in media representations of Italy (here, Rome), and a subtle reference to the death of Ramona, played by the real-life diva Sabrina Ferilli.[13] In either case, the synopsis presents a gendered relation of looking, and reproduces the typical structure of male looker and female to-be-looked-at. This is accentuated by the fact that the text's imagery functions through a metaphor of the Italian figure of spectacular femininity *par excellence*—the diva (Gundle, 2007). In contrast with the male star and male protagonist as active bearers of the look, the female star is, by dint of both her structural relation to him and her role as a fetishised female character, rendered passive.

In relation to Italian cinema, Hipkins (2008, p. 225) highlights the requirement for a diva to be passive, and thus take the position Mulvey describes, in order to be integrated into Italian film history. We witness the same structural relation in the Cannes synopsis: the diva is not only dead (and thus passive), but "splendid and indifferent." Reference to her beauty (splendour) and her indifference (another passive concept) cements the position of the diva as a lifeless fetish object, an image of beauty rather than an active subject. In terms of the synopsis's representation of both the film's, and to an extent its own, perspective, the presentation of Jep as the one who looks, followed by the image of Rome as dead diva to-be-looked-at, is crucial. The position of these words, concluding the text, indicates their importance. Moreover, I would argue that, particularly through the image of the diva as dead, they imply the feminine as a site of trauma – the impossible, structural loss, a key element in the privileged mode of male melodrama that constitutes the Italian film canon. This final technique enacts a masculine-feminine relationship and presents it as the culmination of the synopsis. This move therefore retroactively determines the meaning of *The Great Beauty* through the figuration of a male looking at a feminine figure who signifies loss. The traumatic dead diva occupies the structural absence around which the protagonist's, and implicitly the film's, melancholic perspective is structured. As such, the Cannes synopsis presents *The Great Beauty* in line with typical notions of canonical Italian cinema in which a melancholic male look surveys a feminised and degraded Italy.

13 Although not a concern here, the extent to which Ramona, her name semantically similar to "Roma" or "Rome," symbolises the degradation and loss of Rome—its golden age, its innocence—is relevant to interpretations of *The Great Beauty* in its textual dimension.

Tallinn: Masculinity, Mortality, Universality

While the Tallinn synopsis contains nothing so obvious as a direct reference to looking, it also privileges a masculine perspective, citing only male figures in the text, all of whom it represents as authoritative men through whose points of view Italian and Roman history are figured. *The Great Beauty* is described as viewing Rome from the perspective of a male protagonist, and draws attention to this character's portrayal by the "charismatic male star" whom O'Rawe (2014, p. 1) identifies as a signifier of artistic worth in evaluations of Italian films in the new millennium. Opening on "Jep Gambardella's (Toni Servillo's) birthday," the film takes us "on a dream-like tour of Rome's past and present through Jep's memories, passions and crumbled dreams." On the one hand, the subjectivity and thus partiality of this perspective is highlighted by terms such as "dream-like," "memories" and "passions." On the other, however, the synopsis seems to imply that this perspective also provides insights into Rome—that, even in its oneiric partiality, Jep's viewpoint might reveal to us the authentic Rome. Not only is this subtly implied by the word "tour," placing us in the position of tourists and Jep as our guide, but also through the way in which Jep is described, attributing a certain amount of authority over the city to him. The protagonist is presented as an archetypal Roman, if not Italian, subject; he is the "symbol of Roman decadence." His authority comes, moreover, from his place in a lineage of powerful Italian men who, too, are cast as representatives of the nation. Jep walks "[i]n the footsteps of the Jesuits and the Medicis." Jep is, in other words, the male bearer of Italianness, one in a long line of male figures of power.

This line of Italian forefathers includes, most importantly, male auteurs. The Tallinn synopsis extends Jep's privileged perspective to that of the auteur, slipping between Jep, Sorrentino and Fellini. Here, both the film's and Sorrentino's authority appear to be secured by Fellini's presence in the text. We are given a privileged view of Rome through not only Jep's vision, but that of Sorrentino who, in turn, channels the *grande maestro*. In doing so, the synopsis conjures a canon of Italian cinema constructed in relation to the male auteur. We, passive tourists, are encouraged to give ourselves over to these powerful auteurs and the vision they present. The synopsis states that "[a]nyone familiar with Fellini knows how sometimes one must simply surrender to the film-maker's whims." The auteur holds the ultimate authority over the filmic text. Almost explicitly patriarchal in this respect, the synopsis foregrounds the dominance of the male auteur, emphasising his power over both us and the film. Moreover, this participates in the trope of Italian canonical cinema as a narration of male desire, as well as that of the Romantic male artist on which common tropes of auteur theory are founded (Baumann, 2007, p. 59). The presence of such auteurs, their placement in a lineage of powerful Italian men, and the suggestion of their authoritative vision over Rome evoke the "dominance of popular Italian contemporary films that insistently continue to suture Italian history and the male gaze" (Hipkins, 2008, p. 213). Finally, the slippage between the gender-neutral "film-maker" and its gendered manifestations—Sorrentino and Fellini—should make it clear that the artistic vision presented in the synopsis is a masculine one.

The paratext's insistence on a masculine auteurism culminates when it conflates Jep and Sorrentino: "Paolo Sorrentino turned 43 this year and he has now given us his finest film. Is he also gripped by thought of mortality, like Jep?" In a vulgarisation of auteur theory, the Tallinn synopsis depicts Jep as a manifestation of the director's psyche. With this rhetorical question, Jep becomes the bearer of Sorrentino's privileged vision. Furthermore, this subjectivity is represented as the vehicle for a seemingly universal confrontation with mortality: both Jep and Sorrentino appear to occupy the position of universal subjects. Regarding Jep/Sorrentino's apparent struggle with death, the synopsis concludes "[p]erhaps it is a valuable thing for anyone of us to be reminded of our time and place by the rustle of the reaper." The theme of death, as well as the reference to "anyone of us," positions Jep/Sorrentino as representative of a universal human struggle. The gendered melancholy of an ageing auteur and filmic character is cast as neutral—as part of the film's engagement with "the big, serious themes of existence," to borrow O'Rawe's expression. In fact, this invites a reading in line with notions of canonical Italian cinema as being founded on "the traumatised body of the male auteur [...] read as universal" (O'Rawe 2008, pp. 175–176), only now the baton has been passed from a dead Fellini to an ageing Sorrentino. That this encounter should inspire Sorrentino to deliver "his best work yet" raises the idea of a relationship between creativity and mortality: the film is shown to depict a universal confrontation giving rise to a universal artwork—yet, implicitly, one achieved via the male, *sinthomatic*, auteur.

Both synopses present *The Great Beauty* as a film told from Jep's perspective. We see Rome through Jep's memories or gin-soaked eyes. The Cannes synopsis seems to present a subtle and relatively untroubled relationship between its own implied perspective, that of the film, and that of Jep. Through its slippage between passive verbal constructions and the depiction of Jep's acts of looking, the protagonist is shown to bear the look of *The Great Beauty* and, to an extent, that of the implied reader/viewer. Meanwhile, Tallinn's representation of the film conflates Jep's viewpoint with that of the film's director, Sorrentino, who in turn is constructed in relation to the paradigmatic Italian auteur, Fellini. In this way, the film is presented as providing an artistic view of Rome, a tour through the eyes of both an archetypal Roman, Jep, and an auteur, Sorrentino. Tallinn therefore can be seen to not only privilege Jep's perspective but to highlight the figure of the male artist, the presence of a male artistic look onto—something that will become pertinent when we consider *The Great Beauty*'s characterisation of Jep.

A greater difference between the two synopses lies in the extent to which they either highlight or leave implicit the gendered dimension of their constructions of the film. In some respects, the Cannes text could be read as highlighting its own partiality. It makes a gendered relation of looking explicit: *The Great Beauty* is represented in line with notions of a melancholic male looking over a feminised site of loss and trauma (Jep confronting the image of Rome as a dead diva). It is ambiguous as to whether the splendid indifference of the dead diva challenges the perspectives of Jep, the film and the text. However, given the context of European A festivals' repeated construction of "the art of film" through the *sinthome* of the male auteur and the masculinity of the Italian film canon mobilised across institutions, it seems likely that the text invites us to *enjoy* this partiality in the Lacanian sense of *jouissance*. The synopsis represents the paradoxical gendered universality of its construction of *The Great Beauty* not to critique it, but as part of the senseless enjoyment of ideology discussed in Chapter 2. It is the partiality, the senselessness of the connection between the particular and the empty universal, that we enjoy and that secures our (never total) subjection to ideology—in this case, the ideologically gendered construction of "the art of film." Furthermore, the precise partiality that we are invited to enjoy is grounded in the same structure of sexual difference that governs both Mariani's (2017) and Simor and Sorfa's (2017) interpretations of the film. A crucial law that governs institutional representations of *The Great Beauty*, and with it Italian cinema, therefore appears to be the law of sexual difference, the construction of a gender binary that opposes masculine and feminine while affording the male/masculine superiority.

While the Cannes synopsis may invite the reader to enjoy the partiality of the masculine perspective through its opposition to the feminine, the Tallinn synopsis renders this gender relation implicit as a hidden symbolic law rather than an explicit manifestation of idiotic enjoyment. The Tallinn synopsis downplays its gendered dimension, excluding the feminine completely and presenting Jep/Sorrentino's confrontation with death as universal. The text positions the male figure as universal through its mobilisation of a lineage of male Italian "greats": the Medicis, Jesuits, Fellini, Sorrentino and Jep. The relationship implied between the latter three figures produces the sense of an untroubled relationship between the male auteur and a cinematic vision of Rome. The text also represents the male's confrontation with death as a traumatic encounter with not a feminised, dead figure, but mortality itself. The synopsis universalises the viewpoint of the protagonist and auteur further, as their confrontation with mortality can be related to "anyone." The masculine gaze of the artist—be he Jep, Fellini or Sorrentino—is cast as universal, and thus "art" is given the appearance of a coherent meaning though a structure of gender difference that privileges the masculine and excludes the feminine.

Film Analysis

Portrait of the Artist as a Melancholic Man

The Great Beauty contains several depictions of "Roman decadence" and Jep's status as the "symbol" of it that the Tallinn and Cannes synopses foreground. Likewise, a central facet of Jep's character is his status as an artist, something implied in a metacinematic way through Tallinn's auteurist slippage between the protagonist and Sorrentino. The way in which *The Great Beauty* establishes Jep's status as an artist (moreover, a melancholic male artist) has an important bearing on the film's potential to depict and challenge notions of the universality of the masculine artistic vision mobilised in both festival synopses. Jep is characterised as a writer (the predecessor of the auteur, the author) in the film's opening scenes. Moreover, the technique that effects this characterisation distinguishes the protagonist from his peers, affording him a privileged position in the film—even, perhaps, an auteur-like access to a metacinematic space between the diegesis and the audience. In the party scenes that open the film, Jep initially appears as one among many degraded Roman partygoers, the camera moving through the crowd and cutting between a multitude of anonymous faces. Then, as the ageing showgirl Lorena (Serena Grande) announces "Auguri Jep! Auguri Roma!" we discover the identity of the patron of this bacchanalia, the "symbol of Roman decadence" described by Tallinn.[14] The camera cuts to the back of a man, who slowly turns to reveal himself: another ageing

14 The casting of Grande in this role is itself significant: like her character, Grande is a denigrated ex-showgirl who thus may represent the same ideas of feminine degradation in the popular imaginary.

figure with dark eyes, yellow teeth, and a debauched smile. This slow reveal demonstrates Jep's special status in the film, since no other character receives such treatment, but the reveal otherwise does not yet differentiate him particularly from the other partygoers. Rather, he seems the mirror image of the "disfacimento psico-fisico totale" (total psychological and physical degradation) used to describe Lorena:

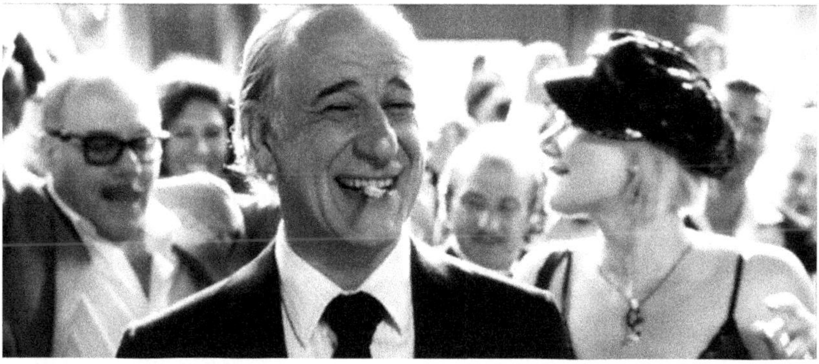

Figure 3: Jep Gambardella, an image of disfacimento psico-fisico totale? *The Great Beauty* (Sorrentino, 2013). Curzon Artificial Eye.

However, while Lorena could be said to remain a symbol of feminised degradation, Jep is elevated to the status of artist.[15] While the rest of the partygoers are dancing *La Colita*, the film slows down, the music becomes muted, and Jep steps out from the crowd to address the audience. The figure we just saw is suspended, and a more distinct one emerges. Not only is he physically separated from the others; he appears to occupy another plane, temporally different. He moves in normal time while the others are frozen, and is also given a different relationship with the viewer. Unlike other characters, he addresses the audience directly, seemingly one level above the diegetic reality that the others occupy.

We might compare this with Moretti/Giovanni's stepping out into a meta-diegetic space in *The Son's Room* (see previous chapter). Seen from this perspective, Jep steps into an extra-diegetic space, possibly as a mouthpiece for the auteur—a special figure who is shown as articulating the auteur's and the film's artistic vision. When we consider that Jep, too, is cast as an artist, this slippage becomes more credible. The monologue with which Jep

15 The last time we see Lorena as she is clutching her bloody nose, having taken too much cocaine. While Jep is also unravelling in this scene, his narrative continues, later culminating in the fantasmatic epiphany discussed below.

addresses the audience and the seriousness of his expression as he does so function to demonstrate his creative sensibility. In an extension of the film's visual distinction of Jep from his peers, the protagonist recounts precisely that which makes him different: his love of the smell of old people's houses. This, he continues, made him realise that he was destined for "sensibility"—to become a writer. The combination of the cinematic techniques already separating Jep from the others, and the absence of any competing perspective encourages the viewer to believe this narrative, to distinguish Jep on the basis of his creative sentiments. In short, this scene casts Jep as privileged protagonist, the vehicle of the film's narrative and thus (in an auteurist reading) the auteur's vision. Crucially, the scene predicates his special status on his characterisation as an artist: Jep's representation as protagonist and artist, occurring at the same time, intertwines the two. We are led to assume that the narrative (and, with it, Rome) will be seen through the eyes of the male author.

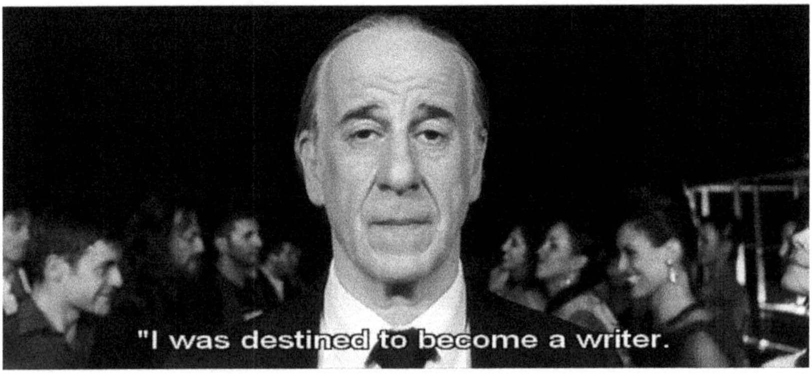

Figure 4: Jep, the artist. *The Great Beauty* (Sorrentino, 2013). Curzon Artificial Eye.

Jep's characterisation has important implications for the kind of perspective foregrounded by *The Great Beauty*. Thus far, the film reinforces, even performs, notions of art as the expression of a masculine vision through its privileging of the figure of a male writer. Indeed, the primary narrative of *The Great Beauty* is Jep's struggle to write due to, we discover, his inability to confront the loss of his first love, Elisa. The film plays with the commonplace notion of art as an expression of male desire for the impossible, unattainable feminine figure—or rather, as a work structured around male melancholy in which the feminine is positioned as the site of traumatic lack, a site of loss.[16]

16 I refer to the tradition of courtly love. Its associations with Italian art—even as Italian culture's foundations—could be said to have its roots in ideas of Dante Alghieri as the "Father" of Italian art, culture and language, and the centrality of his *Divine Comedy*, in which Dante pursues an idealised lover, Beatrice, from Hell, through Purgatory, to Paradise. This is a common trope in discussions of Dante and/or courtly love; see, for example, Boase (1977).

The film moves between staging the partiality, the gendered dimension of Jep's narrative, and Jep's description of his pursuit for art in universal terms. Jep's struggle with writer's block (an obstacle in his identity as an artist) is, he tells Suor Maria, because he has not yet found "the great beauty." In this moment, he appears engaged in a typical, universal search for beauty befitting his artistic sensibility. Yet, in contrast with the seeming universality of this claim, the ending of the film reveals that the "great beauty" Jep has been searching for was, rather, his own memory of Elisa. The film closes on a shot of her looking into the camera (aligned with Jep's point of view), which fades to a black screen with the words *la grande bellezza* (the great beauty) inscribed on it. While it is unclear how ironic this ending is intended to be, the resolution could be interpreted as retroactively determining the film's narrative as a Dantesque quest of the male artist towards the impossible, sacred woman. Therefore, while the Tallinn synopsis presents *The Great Beauty* in terms of a creative confrontation with mortality, we might question its omission of the gendered aspect of such a confrontation as depicted in the film. Its discourse of a male artist's seemingly universal confrontation with death seems to conceal a particular narrative of male melancholy. The extent to which the film can be interpreted as troubling this universalisation depends on the way in which Jep's look, both over Rome and at Elisa, is represented. To what extent is this artist's gaze shown in its partiality—in, we might say, its fantasmatic dimension?

The Irruption of Male Fantasy: Jep's Look, the Object's Gaze

To investigate the film's representation of Jep's perspective, and the notion of melancholic, masculine artistic vision in the film, I now turn to *The Great Beauty*'s depiction of perspective as such. Throughout the discussions and analyses of how European A festivals might represent "the art of film" through notions of an auteur's creative vision and, more precisely, a *male* auteur's vision, the question of perspective has been paramount. It is therefore not surprising that I have made several references to Mulvey's theory of the male gaze, albeit mostly in passing. Both the data on European A festivals awarding Best Picture only to Italian films directed by men, as well as the Cannes and Tallinn synopses' representation of a highly successful Italian prize-winner suggest that such festivals privilege the male gaze in a typical, Mulveyan sense. They seem to position the male auteur as active subject. A brief analysis of *The Great Beauty*'s representation of Jep as a melancholic male artist indicates that the film performs and participates in this process. However, in order to understand how this might be disrupted in the film, we must delve more deeply into the structures of the male gaze, the process of "suturing" perspective via a male figure, and the intrusion of the Real of the gaze (the capitalised Gaze) that makes manifest the ultimate failure of this operation. Although *The Great Beauty* initially appears to suture its narrative perspective to Jep, and thus privilege and universalise the "male gaze" in its meta-discourse on art, it also contains techniques that represent the disruption of suture. Such techniques highlight the intrinsic non-totality, and thus non-universality, of Jep's perspective as such. Identifying and interpreting them is thus essential to an analysis of the film that aims to disrupt the ideological workings of the festival synopses that either stage this universality or invite us to enjoy its gendered partiality.

I will not rehearse Mulvey's well-known theory of male gaze here but move straight to the theoretical developments that take it as their spur. For clarity, I will also refer to Mulvey's gaze as "look" (a closer translation of the Lacanian *voir* on which Mulvey draws, in contrast with *le regard* used in Lacan's later seminars to refer to the Gaze). Copjec (1994) responds to criticisms that Mulvey's notions of the look are too totalising in their suggestion that films might successfully suture a film's meaning to the male perspective. Copjec instead argues for the inherent failure of suture. She posits that the suturing of a field (e.g., the field of on-screen perception) through a supplementary element (e.g., a character's perspective) is never total since it always bears the trace of this process:

> Suture, in brief, supplies the logic of a paradoxical function whereby a supplementary element is added to the series of signifiers in order to mark the lack of a signifier that could close the set. The endless slide of signifiers (hence deferral of sense) is brought to a halt and allowed to function "as if" it were a closed set through the inclusion of an element that acknowledges the impossibility of closure. (p. 174)

For example, if a spectator is encouraged to interpret the events on screen via the perspective of a male character, thus halting the "deferral of sense" (i.e., allowing the spectator to make sense of the film), they can respond at best "as if" they fully share character's perspective—the character remaining nonetheless a "supplementary element" that bears the trace of the impossibility of a full interpretation of the film. Moreover, "the impossibility of closure" also determines the impossibility of the male character's totalising perspective on a scene and thus his mastery over the image and its contents (e.g., the objectified woman).

The manifestation of such impossibility of closure is what Lacanian film theory discusses as intrusions of the Real or, in relation to perspective, the Gaze. For example, Žižek (2001b) reinterprets the process of cinematic suture, theorising it through this notion of the Gaze. Initially he describes the typical process of suture which follows the shot reverse shot structure (a process we will see at work in *The Great Beauty*'s representation of Jep's perspective). First, the viewer is presented with a shot of a scene in which the point of view of the shot is not registered. The origin of the image is not shown, producing a traumatic "decentering gap" or "absent cause" (Žižek, 2001b, p. 33). The lack of a cause means that sense is deferred once more; suture's power to secure meaning is disrupted. This is remedied by a reverse shot that shows the point of origin of the previous image; it often shows a character looking at the image just seen. The move from shot to reverse shot can be thought of as "suturing" the image into a perspective—usually, following Mulvey, that of the man. This provided the dominant perspective on the film: man as master of the image. The second shot "represents (within the diegetic space of representation) the absent subject for/of the first shot," apparently closing the diegetic field, enclosing it within a character's perspective (Žižek, 2001b, p. 32). If that character is male, the diegesis is thus to be sutured, enclosed, within a masculine perspective. However, if suture simultaneously "acknowledges the impossibility of closure," as Copjec argues, such a "stitching up" of meaning is not possible. This is what I have referred to in general as film's potential to make manifest the Real of ideology, and thus its radical potential.

Several film techniques make this impossibility manifest, re-inscribing the Real in the text. Particularly relevant to the film analysis below is Žižek's (2001b) argument that films that show images from an impossible perspective—for example, the "point of view" of an object—disrupt the suturing operation. In such moments, the Real appears in the form of "the Gaze of an impossible subjectivity which cannot be located within the diegetic space" (Žižek, 2001b, p. 34). This not only disrupts the presentation of events on screen as being from a character's point of view but represents the impossibility of the character's total perspective on a scene; it shows, through the object's impossible perspective, the "blind spot" in the character's vision, occupying a position inaccessible to the character (Žižek, 2001b, p. 34).

McGowan (2007) also analyses the intrusion of an object out of place in the film world as another means by which the Real can be made manifest. Writing on David Lynch's films, he argues that strange ("uncanny") objects appear at the exact moment a sexual union seems possible, throwing the characters' worlds "out of joint" (p. 205). This object alludes to the impossibility of the sexual relationship in both the romantic sense and in the psychoanalytical sense of the fantasy that the subject can fill in their own lack if they attain the object of their desire.[17] The intruding object is usually a strange, traumatic thing, underscoring some fundamental otherness at the heart of reality. In both the techniques discussed by Žižek and McGowan, the split between some kind of surface reality and its ultimate impossibility, or that "reality's" status as fantasy, is signified in some way. Combining the two scholars' theories about how the Gaze can be made manifest in film indicates two techniques through which *The Great Beauty* may disrupt the synopses' suturing of the film to Jep's (and, in the Tallinn synopsis, Sorrentino's) masculine viewpoint: the inclusion of scenes shot from an impossible perspective, which disrupts the very notion of the point of view shot, and the appearance of strange, traumatic objects that resist meaning. Both make manifest the Real of the film, the impossibility of the closure of the diegetic space and, perhaps along with it, the film's meaning. In doing so, they may also challenge the suturing of meaning not only though a masculine perspective, but the possibility of a suturing perspective as such, highlighting its inherent partiality.

Early scenes in *The Great Beauty* appear to privilege Jep's vision of Rome, following him and his look through the city. In such moments, it seems that the film does in fact take us on "a dream-like tour of Rome's past and present through Jep's memories, passions and crumbled dreams." The scenes that achieve this are structured around a series of shot reverse shots that alternate between Jep's point of view and shots showing his reaction to the things he sees, reproducing the structure of cinematic suture described above. In this way, the film's meaning is sutured through Jep's perspective both visually and affectively: the images of Rome are, on a basic level, shown to emanate from Jep's point of view, and their meaning is suggested by the presentation of his emotional responses to them.

His first walk through the city opens on a shot of young children dressed in white, playing in a convent. The film then cuts to Jep's face moulding into a smile, his eyes (we are led to assume) fixed on the scene we have just been shown. This structure continues throughout Jep's walk, culminating in a sequence of: a moving long shot of a nun picking oranges in a convent garden (Fig. 5); a mid-shot of Jep through the bars of the garden, slowing to a stop, his face beginning to register awe at the scene in front of him (Fig. 6); another long shot of the garden, now static and framed not only

17 On the fantasy of the sexual relationship, see the next chapter.

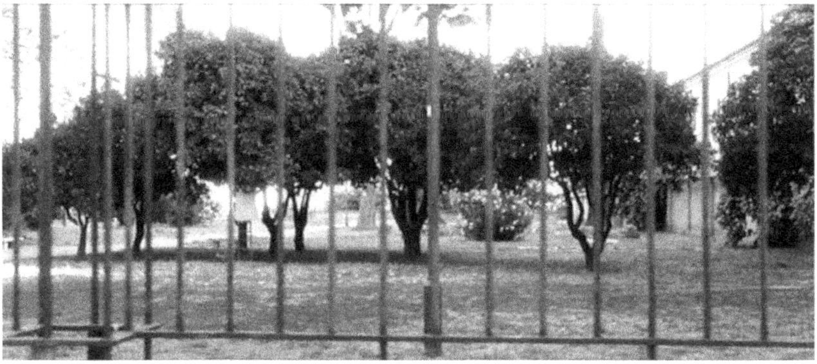

Figure 5: Suturing Jep's perspective on Rome (1): garden through bars. *The Great Beauty* (Sorrentino, 2013). Curzon Artificial Eye.

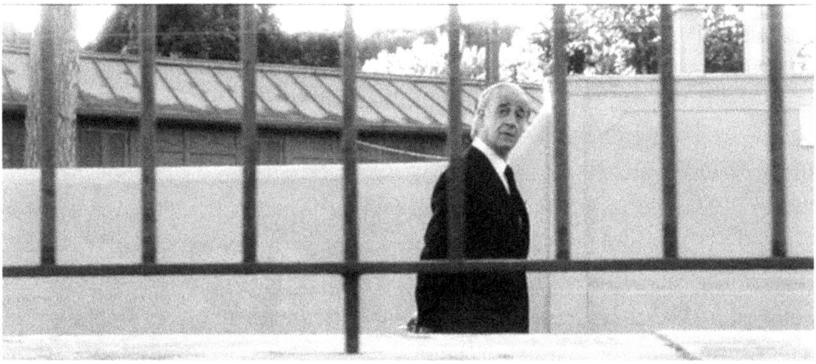

Figure 6: Suturing Jep's perspective on Rome (2): reverse shot of Jep through bars. *The Great Beauty* (Sorrentino, 2013). Curzon Artificial Eye.

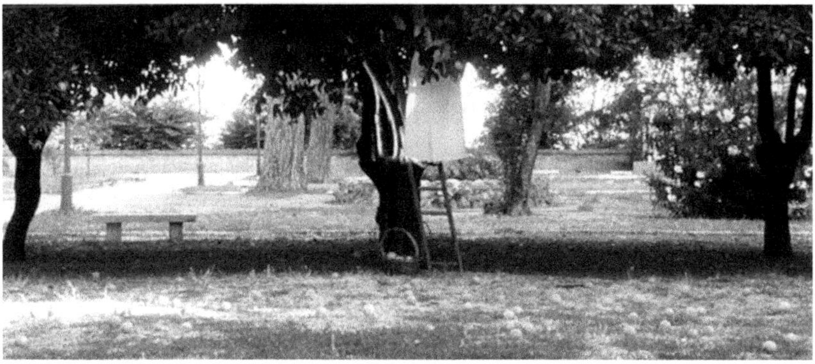

Figure 7: Suturing Jep's perspective on Rome (3): orange trees in garden. *The Great Beauty* (Sorrentino, 2013). Curzon Artificial Eye.

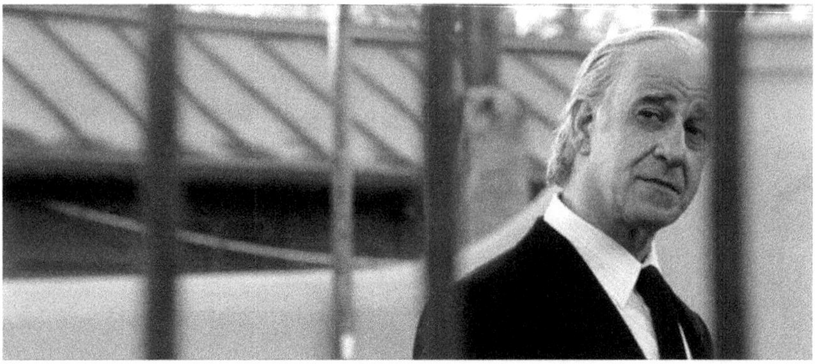

Figure 8: Suturing Jep's perspective on Rome (4): final reverse shot of Jep. *The Great Beauty* (Sorrentino, 2013). Curzon Artificial Eye.

from Jep's perspective but also in an artistic, stylised fashion (Fig. 7); and a close-mid-shot of Jep's appreciative expression (Fig. 8).

In the first shot, the camera is mobile, matching the speed of Jep's walk (presented seconds before). It thus already gives a sense that the scene is being viewed from the protagonist's perspective. This is confirmed when the camera cuts back to Jep (Fig. 6). At this point, the camera moves in to register Jep's look of awe and then cuts back to an artistically framed shot of the scene (Fig. 7). The image is symmetrical, with an aesthetically pleasing interplay of colours, such as the orange and green, combined with an intriguing image of a truncated nun. The content of the shot indicates that Jep might be its origin within the diegesis, since its stylisation suggests an artistic vision over the scene (a vision that would be interpreted as a signature of the auteur, perhaps, but can also be seen in the context of Jep's characterisation as a cultivated artist constantly in search of beauty). This is confirmed once more as the film cuts back to Jep, shown appreciating the aesthetically pleasing scene just shown. *The Great Beauty* repeats this procedure, frequently cutting between a scene and Jep looking upon it, his reaction potentially providing an affective model for the viewer to follow. The reading just given suggests that the film text, like the synopses, sutures the film's meaning through Jep's perspective. Combined with the appearance of an artistic sensibility influencing the representation of the images, this produces the impression that we are being shown Rome through the point of view of the male artist.

This procedure is, however, disrupted by intrusions of the Gaze through the film's use of the two techniques described above: the presence of senseless traumatic objects and shots that appear to emanate from an impossible perspective. I highlight these moments to antagonise the Cannes and Tallinn synopses' representation of *The Great Beauty* as a film narrated by Jep's masculine look. While scenes such as those described above are overall structured around Jep's perspective, they also frequently include out-of-place shots that undermine this structure. For example, the interplay of shots of children playing in a convent and Jep's look is disrupted by images that appear to be from no diegetic perspective, such as this close-up of a grotesque fountain:

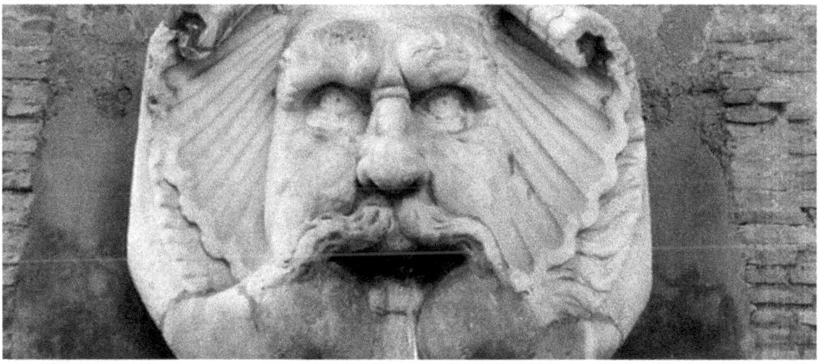

Figure 9: Irruption of the Real: a grotesque fountain Gazes on Rome. *The Great Beauty* (Sorrentino, 2013). Curzon Artificial Eye.

We first see the fountain to the right-hand side of Jep as he is walking away from it. Furthermore, the scene's cinematography highlights the shot's disconnection from Jep's perspective, as the camera moves in on a low arc, finishing impossibly (and uncomfortably) close to the fountain. The framing and camera movement in this shot thus establishes that it cannot be from Jep's or any other character's perspective. Such shots thus appear to disrupt the flow of the suturing procedure I have described above, since the image cannot be incorporated into a perspective that has been represented on screen. Moreover, they appear to be senseless. Both are examples of the strange objects that McGowan (2007) argues disrupt the surface of reality in some films—interruptions of the Real. Not only does this image momentarily disrupt the film's representation of Rome via Jep's perspective, but it also confounds the film's sense. The fountain is out of place with the images of playing children, nuns, and Jep's sentimental appreciation of such scenes. It also does not fit into any of the interpretations contained in the paratexts. A fountain has little to do with the Tallinn synopsis evoking Jep's confrontation with death, for example. One might argue that the shot of the fountain shows Rome stare back in a manner similar to Cannes's representation of *The Great Beauty*. However, this interpretation also does not quite fit, since it does not resemble the image of a "dead diva" through which Rome is symbolised in the synopsis. The image of the fountain is closer to grotesque; it is neither splendid nor, perhaps, indifferent. One could therefore read shots such as this as retaining the senseless quality that McGowan describes.

Such disruptions, these momentary appearances of the Real, ultimately contribute to the film's climax: Jep's "epiphany" that makes up the final moments of the film. At this crucial moment, the film disrupts the shot reverse shot sequence through which it showed Jep's encounter with Elisa, inserting a shot of both characters disconnected from any figure's perspective:

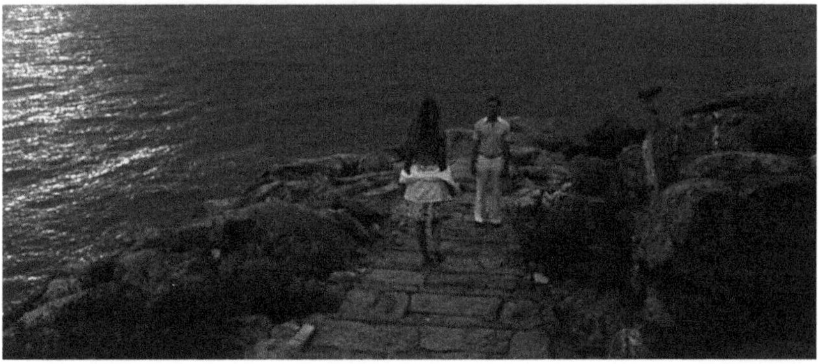

Figure 10: The Real of Jep's masculine fantasy (1): impossible POV shot of encounter with Elisa. *The Great Beauty* (Sorrentino, 2013). Curzon Artificial Eye.

The camera is positioned slightly up the path towards the lighthouse, appearing to capture the scene from the perspective of the rocks on which the lighthouse is built. As well as disrupting the shot reverse shot sequence with the intrusion of an impossible POV shot, the film alludes to the Gaze with the intrusion of an uncanny object: the lighthouse. The lighthouse is shown before and after the exchange of looks between Jep and Elisa, framing the sequence and highlighting its fantasmatic dimension. It appears first as Jep travels to the cliff, where he looks towards it uneasily, and then again after Elisa has shown (young) Jep her breasts. Moreover, during this moment, the lighthouse produces a curious effect of lighting in which the characters' faces are lit up and then plunged into darkness as the lamp of the lighthouse rotates around. This interplay of light and dark gives the scene a dream-like quality and, perhaps, visually registers the interplay of seeing and not seeing—of illumination and darkness, the image and the void, the object of desire and the Real absence underlying it. Finally, the lighthouse itself appears strange; it is a large, out-of-place object that lurks in the background of the scene.

As such, the film appears to manifest the gaze not only through the use of the impossible POV shot described by Žižek (2001b, pp. 33–36), but also by presenting the intrusion of a traumatic object at the moment of sexual union, precisely as described by McGowan (2007, p. 205). These techniques, along with the lighting effects used in the scene (also emanating from the lighthouse), underscore its fantasmatic dimension. In so doing, the film's ending can be read as showing the ideological partiality of Jep's perspective, its being a product of fantasy. While one might question whether *The Great Beauty* itself invites us to enjoy this partiality, a crucial difference between the Cannes synopsis and the film is the presence of a traumatic *third* element that disrupts the binary relation of looking that the paratext presents. Rather than depicting a masculine look at a traumatic feminine figure, the film alludes to the site of trauma being internal to Jep's fantasy (and, with it, the notion of art that Jep, as a character, represents)—the Gaze, or blind spot, that his perspective cannot take into account. The disruption appears not through the appearance of some traumatic feminine, but rather through the Real of Jep's perspective itself. The film text can be seen to disrupt the gender binary as it locates antagonism *within* a gendered subject position, within Jep's masculine point of view. As such, I would argue that the film as it alludes to the destabilising, Real absent cause—the void at the centre of *The Great Beauty*'s masculine fantasy (shown via the lighthouse)—can, in its radical and threatening nature, thwart even a cynical enjoyment of ideology.

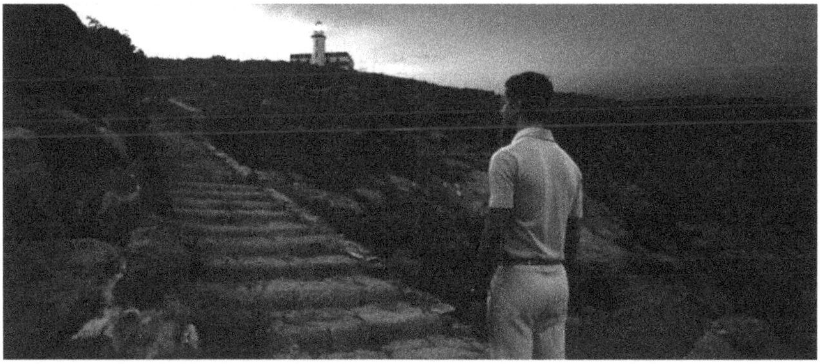

Figure 11: The Real of Jep's masculine fantasy (2): uncanny intrusion of the lighthouse. *The Great Beauty* (Sorrentino, 2013). Curzon Artificial Eye.

Conclusion

The interplay of perspectives undercut by fantasy in *The Great Beauty* underscores the ideological functioning of European A festivals' representations of the film which, in turn, may be expressive of the ideology conditioning such festivals' representation of Italian and art cinema more generally. The Tallinn synopsis conflates Jep with Sorrentino, presenting the latter as the film's auteur, and signals that both artists might have a productive confrontation with mortality. While this fits with *The Great Beauty*'s characterisation of Jep as a writer in the throes of some kind of confrontation with death, Tallinn's representation of the film disavows the gendered aspect of this narrative. The synopsis attempts to construct an artistic universality centred, implicitly, on the male artist (be it auteur or protagonist), whose inspiration comes from the seemingly gender-neutral question of death per se. However, *The Great Beauty*'s focus on Jep's struggle not so much with death as such, but with the death of Elisa, highlights the gendered dimension of this universality. While the film text may articulate the seemingly universal message of creativity and mortality that Tallinn ascribes to it, *The Great Beauty* also appears to self-consciously underline this through the figure of a melancholic male artist pursuing an idealised, lost female lover.

This imagery is central also to the Cannes synopsis, which describes *The Great Beauty* as an encounter between Jep's melancholic perspective and the traumatic figure of the dead diva. In contrast, *The Great Beauty* depicts several points of antagonism within Jep's look, and as such has the potential to disrupt the masculine/feminine binary according to which the Cannes synopsis of the film is structured. The appearance of traumatic, senseless objects (the fountain and the lighthouse), and shots from an impossible "objective" (as in pertaining to the object) point of view, can be understood as irruptions of the Gaze, antagonistic elements in the film text that destabilise the process of suture and any illusion of perspectival mastery. In so doing, the film text locates antagonism *within* the masculine perspective rather than as external to it (as in an antagonism between the masculine and feminine).

These aspects of the film text highlight how the Cannes synopsis locates antagonism, in contrast, between two genders—between the male looker and dead diva—rather than as internal to gender itself. In doing so, it reproduces a fantasy of sexual difference, the fantasy that there should be a stable gender on each side of the binary, which disavows the antagonism internal to gender as such. Therefore, while the Tallinn synopsis disavows the partiality of its gendered construction of *The Great Beauty* (masculinity functioning on the level of implicit symbolic law), the Cannes synopsis presents and invites us to enjoy this partiality without undermining the structure on which such enjoyment is predicated. These synopses evidence two interrelated approaches to the construction of the ideological universal "art of film." First, Tallinn conceals the gendered particularity of the ideological universal "art of film" by moving it to the implicit level and presenting the masculine artistic vision as universal. Second, Cannes encourages a cynical enjoyment of this particularity that, while highlighting it, does not fundamentally undermine it. Both Cannes and Tallinn construct *The Great Beauty*'s artistic merit, its status as exemplary of "the art of film," through notions of art as the product of male artists and expressing a masculine vision over their subject matter. Italian cinema may be constructed by European A festivals on the basis of a false universality that disavows its fixation on specifically gendered creativity.

This theorisation of film festivals' preoccupation with authorship suggests that a more pertinent risk, inherent to the figuration of the auteur as *sinthome*, remains: the fetishisation of identities in order to "brand" the auteur and, in turn, art cinema. As I propose above, the inclusion of the excluded, such as the feminine, into the order of European A festivals does not resolve the contradiction inherent to the universality mobilised by these institutions. It cannot *not* resolve the contradiction of the auteur's status as a signifier of artistic freedom that nonetheless delimits films' meanings for commercial purposes, particularly when that delimitation takes on a gendered dimension. While the presence of a greater diversity of directors at European A festivals is welcome, we must remain attentive to how such inclusion could reinforce, rather than disrupt, festivals' ideological functioning. With the fundamental structure of auteurism left untouched, the female auteur may come to stand for both artistic universality in her status as auteur, and perhaps a political universality in her status as "other," without resolving the contradictions that each would entail.

Bibliography

Balicco, D. (2013). Il film in questione: *La grande bellezza* (2013). *Allegoria*, *68*, 205–212.

Baumann, S. (2007). A general theory of artistic legitimation: How art worlds are like social movements. *Poetics*, *35*(1), 47–65.

Bianchi, P. (2018). La spada di Lazzaro. *Doppiozero*. 15 May. [Online]. Available from: https://www.doppiozero.com/materiali/la-spada-di-lazzaro

Boase, R. (1977). *The origin and meaning of courtly love: A critical study of European scholarship*. Manchester University Press.

Box Office Mojo. (2018b). *The Great Beauty: International box office results*. [Online]. Available from: http://www.boxofficemojo.com/movies/?id=greatbeauty.htm

Brunetta, G. P. (2007). *Il cinema italiano contemporaneo: da* La dolce vita *a* Centochiodi. Laterza.

Copjec, J. (1994). *Read my desire: Lacan against the historicists*. Verso Books.

Cucco, M. (2014). Che cosa è un film? *La grande bellezza* in una prospettiva di economia e politica di media. In M. Cucco (Ed.), *La trama dei media. Stato, imprese, pubblico nella societa dell'informazione* (pp. 101–119). Carocci editore.

De Lauretis, T. (1984). *Alice doesn't: Feminism, semiotics, cinema*. MacMillan.

De Marco, C. (2015). Moretti, Sorrentino, Garrone: "In it together for Italian film." *Cineuropa*. [Online]. Available from: http://cineuropa.org/nw.aspx?t=newsdetail&l=en&did=289826

Donadio, R. (2013). La dolce vita gone sour (and this time in color). *The New York Times*. 8 September. [Online]. Available from: https://www.nytimes.com/2013/09/09/movies/paolo-sorrentinos-great-beauty-explores-italys-decline.html

Elsaesser, T. (2016). The global author: Control, creative constraints, and performative self-contradiction. In S. Jeong & J. Szaniawski (Eds.), *The global auteur: The politics of authorship in 21st century cinema* (pp. 21–41). Bloomsbury.

Festival de Cannes. (2013). *La Grande Bellezza* (*The Great Beauty*). [Online]. Available from: http://www.festival-cannes.com/en/films/la-grande-bellezza

Gordon, R. (2015) Inside-out. History, beauty and the cultural currents of Italianness within and across borders. *Studi culturali, 12*(3), 325–338.

Gundle, S. (2007). *Bellissima: Feminine beauty and the ddea of Italy*. Yale University Press.

Hayward, S. (2013). *Cinema studies: The key concepts* (4th ed.). Routledge.

Hipkins, D. (2008). Why Italian film studies needs a second take on gender. *Italian Studies, 63*(2), 213–234.

Jaikumar, P. (2016). Feminist and non-Western interrogations of film authorship. In K. Hole, D. Jelača, E. Ann Kaplan, & P. Petro (Eds.), *The Routledge companion to cinema & gender* (pp. 205–214). Routledge.

La Porta, F. (2013). Il film in questione: *La grande bellezza* (2013). *Allegoria, 68*, 213–216.

Loist, S., & Verhoeven, D. (2019). Complex not complicated: Gendered media industries in the wake of #MeToo. *Media Industries, 6*(1), 67–71.

Marcus, M. (1996). *Caro Diario* and the cinematic body of Nanni Moretti. *Italica, 73*(2), 233–247.

Mariani, A. (2017). The empty heterotopic (non-)space of Sorrentino's characters in *The Great Beauty* and *The Consequences of Love*. In S. G. Byer & F. Cecchini (Eds.), *Representations of female identity in Italy: From Neoclassism to the 21st Century* (pp. 170–186). Cambridge Scholars Publishing.

Martin, A. (2016). Refocusing authorship in women's filmmaking. In J. Levitin, J. Plessis, & V. Raoul (Eds.), *Women filmmakers: Refocusing* (pp. 29–37). Routledge.
Martini, A. (2015). Concept city: Roma ri-vista e vissuta ne *La dolce vita* e *La grande bellezza*. *Carte Italiane*, *2*(10), 107–119.
Maule, R. (2014). Women's festival 2.0 between grassroots globalization and neoliberal feminism: The birds eye view festival. *Comunicazioni sociali*, *1*(3), 368–374.
McGowan, T. (2007). *The real Gaze: Film theory after Lacan*. State University of New York Press.
Minuz, A. (2013). Il film in questione: *La grande bellezza* (2013). *Allegoria*, *69*, 217–220.
Mori, G. (2016). Il cinema del godimento: lo sguardo come fattore politico da Fellini a Sorrentino. *L'avventura*, *61*(1), 149–169.
Mulvey, L. (1975). Visual pleasure and narrative cinema. *Screen*, *16*(3), 6–18.
O'Healy, Á. (2000). Theatre and cinema: 1945–2000. In L. Panizza & S. Wood (Eds.), *History of women's writing in Italy* (pp. 254–265). Cambridge University Press.
O'Leary, A. (2017). What is Italian cinema? *California Italian Studies*, *7*(1), 1–26.
O'Rawe, C. (2008). "I padri e i maestri": Genre, auteurs, and absences in Italian film studies. *Italian Studies*, *63*(2), 173–194.
O'Rawe, C. (2014). *Stars and masculinities in contemporary Italian cinema*. Palgrave Macmillan.
Priimägi, T. (2013). *The Great Beauty*. Tallinn Black Nights Film Festival. [Online]. Available from: http://2013.poff.ee/eng/films/programmes.p/official-competition-eurasia-1/the-great-beauty
Rich, B. R. (1998). *Chick flicks: Theories and memories of the feminist film movement*. Duke University Press.
Romney, J. (2018). "Happy as Lazzaro": Cannes review. *Screen Daily*. [Online]. Available from: https://www.screendaily.com/reviews/happy-as-lazzaro-cannes-review/5129305.article
Silverman, K. (2003 [1988]). The female authorial voice. In V. W. Wexman (Ed.), *Film and authorship* (pp. 50–75). Rutgers University Press.
Simor, E., & Sorfa, D. (2017). Irony, sexism and magic in Paolo Sorrentino's films. *Studies in European Cinema*, *14*(3), 200–215.
Tarr, C. (1999). *Diane Kurys*. Manchester University Press.
Verhoeven, D., Coate, B., & Zemaityte, V. (2019). Re-distributing gender in the global film industry: Beyond #MeToo and #MeThree. *Media Industries*, *6*(1), 136–155.
White, P. (2015). *Women's cinema, world cinema: Projecting contemporary feminisms*. Duke University Press.
Žižek, S. (1999). *The ticklish subject: The absent centre of political ontology*. Verso.
Žižek, S. (2001b). *The fright of real tears: Krzysztof Kieślowski between theory and post-theory*. British Film Institute.

Filmography

Alcarràs (2022). Simón, C. dir. Spain.

Anatomy of a Fall (*Anatomie d'une chute*) (2023). Triet, J. dir. France.

The Dark Sea (*Mare nero*) (2005). Torre, R. dir. Italy.

Daughter of Mine (*Figlia mia*) (2018). Bispuri, L. dir. Italy.

Dolce Vita (*La dolce vita*) (1960) Fellini, F. dir. Italy.

Don't Tell (*La bestia nel cuore*) (2005). Comencini, C. dir. Italy.

The Great Beauty (*La grande bellezza*) (2013). Sorrentino, P. dir. Italy.

Happening (*L'Événement*) (2021). Diwan, A. France.

Happy as Lazzaro (*Lazzaro felice*) (2018). Rohrwacher, A. dir. Italy.

Honey (*Miele*) (2013). Golino, V. dir. Italy.

Il Divo (*Il divo: La spettacolare vita di Giulio Andreotti*) (2008). Sorrentino, P. dir. Italy.

Mia madre (2015). Moretti, N. dir. Italy.

Non è giusto (2001). De Lillo, A. dir. Italy.

The Piano (1993). Campion, J. dir. UK.

Quo Vado? (*Quo vado?*) (2016). Zalone, C. dir. Italy.

Shooting the Moon (*L'albero delle pere*) (1998). Archibugi, F. dir. Italy.

Shoplifters (*Manbiki kazoku*) (2018). Koreeda, H. Japan.

Tale of Tales (*Il racconto dei racconti*) (2015). Garrone, M. dir. Italy.

Titane (2021). Ducournau, J. dir. France.

Touch Me Not (2018). Pintilie, A. dir. Romania.

Via degli specchi (*Via degli specchi*) (1983). Gagliardo, G. dir. Italy.

The Vesuvians (*I vesuviani*) (1997). Capuano, A., Corsicato, P., de Lillo, A., Incerti, S., & Martone, M. dirs. Italy.

When the Night (*Quando la notte*) (2011). Comencini, C. dir. Italy.

The Wonders (*Le meraviglie*) (2014). Rohrwacher, A. dir. USA.

The Young Pope (2016, television series). Sorrentino, P. dir. Italy/USA.

Youth (2015). Sorrentino, P. Italy.

Section II

Political Universality

4. There Is No Sexual Relationship: *Facing Window* at Karlovy Vary

Abstract: Moving from art to politics, this chapter examines European A festivals' claims to a political-humanist universality. I investigate how such claims are underpinned by their construction of, and contradictory attempts to integrate, figures of the social other. I consider this as a kind of product differentiation: a mode of distinction from film festivals' nominal opponent, Hollywood. The chapter investigates the status of gay, Turkish-Italian director Ferzan Özpetek as not only an auteur, but figure of "acceptable otherness," as well as Karlovy Vary's representation of *Facing Window* (2003) as a narrative of closure through the integration of a queer, Jewish "other," Davide. The chapter concludes that European film festivals' promotion of social inclusion is undercut by their investment in structures of difference.

Keywords: otherness, art cinema, Italian cinema, film festivals, Ferzan Özpetek, queer cinema

Giovanna has not yet reached thirty but she already has several years of a somewhat "tired" marriage with Filippo behind her. She divides her time between a tedious job, two small children and extra work as a baker for a local café. The only way for her to relieve her stress is the occasional night-time observation of an attractive young man living in the flat opposite and the fabrication of dreams. Giovanna's stereotypical life is disturbed by an old man Filippo brings home one evening. Her initial mistrust turns to increasing fascination with a person swathed in mystery whose layers she gradually begins to peel away. The strange life of the eighty-year-old Davide influences Giovanna's life more than she is prepared to admit. Özpetek's new film, depicting the force of an unusual encounter which offers hope for a new and happier life, won five Davids at the Italian National Film Awards, including one for Best Film,

Johnson, R., Film Festivals, *Ideology and Italian Art Cinema: Politics, Histories and Cultural Value.* Taylor & Francis Group, 2024
DOI 10.5117/9789463720366_CH04

Best Actress (Giovanna Mezzogiorno) and Best Actor (Italian film legend Massimo Girotti, who died in January 2003).
– *Synopsis of* Facing Window *in the Karlovy Vary 2003 print and online programme*

Introduction

In the previous chapters, I discussed the claim that European A festivals select and award films on the basis of artistic value alone. Such a claim disavows the contingency of not only film festivals' selection and awarding of films, but the (often gendered) standards of artistic merit that these film festivals claim to uphold. We encountered a key ideological figure: the figure of the auteur, the ultimate expression of the notion of "the art of film" as transcending historical and industrial conditions. Yet this figure is a knot of contradictions, its universality continuously undercut by the contingencies of commerciality and identity. Our next case study, *Facing Window* (*La finestra di fronte*, Özpetek, 2003), won the Crystal Globe at Karlovy Vary in 2003. The award drew upon and reinforced the status of the film's director, Ferzan Özpetek, as an auteur. By the time that *Facing Window* premiered at Karlovy Vary, several of Özpetek's films had been selected at A-list film festivals, with some winning specialised awards, usually in LGBTQ* categories. His first feature, *Harem Suare*, an Italo-French-Turkish co-production set in Istanbul in 1904, premiered at Cannes and was nominated for the "Un Certain Regard" award. *Hamam* (1998) followed, a film that moves between Italy and Turkey to recount a burgeoning romance between an Italian heir, Francesco, and Mehmet, the son of the Turkish couple that manages his property. The film premiered in the official selection at the Mar del Plata film festival, was shown at the Istanbul international film festival and later won a GLAAD award for its depiction of the relationship between the two men. Finally, *Ignorant Fairies* (*Le fate ignoranti*), the film that immediately preceded *Facing Window*, premiered in the official selection at the Berlinale and won the Sebastiane LGBT film award at the San Sebastian film festival. Beyond the A circuit, the film also won Best Feature at NewFest: The New York LGBTQ+ film festival and the GLIFF award at the Austin Gay and Lesbian Film Festival.

The celebration of Özpetek and his films highlights another dimension of the institutional legitimation of certain kinds of films and their directors. Film festivals, critics and scholars promote Özpetek's identity as a gay, migrant filmmaker above all, such that he has been perceived as "the acceptable face of queer Italy," and his filmmaking as "attuned to the multiculturalism, identity politics and aesthetics of postmodern contemporaneity" (Hipkins & Renga, 2016, p. 378; Gordon, 2012, p. 106). Özpetek's auteur status is intertwined with his construction as an "acceptable" other figure, his identity mobilised as representative of a queer, multicultural Italy.

The reception of the director and his films reflects the "various regimes of taste" that Antoine Damiens (2018, p. 37) identifies in queer cinema and film festivals. In the case of queer cinema and its auteurs, "generalist" discourses of quality complement "specialised" discourses of queer cinema, creating a "relay" between art and identity in the legitimation of certain films (Damiens, 2018, pp. 36–37). While these discourses may be strategically mobilised in different contexts—the artistic value of a film emphasised over its queer politics, or vice versa—the two remain operative within European A festivals' representation of their prize-winners. Given the foundational importance of the "art of film" to such festivals' ideological functioning, their emphasis on quality is ever-present. Meanwhile, celebrations of certain films and their directors as (acceptably) queer can either take the form of the explicit promotion of LGBTQ* identities, as in the Sebastiane LGBT award won by *Le fate ignoranti*, or be subsumed into a more ubiquitous ideological formation of "difference," as we will find below.

I consider European A festivals' construction of specific marginalised identities, for example that of the migrant, in the next chapter of this book. This chapter, meanwhile, seeks to identify fundamental ideological structures operative in festivals' awarding and representation of art cinema. As such, rather than focusing on these institutions' engagement with queer or racialised identities, I investigate their relation to the broader category of difference and figures of the marginalised other more generally. The dynamic of artistic legitimation and acceptable otherness is central to European A festivals' ideological functioning, their self-representation as institutions that, although prising artistic merit above all, also nominally pursue politically progressive agendas of integrating "difference." While more overtly colonialist constructions of the other in cinema are well documented—perhaps most famously in Ella Shohat and Robert Stam's (1994) *Unthinking Eurocentrism*—this "progressive" orientation is under-studied, particularly in film festival research. Yet the relationship between European art cinema, its institutions and the construction of otherness along broadly humanist lines has a long legacy. Mike Wayne (2002, p. 1) has argued that "cultural difference" has historically been the "master signifier" of European cinema, above all in the production, distribution and exhibition of such filmmaking. He locates this nexus of cinema and difference in European traditions of post-Enlightenment liberalism, which posit Europe as "the source and guarantor of Enlightenment ideals" through the celebration of cultural diversity (Wayne, 2002, pp. 1–2). This cultural diversity, we should add, is only legible within a post-Enlightenment epistemological framework that places Europe at the centre, the "source" of ways of knowing and being.

Another strand of this legacy is art cinema's origins in the European "cinema of the other," out of which dominant forms of art cinema have emerged. *This* "otherness" refers to a stylistic difference from Hollywood filmmaking (long takes, psychological realism, experimental techniques, etc.) as well as the recurrent engagement with themes of social otherness. Here, as in film festivals, the aesthetic and the social intertwine. Randall Halle (2010, p. 303) has observed the prevalence of this dynamic in institutional representations of art cinema, which, he argues, continue to be animated by such traditions. Through a content analysis of film programmes, Halle (2010) identifies the prevalence of tropes of cultural otherness in cinematic institutions' promotion of European co-productions. He concludes that such paratexts enable these institutions maintain their image as sites where one can discover and "learn" about the other:

> The point is that something happens in films and in the institutions of promotion and criticism to establish a (cultural) distance between the viewer and viewed, to establish a differential on one side of which the story is about another culture through which I learn. (p. 316)

Halle writes specifically of institutions' framing of some cinemas and places as outside Europe, as therefore being culturally distant or "other," a theme I explore in relation to migration cinema and colonialism in Chapter 5, and regarding Orientalism and representations of the Global South in Chapter 6. Generally speaking, however, this cultural distance enacts the cultural difference that Wayne also identifies in traditions of European cinema. It suggests that such a framework inscribes a subtle binary between the implied "universal," Enlightenment subject and the culturally "different" figure or film. Examining European A festivals' construction of a variety of other figures through their programming and representation of films, we can observe a structural preoccupation with difference. Festivals' foregrounding of difference instantiates their claim to include the other within their symbolic order. Another performative contradiction, this claim is in tension with the means used to make it: such a claim's reliance upon the reproduction of categories of difference and the production of distance between their implied audiences and the others that festivals construct.

European A Festivals' Others

The Fantasy of the Sexual Relationship, or, the Promise of Integration

European film festivals' engagement with themes of difference and figures of the other is embedded in common strategies of festival branding and soliciting media attention. As Cindy Hing-Yuk Wong (2011, p. 1) observes, festivals commonly court controversy, "catalysing debates over issues ranging from technical achievements to human rights and sexual identities." This is central to such events' perceived topicality: their cultural relevance as sites for the cultivation of both "the art of film" and the cultivation of political or social awareness. In his guide to programming cinemas and film festivals, Peter Bosma (2015, p. 72) identifies two poles of film festival curation: "contributing to innovative cinema poetics," on the one hand, and "expressing persuasive opinions about social problems," on the other. While initially separating these elements, Bosma underlines the "overlap" between the two positions within festival curatorship: both the aesthetic and the political are crucial for the creation of a festival's programme and "curatorial profile" (pp. 71–72).

This is particularly the case for A-list festivals, which trade on their reputation for exceptional cultural importance. Returning to Wong (2011), we find several occasions on which European A festivals engaged with topical political issues through their programming and awarding of films. Cannes awarded the Palme d'Or to anti-war film *Fahrenheit 9/11* (Michael Moore, 2004) at a time when George Bush faced widespread condemnation for his pursuit of wars in Iraq and Afghanistan, for example. Wong also points to Venice's exhibition of *Still Life* (*San xia hao ren*, Jia Zhangke, 2006), a film about China's state-sponsored Three Gorges Dam, at a time when the dam was under increasing scrutiny in the West.[1]

The Berlinale's commitment to engaging with political issues is perhaps the most renowned among the "big three" European A festivals. This was intentional, aiming to create a curatorial profile that would enable the Berlinale to compete with Cannes and Venice, despite taking place in the sub-zero environment of Berlin in February. Dieter Kosslick, festival director from 2001 to 2019, oversaw a programming strategy that focused on political

1 The relationship between Venice and political dissident Jia Zhangke has recently been cemented by his collaboration with festival director Marco Müller in launching the Pingyao Film Festival in October 2017, apparently one of only a few major film events in China not controlled by the government (Frater, 2018).

issues such as migration, climate change and LGBTQ rights. In a recent interview, Kosslick (in Boutsko, 2021) highlights the importance of this strategy to the festival's reputation, pointing to the awarding of the Golden Bear to *Grbavica: The Land of My Dreams* (*Grbavica*, Jasmila Žbanić, 2006), a film that exposed war crimes committed during the Srebrenica massacre in Bosnia. As well as programming films about the Bosnian war, the Berlinale has repeatedly screened films that engage with German-Turkish migration and, as we will explore in Chapter 5, the so-called "European refugee crisis." In 2022 the festival introduced a non-binary acting award, marking a new era in its engagement with gender politics.

Karlovy Vary, the festival this chapter focuses on, has also cultivated a reputation for socially engaged programming and prize-giving. In its post-Soviet iterations, the festival is known for programming Eastern European films that dissect and critique "the nightmare of Communism's official vision," engaging with the politics and legacies of shared trauma that haunt the region and its cinemas (Vimercati, 2012, para. 3). More recently, the festival has followed other A-listers by taking a broadly humanist stance on migration, awarding its top prize in 2021 to *As Far as I Can Walk* (*Strahinja Banović*, Stefan Arsenijević, 2021), a film about a Ghanaian married couple confined in a Serbian refugee camp.

This list is far from exhaustive; as recent examples show, every year brings further instances of European A festivals' engagement with topical social issues. In each case, the festival represents itself as an institution that offers a platform for filmmakers to intervene against a dominant, usually right-leaning or authoritarian political power, be it the Bush administration, the Chinese government, war criminals or a xenophobic far right. Such interventions are often mediated by the festivals' and films' staging of a figure of the other. In the aforementioned examples, our attention is directed towards the political dissident, the exile, the survivor of war, the migrant, the non-binary actor. Film festivals present themselves as institutions capable of representing that which is other, as an alternative symbolic order in which the other can be included.

The notion of film festivals as an alternative space and as capable of representing that which is other (as, perhaps, the "real" universal symbolic order that can include the excluded) has also been suggested by Marco Müller's assertion that film festivals function to "reveal what the markets hide" (Müller, cited in Cousins, 2009, p. 156). This statement, from the former director of Venice, one of the most significant film festivals on the A circuit, encompasses the anti-commercial and revelatory rhetoric through which film festivals represent themselves and the films they award. It can be taken quite literally to mean that festivals show films that would not otherwise be shown due to their lack of competitiveness on the international film market. However, Müller's comments also point towards wider notions of the alternative. The "market," in other words, is not only commercially dominant but discursively dominant, and film festivals provide an alternative space for that which is "hidden" or excluded by the regime of the market. The "market" is implied to be a dominant, even oppressive, force that "hide[s]" certain narratives, while film festivals are, in contrast, positioned as a symbolic order capable of revealing that which remains hidden—narratives and identities that may have been "othered" in more commercial contexts. In a manner that complements the claim to operate under the sign of artistic universality, these festivals posit themselves as being able to construct a *humanist universality*, a symbolic order in which everything, and everyone, can be included.

Applying a psychoanalytical lens, we might note that European A festivals' self-promotion as sites of humanist universality follows the logic of the sexual relationship:

> In the imaginary relation, the two poles of opposition are complementary; together they build a harmonious totality; each gives the other what the other lacks—each fills out the lack in the other (the fantasy of the fully realised sexual relationship, for example, where a man and a woman form a harmonious whole). (Žižek, 1989, p. 193)

Here, the two complementary poles of opposition are film festivals and the figure of the other: each reciprocally provides meaning. Festivals present themselves as giving the other meaning through their promotion of othered identities, from directors of marginalised identity such as Ferzan Özpetek to characters within films. In a reciprocal but not necessarily equal relationship, these figures also give festivals meaning: they are crucial to these institutions' self-promotion as those which "reveal what the markets hide," as politically progressive, humanist and topical events.

The potential inequality of this structure is suggested by Olúfemi O. Táíwò's (2022) theorisation of "elite capture," a process by which powerful institutions "capture" forms of political struggle and redirect resources to their own benefit. As European A festivals seek to incorporate marginalised others and their struggles for liberation, they take up such causes in a way that ultimately benefits the festival, securing their cultural relevance and, with it, financial resources and media attention. Moreover, these institutions, in positioning themselves at the centre of such struggles, leave the structures of power they claim to challenge fundamentally untouched. As I analyse at length in the next chapter, European A festivals' appropriation of "topical" social issues, particularly those touched by colonialism, ultimately reinforces the unequal geopolitical and discursive positioning of Europe as "centre" and all regions beyond as "periphery." This also reinforces the hierarchy of the festival network, in which A festivals maintain dominance, while grassroots and specialised "social issue" festivals remain financially and discursively marginalised.

The relative power of European A festivals is secured through their establishment of these two poles of opposition, underpinning their claim to offer complete orders of meaning. In representing the other, such festivals appear to form "a harmonious totality," a site of inclusion capable of achieving universality. However, the notion of a "harmonious totality" disavows the fact that any socio-symbolic order is "always traversed by an antagonistic split which cannot be integrated" (Žižek, 1989, p. 126). The fantasy of the sexual relationship is dependent upon a structural, often binary, opposition such as the heteronormative man-woman gestured to above. It is, in short, structured around an incommensurable difference. The paradox of this fantasy—one which, I argue, conditions European film festivals' awarding and representation of films—is that it posits a cancellation of the very difference that it simultaneously constructs. To posit universality, then, European A festivals must, repeatedly and paradoxically, reinforce structures of difference, reproducing figures of the other whom they claim to integrate.

Symbolic Opposition: The Performed Opposition to Hollywood

If European A festival ideology is organised around the fantasy of a harmonious relationship with the marginalised other, it is also organised around a second, opposite fantasy structure: that of conflictual opposition to the mainstream (the "market" to which Müller refers). At this point, it becomes necessary to distinguish between imaginary and symbolic orders of meaning. As outlined above, the imaginary level is one of identification, the complementary relationship that underpins the fantasy of the sexual relationship. In contrast, the symbolic level is founded on conflict:

> The symbolic relation is, on the contrary, differential [...] A given element does not fill the lack in the other, it is not complementary to the other but, on the contrary, takes the place of the lack in the other, embodies what is lacking in the other: its positive presence is nothing but an objectification of a lack in its opposite elements. (Žižek, 1989, pp. 193–194)

In contrast with the imaginary relation, the other in the symbolic is not complementary, but rather oppositional. This element is a symbolisation, "an objectification of a lack" through opposition. The symbolic order's fundamental antagonism, its "lack," is displaced onto an "opposite element."

Žižek (1989, p. 142) argues that is element is, most often, a figure that the symbolic order constructs as being external, opposed to it. The symbolic relation follows the logic of suture, the "fundamental ideological operation" of covering up the symbolic order's inherent lack by displacing it onto another, externalised element (Žižek, 2001b, p. 33). In its oppositional form, suture is the process by which a social order's failure to integrate all elements is compensated for through its creation of a figure of opposition—a "constitutive Outside" (Žižek, 2004a, p. 102). This figure is the "excessive element which 'sutures' it precisely insofar as it does not belong to the series" (p. 102). Rather than an acceptable other to be integrated, this "excessive element" is an opponent, an other to be excluded. Positioning the excessive other as outside the symbolic order also "produce[s] the effect of self-enclosure," another fantasy of totality (p. 102).

Film festivals are also discursively constituted through outside, oppositional elements; they are defined through opposition to an "external" figure. Elsaesser (2005) has noted that European A festivals are in fact founded on opposition:

> Most film festivals, as we saw, began as counter-festivals, with a real or imagined opponent: Cannes had Venice, Berlin had the Communist East, Moscow and Karlovy Vary the Capitalist West. All have Hollywood, and (since the 1970s) the commercial film industry, as both their "significant other" and their "bad object." (p. 100)

European A festivals can be considered as mobilising an oppositional status since their inception—a status as "counter-festivals." They have, discursively at least, come into being through a procedure of suture. Since the 1970s, the A circuit has become characterised by festivals' shared opposition to one particular "significant other" and "bad object"—"Hollywood" and "the commercial film industry." The European A festival circuit's common image is marked by the logic of symbolic opposition, with Hollywood taking the place of the external element. European A festivals suture themselves through a constitutive opposition to Hollywood as their "bad object."[2]

2 This structure is in fact the dialectic proper to art cinema, highlighting once again the intimate relationship between the two. As Harbord reminds us (2002, p. 43), "[i]f arthouse cinema functions through a notion of independence, implicit to its identity is that which it is independent

European A festivals are not, in practice, independent from Hollywood. However, they mobilise a rhetorical distinction from Hollywood in order to give the impression of a coherent identity, both for themselves and the category of "art cinema." Marijke de Valck (2007, p. 58) has argued that "the success of the international film festivals has benefited from its ambiguous relationship to Hollywood, as it both counters and emulates its practices." For example, competitive film festivals depend on "Hollywood stars, products, and glamour," and the appearance of any of these affords a festival "immediate endorsement and attention" (Wong, 2011, p. 5). Film festivals' potential to offer "an 'alternative distribution network' for world cinema beyond Hollywood" depends, in fact, on Hollywood—its star power, its funding and even its films being used to secure attention and endorsement for cinema made outside of such a system (Iordanova, 2009, p. 23).

Kenneth Turan (2002, p. 13) describes Cannes as in a "love-hate" relationship with Hollywood. The festival emulates Hollywood's glamour and depends on its productions for prestigious premieres. However, Cannes consistently excludes from its official selection not only Hollywood productions, but films perceived as overly commercial. This is common practice among the festivals on the European A circuit, rendering their main competitions an arthouse "erudite salon" (Wong, 2016, p. 86). Hollywood's presence elsewhere in the festival is compensated for in the main competition, which privileges films on the basis of artistic (and, I add, political) differentiation. If the main competition is an A festival's defining section, the exclusion of films perceived as commercial enacts a powerful rhetorical rejection of the US mainstream.

De Valck (2007) highlights the contrast between rhetoric and practice, again referring to the French festival:

> Cannes will continue to use anti-Hollywood rhetoric and foster anti-American sentiments to cultivate its self-image as an independent, politically correct, and leading center for "alternative" film culture, while, at the same time, knowing better than to damage the relation and risk a lethal exsanguination of the festival network's coronary artery. (pp. 206–207)

While Hollywood in fact constitutes "the festival network's coronary artery," festivals such as Cannes mobilise a rhetorical opposition to the American

of. Thus, inscribed in its own programme is the dialectic of mainstream, monopolised filmic culture and a tradition separate from and acting against its definition of film. This dialectic suggests that the mainstream is homogeneous, coherent and consistent in its production of a film culture."

commercial film industry in order to forge their "self-image." In short, European A festivals, despite their practical reliance on Hollywood, suture their identity through a symbolic opposition to it.

This opposition also generates the appearance of a positive identity for festivals. As de Valck argues, the "anti-Hollywood rhetoric" deployed by festivals also serves to produce a positive identity, such as Cannes's "self-image as an independent, politically correct, and leading center for 'alternative' film culture." Given Cannes's status as the premier A festival on the circuit, film festivals on this circuit likely emulate its rhetoric and may define themselves, therefore, as "not-Hollywood," "independent" and "alternative." Here, a negative identification (opposition) complements a positive one, designating a set of features constructed out of such opposition. Elsaesser (2005) goes on to describe the same process:

> The ritualised appeals are to originality, daring, experiment, diversity, defiance, critique, opposition—terms that imply as their negative foil the established order, the status quo, censorship, oppression, a world divided into 'them' and 'us.'" (p. 100)

Thus, we can identify a dialectical process in which festivals' performance of a certain identity—daring, experimental, diverse and so on—is caught in an oppositional relation between "them" and "us." Each implies the other: "defiance" implies "oppression," for example. This follows precisely the logic of symbolic differentiation, as each element is symbolised through its difference to the other. Here we come full circle: European A festivals construct themselves through an oppositional relation to a "constitutive Outside," Hollywood, which in turn generates their image as alternative and able to integrate that which is other (in particular, that which is considered to have been rendered other by Hollywood). In short, the festivals present themselves as a harmonious totality in opposition to the "oppressive," exclusionary order of Hollywood; they disavow their status as ideological, subject to an exclusionary logic precisely by displacing this status onto Hollywood.

Structural difference is fundamental to the ideological operation of European A festivals and can take two interrelated forms. Through their self-promotion as institutions capable of integrating marginalised others, European A festivals appear to be structured according to the logic of the sexual relationship—the fantasy of an "harmonious totality" (Žižek, 1989, p. 193). However, this procedure is marked by a fundamental antagonism: the inherent impossibility of representing every element (the limit to signification, the Real). In this case, the antagonism is manifest in European

A festivals' foregrounding of the difference of the other while claiming to integrate them, a procedure that suggests a form of "elite capture" of political struggles. These festivals are also engaged in constructing a symbolic antagonism between themselves and Hollywood, a "bad object" in contrast with the "good object" presented in the figure of the social other. As we have seen, European A festivals attempt to mask their fundamental fissure through their claim to represent the other, and their symbolic opposition to Hollywood.

Facing Window: A Film Capable of Integrating the Other?

Scholars have most frequently analysed *Facing Window* in relation to the question of otherness, as part of "an idiom of filmmaking acutely attuned to the multiculturalism, identity politics and aesthetics of postmodern contemporaneity" (Gordon, 2012, p. 106). Indeed, the film's representation of marginalised identities, from migrant to queer, appears to be one of its defining features, although scholars disagree on how far these identities are shown to be assimilable into various social orders. Wood (2005, p. 80) highlights the centrality of othered identities to *Facing Window*'s representation of history, arguing that the film is above all a "quest narrative that uncovers a lost 1940s history of racial and sexual persecution in the Jewish ghetto of Rome." *Facing Window* is considered to represent that which is other—a "lost" history in which social ("racial and sexual") others were persecuted. Wood argues that, beyond representation of the past, the film also posits a "multicultural present" (2005, p. 80). This is part of a broader attempt to integrate others in both epochs: "excavating the past results in acceptance of diversity and an alternative 'family' that represents the nation" (p. 80). Wood's reading of the film raises the possibility of it being mobilised in line with a fantasy of the successful integration of the other into the social order of the nation.[3]

Alberto Zambenedetti (2006, p. 110) uses *Facing Window* as an example of Özpetek's "other's cinema" but, unlike the scholars above, posits that a radical otherness is suggested in the film's treatment of the migrant other. Reading

3 The parallel between the nation as symbolic order and European A festivals as symbolic orders has further implications precisely due to the "European" aspect of these festivals. We might ask to what extent European A festivals mobilise a rhetoric in line with that of a supranational, European identity, and what effect this has on the construction of both Italian cinema and the figure of the other. For a further discussion of this, see chapters 4 and 5.

the film through the idea of Özpetek as an "exilic director," he highlights *Facing Window*'s narrative of migrants Eminè and Giambo. Notably, this reading reproduces the auteurist logic I discuss above via the legitimation of *Facing Window* through its director's status as other. However, of more interest here is where such logic leads Zambenedetti's argument. Although his analysis is brief, Zambenedetti (2006) indicates that the film represents the predicament of the "non-white" migrant in Italy, forced to assimilate in a way that involves "the suppression of the influence of the cultures of origin of their own parents on their new, hyphenated identity, and the distancing from their heritage" (p. 112). This is suggestive of the violence that often accompanies integration, the castration of the heritage of the other on which their inclusion is predicated—assimilation as castration. Considered in relation to the fantasy of social totality, this would signal a point of failure in the symbolic order, presenting an element that the social order cannot integrate or that must be "suppressed." We therefore might consider the extent to which *Facing Window* suggests a radical otherness that contradicts the notion of social totality, and thus European A festivals' self-representation as a coherent socio-symbolic order.

Interpretations of *Facing Window* as an example of commercially successful Italian queer cinema investigate the film's capacity to integrate the queer "other." These analyses also foreground the complex relationship between representations of the other and the mainstream, such as Hollywood. Duncan (2013, pp. 258–259) identifies the criticism that the "relatively unchallenging narrative and aesthetic structures" mean that films directed by Özpetek "do little of the work that queer as a contestational category aspires to carry out." However, he argues that the films can challenge heteronormativity on both a textual level and an industrial one. First, they "can be read in ways that challenge the heteronormative bias of commercial cinema" (p. 259). Secondly, the casting of major Italian stars such as Riccardo Scamarcio and (I add) Raoul Bova "suggests a very different economy of male stardom to that dominant in Hollywood" (p. 259). In this reading, both the film texts and the alternative economy of male stardom suggested by the casting of Italian "heartthrobs" offer the potential to queer "commercial cinema" and/or Hollywood, to queer that which is taken to be dominant.

Bauman (2015) develops this line of reasoning with her analysis of male stardom in Özpetek's oeuvre. She argues that films such as *Ignorant Fairies* and *Facing Window* mobilise a queer gaze towards heterosexual male stars, placing them in the feminised position as "bearers of the gaze," sexualised objects whose primary function is to be looked at (p. 389). She concludes that, while these films are "by no means radical," since they reproduce structures of masculine beauty typical to Italian male stardom, the queering of these stars opens a space for the contradictions between "mainstream" virile masculinity and "alternative" queer identity to emerge (p. 401). Taking Duncan's and Bauman's interpretations together, it appears that *Facing Window*'s status as, if not radical, then alternative, is secured through the film's legitimation via the figure of Özpetek as a queer auteur, perhaps appearing as a counterpoint to stars such as Bova. (Bauman implies that such stars are queered by the auteur's homosexual gaze.) We might consider, then, the extent to which *Facing Window*'s differentiation from Hollywood is predicated on its privileging of othered identities (including that of the auteur), and the extent to which queerness is shown to be either assimilable into or disruptive of dominant cinematic and/or social orders.

Marcus's analysis of *Facing Window* brings together the threads of Holocaust memory, the relationship with the other and the implication of a "moral" opposition to the "mainstream" (2007, p. 143). The latter question seems to form an assumption on which her interpretation of the film rests. I engage with this text in more depth both here and throughout the chapter, since it will prove most relevant to my analysis of the synopsis and, later, the film. Her piece is useful as a means of identifying aspects of the film to analyse and is particularly valuable when taken as an instantiation of the ideology that structures the institutional construction of Italian cinema.

Marcus's interpretation of *Facing Window* is structured around an opposition between two relationships: Giovanna's with Lorenzo, and Giovanna's with Davide. She places the first on the level of "narcissis[m]" and "romantic escape" (p. 152), and the second on the level of "conscious and morally responsible choices" (p. 143). Marcus demonstrates that *Facing Window* depicts Giovanna's desire for Lorenzo as a narcissistic fantasy, in which "the lover's idealised self-image is mirrored in the eyes of the beloved" (p. 149). In contrast, the scholar claims that Giovanna's refusal of this relationship in favour of a non-romantic relationship with Davide provides a model for Italian cinema and memory to work through the traumatic past of the Holocaust (p. 143). Marcus claims that the "bond" between the two characters facilitates "Davide's success in coming to terms with his past" as a queer Holocaust survivor, as well as "Giovanna's internalisation of Davide's example and decision to live out the lesson of his suffering" (p. 143). This fulfilling relationship between the two provides hope for both "Italian cinema" and "the current generation [...] to acknowledge and mourn a traumatic past" (p. 143). Notably, this interpretation follows a reading of Freud's (1917) *Mourning and Melancholia* that implies that mourning's success is marked by the integration of the other into a symbolic order (either the subject's psyche or the symbolic order of memory, as in the collective mourning posited by memory studies). This success is represented, Marcus argues, by Giovanna's ability to "appropriate the perspective of Davide, [...] to entertain a perspective that was truly other" (p. 152).

When we view this interpretation from the perspective of European A festivals' representation of themselves and the films they award, understood through the theory of the sexual relationship, a contradiction emerges. Marcus's reading highlights the fantasmatic aspect of the sexual relationship through her analysis of the film's less "worthy" romantic narrative (she compares it to a *telenovela*), associating it with narcissistic desire to fill in one's lack through a relationship with the (romantic) other. However, we might also note that Marcus's account of the film's narrative of a supposedly more morally acceptable relationship with the social other implies that it is structured according to the logic of the same fantasy. The notion of Giovanna's ability to "entertain a perspective that was truly other" implies, in fact, that the integration of the other is possible. As in the fantasy of the sexual relationship, the other is fully "appropriated," integrated. Marcus's interpretation implies that the film's depiction of mourning through Davide and Giovanna follows the logic of the successful sexual relationship in which each fills out the lack in the other. It follows the same logic apparently refuted in the romance narrative.

Significantly for this chapter's analysis of European A festivals' ideological representation of cinema, this interpretation suggests that the queer, Jewish other is integrated into the order of the film's narrative and the larger orders of meaning with which it engages, such as Italian cinema and Holocaust memory. Looking somewhat awry at Marcus's interpretation, then, it appears that her reading reproduces the structure I have identified: the fantasy of the successful integration of the other complemented by an opposition to mainstream forms (if not Hollywood, then the *telenovela*). It remains to be seen whether this ideology is also at work in Karlovy Vary's representation of the film, and the extent to which the *Facing Window* follows this logic or, rather, contains elements that disrupt it.

Synopsis Analysis

The Karlovy Vary paratext contains several terms and rhetorical constructions that foreground the presence of two mysterious figures, with one privileged as a figure of the other. Throughout the analysis, it will become clear that the Karlovy Vary synopsis represents the film in relation to a vaguely defined otherness that offers a source of "hope" for the protagonist, while positing the film's romance narrative as one of escapism. As I investigate further below, this signals a crucial aspect of the synopsis's representation of *Facing Window*: the displacement of closure from a narrative of a romantic relationship onto one of a relationship to a marginalised other.

Uncannily similar to Marcus's interpretation of the film, the Karlovy Vary synopsis constructs *Facing Window* through the opposition between the escapist illusion of a romantic relationship and the emancipatory potential of a relationship with the other.[4] The synopsis implies that the non-romantic relationship between Giovanna and Davide can not only render the other (Davide) legible but afford "hope for a happier life" for the subject (Giovanna). The text manifests the logic of the sexual relationship as a fantasy in which the other can be integrated into the symbolic order as it simultaneously describes and enacts Davide gradually being rendered legible. In contrast with Giovanna, whose name constitutes the first word of the text, Davide is initially anonymised as "an old man." Davide's gradual integration into the symbolic order is most clearly suggested through the text's representation of his relation to Giovanna. He is initially an object of "fascination" and "mistrust" for her. His appearance in her life "disturbs" it and is described as "an unusual encounter." In contrast, Giovanna's life is "stereotypical." While her existence is presented as the status quo, Davide's is defined in opposition to it—a fascinating, unusual disturbance. Although subtle, this presentation of *Facing Window* produces an opposition between the norm and the other. Moreover, Giovanna's fascination is shown to stem from to Davide being "swathed in mystery." This further evokes notions of illegibility, a veil that conceals the truth of the character. This is reinforced, particularly in its normative dimension, by the notion of Davide having had a "strange life." Overall, notions of illegibility and non-normativity overlap: Davide is represented as abnormal and (thus) illegible.

Then, as Giovanna is said to "gradually begin to peel away" Davide's "layers," the synopsis also begins to reveal more about his identity, describing him no longer as an "old man" but "eighty-year-old Davide." This shift suggests Davide's entry into the symbolic: although still "strange," he is gradually integrated into the symbolic order of both the synopsis as it reveals more about him, and the film as Giovanna discovers the hidden "truth" of Davide's identity. The paratext structurally instantiates the fantasy of gradually

4 I mean uncanny here in the sense of the resurfacing of a symptom—a stain of the Real of ideology. See Žižek (1992).

integrating the other and rendering them legible on both the level of the text itself and its representation of *Facing Window.*

The synopsis also presents the idea that Giovanna's relationship with Davide is fulfilling—that each can "fill out the lack in the other"—while displacing the notion of the failure of the sexual relationship onto the film's romance narrative. The "fabrication of dreams" that describes the film's representation of Giovanna's romantic attachment to Lorenzo is opposed by the "force of an unusual encounter that brings hope for a happier life." This phrase, occurring at the end of the synopsis, retroactively conditions the meaning of the film; its location at the conclusion of the description implies its importance as a summary of the film's significance overall. Giovanna's relationship with Davide is powerful, and emancipatory (a "force" that gives "hope"), resulting from an "encounter" with the other. In contrast, Giovanna's romantic attachment to Lorenzo is depicted not as leading to a transformative relationship, but as a form of escapism. She observes him to "relieve stress" and as part of "the fabrication of dreams."

The synopsis depicts Giovanna's attraction to Lorenzo as contrived. Not only does this align with Marcus's association of romantic closure with mainstream forms that limit moral agency, such as the *telenovela*, it also subtly reinforces the stereotype of Hollywood cinema as a cinema of escapist fantasies emblematised through the trope of the "happy couple" (MacDowell, 2013, p. 1). Moreover, Lorenzo remains nameless in the text, implying the failure of the sexual relationship between him and Giovanna. While in the case of Davide this namelessness combines with the repetition of terms that emphasise his strangeness to render him other, Lorenzo is described as "an attractive young man"—not a social other so much as a good-looking yet mysterious man. Therefore, the relationship that would have been between him and Giovanna is depicted as the coming together of two representatives of the status quo, the "stereotypical" woman and "attractive" man. The synopsis's representation of their narrative stops here. In omitting any reference to the development of Giovanna and Lorenzo's affair, a crucial plotline in the film, the synopsis disregards *Facing Window*'s romance narrative and refuses the possibility of a successful sexual relationship in its erotic form. The synopsis implies that closure is afforded by an apparently more progressive relationship between the protagonist and the other, while the romantic one is implicitly depicted as fantasmatic and doomed to failure.

In this way, the synopsis refuses to render the attractive, romantic other legible, and legitimises *Facing Window* in relation to the notion of rendering the social other legible instead. That this occurred in the context of an institution that has been shown to promote films on the basis of their constructed difference from Hollywood suggests that this may instantiate an ideological procedure in which a cynical rejection of romantic closure becomes a marker of distinction. The refusal of romance as a means for closure, and displacement of this closure onto the representation of a narrative about the other, is crucial to the synopsis's, and Karlovy Vary's, constructed opposition to Hollywood. The text enacts a refusal of a narrative structure associated with the mainstream—the successful romance narrative—as a means of differentiating *Facing Window* and, in turn, the festival exhibiting it. However, it nonetheless maintains the logic of the fantasy of the sexual relationship, the harmonious totality promised by the integration of the other. It subtly displaces this fantasy onto Giovanna and Davide, privileging this narrative while casting that between Giovanna and Lorenzo as the sole site of an illusory fantasy. This constructs *Facing Window* in a way that symptomatically manifests ideas of European A festivals' opposition to Hollywood, and reproduces the underlying ideological structure of the fantasy of totality—the integration of the other. The impossibility of this closure, and thus the ideological procedure instantiated by the synopsis, become yet clearer when contrasted with the film text.

Film Analysis

"There Is No Sexual Relationship": Giovanna and Lorenzo

While the synopsis positions *Facing Window*'s romance narrative as secondary, Giovanna's pursuit of a romantic relationship with Lorenzo is central to the film's plot and, moreover, its potential to challenge the fantasy of the sexual relationship at the structural level. The film explores this fantasy through the would-be affair between the neighbours, raising the possibility of Giovanna achieving self-fulfilment by attaining her love object. However, it ultimately rejects resolution in this narrative line, suggesting the impossibility of closure. At first glance, the film appears to portray romance in a similar manner to the Karlovy Vary synopsis, seeming to refuse it as a dream fantasy, and thus perhaps performing its own difference from tropes and narrative structures associated with Hollywood cinema. However, examining the form that this refusal takes opens up another interpretation that will assist us in analysing the ideology instantiated in the Karlovy Vary synopsis. *Facing Window*'s potential to signal the sexual relationship's fantasmatic, and even narcissistic, dimension will become clear through the film's use of the technique of interface, the uncanny doubling of a character's image on screen (Žižek, 2001b, p. 39).

This technique, I argue, is not only used when Giovanna is shown to voyeuristically observe Lorenzo, thus signalling that her desire for him is a fantasy; rather, the logic of narcissistic desire culminates when Giovanna rejects Lorenzo for a desire for her own image and the impossible fullness that it represents, which is highlighted in its fantasmatic dimension again through interface. In contrast with the notion that Giovanna somehow transcends the narcissistic logic of the sexual relationship by rejecting Lorenzo and pursuing an implicitly more "moral" relationship with the other, the film suggests the continuation of this logic. This has important implications for an alternative reading of *Facing Window* that can highlight the film's potential to disrupt the fantasy of the sexual relationship as such. In particular, the film's representation of this logic beyond its governing of solely romantic pursuits informs my interpretation of *Facing Window*'s portrayal of the other in the second half of the film analysis.

Facing Window initially depicts Giovanna's desire for Lorenzo in a way that supports descriptions in festival and scholarly paratexts. As Marcus (2007, pp. 148–149) argues, the casting of Bova, an Italian "heartthrob" known for his roles in romantic comedies, not only characterises Lorenzo as a love object for Giovanna, but also indicates the metacinematic dimension of the film's illustration of the protagonist's, and audience's, desire. The film's emphasis on voyeurism and technique of "screening" Lorenzo through windows adds to this metacinematic effect, and we might begin to perceive the presence of a romantic fantasy in frames such as this one:

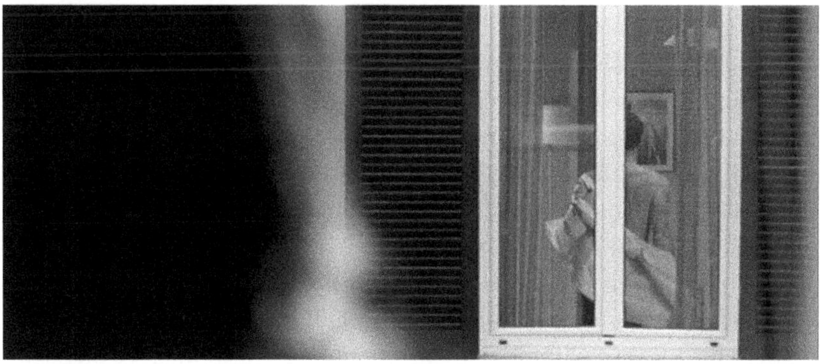

Figure 12: Screening Lorenzo through the *finestra di fronte*. *Facing Window* (Özpetek, 2003). Sony Pictures Classics.

Working within the framework of Mulvey's (1975) gaze theory, Marcus compares the window to the cinematic "screen for the projection of romantic desire" (p. 149). She also positions Giovanna as spectator-voyeur, who "is given to displacing all of her unrealised desires onto the imagined world so tantalisingly glimpsed through the *finestra di fronte* [facing window]" (p. 147). Read symptomatically, Marcus's use of the word "imagined" seems significant, signalling the presence of the "imaginary relation" that structures the fantasy of the sexual relationship. In this case, the relation between the two does not initially appear as reciprocal, but rather implies that Giovanna's fantasy is one in which Lorenzo can give her what she lacks, fulfilling her "unrealised desires."

This suggests the "narcissistic" dimension of sexual desire that Marcus describes. However, I add a consideration of another aspect of the film's depictions of Giovanna's desire for, and eventual refusal of, Lorenzo: its potential to expose the failure of the sexual relationship in its social, as well as romantic, manifestation. To do so, we must re-introduce the notion of fantasy as pertaining not only to the romantic relationship, but the sexual relationship in its social form: a fundamental structure in which the lack in the social order is imagined to be filled by an other, creating a "harmonious totality." This idea (though not always in its Lacanian delineation) is common in film scholars' interpretations of the ideological function of on-screen romance. James MacDowell (2013) identifies the illusion of social closure produced by a film's portrayal of romantic closure as a common trope in criticisms of mainstream romance narratives' perceived "ideological conservatism" (p. 3). Such criticisms, he argues, rest on the notion that the "happy couple" stands in for the resolution of social antagonism, with such resolution, in turn, being considered a marker of conservatism. Writing from a Lacanian standpoint, McGowan (2007, pp. 203–205) has theorised this kind of resolution, but also its reverse: a film's depiction of the impossibility of the romantic relationship having the potential to signal the impossibility of resolving social antagonism.

When we recall that the sexual relationship is precisely a fantasy in which the subject aims (and fails) to fill their own inherent lack, we can interpret the window that frames Lorenzo as a screen onto which Giovanna projects her desire for herself—an unattainable fullness of self, promised only on the level of fantasy. A crucial technique for *Facing Window*'s depiction of fantasy in this way is its use of interface, the redoubling of a character's image on screen. Žižek (2001b, p. 39) has theorised interface as a cinematic technique that disrupts illusions of totality or closure exemplified by techniques that privilege cinematic continuity (for example, the experience of a continuous perspective afforded by the shot reverse shot). The disruptive aspect of interface lies in its potential to represent the "object-cause of desire," the inherent lack in an order of representation (in this case, the order of the film) (Žižek, 2001b, p. 54). While Žižek has theorised this only in relation to metadiegesis (a film's own representational logic), I argue that interface can also disrupt the fantasy of the sexual relationship within a film's diegesis. Shots of Giovanna watching Lorenzo through his window often feature a ghostly reflection of the protagonist herself:

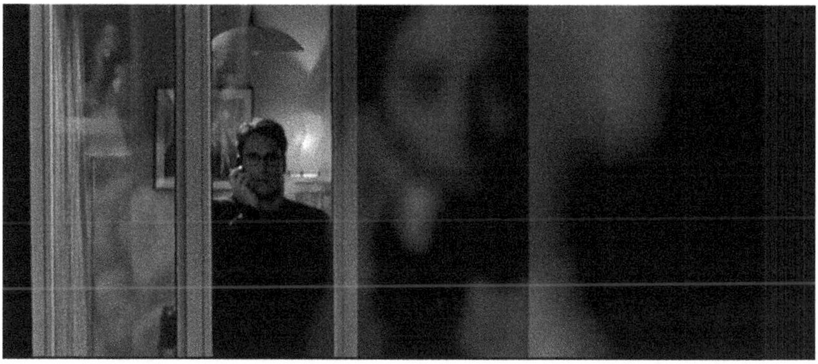

Figure 13: Interface: Giovanna's ghostly desire. *Facing Window* (Özpetek, 2003). Sony Pictures Classics.

Through the notion of interface, this reflection can be interpreted as the uncanny appearance of Giovanna's object-cause of desire—that is, the inherent lack that she fantasises will be filled by Lorenzo. While Giovanna appears to desire Lorenzo, the appearance of her image in the frame indicates the presence of the unattainable object-cause of desire, referring to the lack that defines the subject and that the subject continually attempts to fill by pursuing externalised objects of desire such as romantic partners (Žižek, 1992, p. 6). Thus, *Facing Window* can be interpreted as manifesting the logic of the sexual relationship through Giovanna's desire for Lorenzo: he signifies the attainable object of desire, an other onto which the impossible object-cause of desire is displaced. The image reflected back to Giovanna is the true object (object-cause) of her desire, herself, or, more precisely, the impossible fullness of self signified by her own ghostly image.

Such scenes foreshadow the breakdown of Giovanna's desire for Lorenzo, the failure of their sexual relationship, suggesting the contradictory fantasy on which it is premised. This logic is brought to its culmination in the way that *Facing Window* depicts Giovanna's eventual rejection of her lover, and her motivations for it. Viewed through the notion of interface, we can interpret the film as showing Giovanna's refusal of romance not as a traversal of fantasy, the full acceptance of the lack on which fantasy is predicated, but rather a further delineation of it—the continuing displacement of that lack (Žižek, 2002, pp. 17–18). This begins when Giovanna breaks away from Lorenzo to go to the window through which he used to spy on her. Looking from this vantage point, her own apartment and her own life become the sites of fantasy; she views them through the window-screen, projecting her desire onto them. Giovanna sees her husband, her children, Eminè, and then, finally, an apparition of herself:

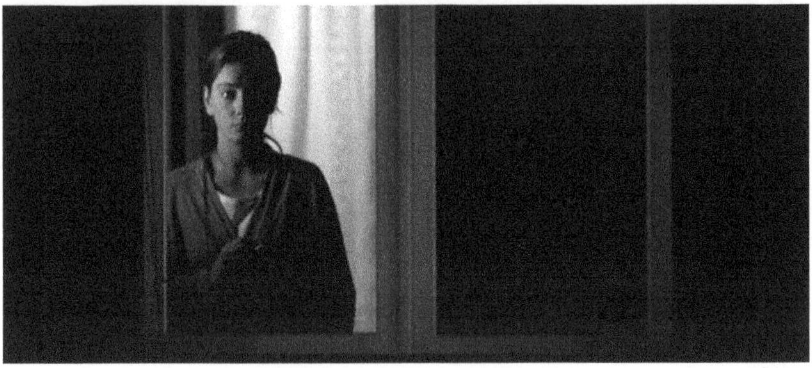

Figure 14: The desire for one's self: Giovanna views herself through the *finestra di fronte*. *Facing Window* (Özpetek, 2003). Sony Pictures Classics.

The film emphasises the appearance of Giovanna's own image, the music heightening, the camera pausing on her apparition, and then cutting back to show her reaction to it. At this juncture, Giovanna's desire for Lorenzo wanes, and she begins desiring herself—or, rather, the fullness that her spectral image represents. If interface signifies the "purely fantasmatic dimension" of a scene, the continuing use of interface, the doubling of Giovanna's image, suggests the continuing presence of a structuring fantasy (Žižek, 2001b, p. 39). As she sees herself through the window-screen of fantasy, she appears to reject Lorenzo in pursuit of the fullness that her spectral image represents. In contrast to the realisation that the object-cause of desire is a lack, the film shows Giovanna continue to desire an illusory fullness; she displaces her fantasy onto another screen. *Facing Window* thus continues to narrate Giovanna's pursuit of the object-cause of desire beyond her tryst with Lorenzo while, through the romantic narrative, highlighting the impossible, fantasmatic dimension of such an undertaking.

The doubling of Giovanna's image in this scene can be interpreted as signalling not the traversal, but the continuation of the fantasy of the sexual relationship. In this way, the film can be interpreted as making manifest the fantasy of the sexual relationship beyond the romantic level, showing Giovanna to be motivated by the impossible desire to fill her constitutive lack. Giovanna's other desires in the film may also be interpreted as following this logic: she is not shown to have traversed fantasy and accepted her inherent lack as a subject, but to continue to displace this lack onto other objects and/or images.

This has implications for the question of *Facing Window*'s depiction of closure more broadly, and above all of whether the film depicts the possibility or impossibility of integrating the other into the social order. Moreover, the way in which *Facing Window* seems to make manifest the logic of the sexual relationship per se can also assist an interpretation of the Karlovy Vary synopsis. *Facing Window* helps us to view the way in which the synopsis displaces the fantasy of closure from romance onto another object. Analysing *Facing Window* as an ambivalent artwork that can make manifest the Real that at once conditions and confounds its ideological construction by Karlovy Vary, we can begin to see how the film text's depiction of fantasy also highlights the fantasmatic dimension of the Karlovy Vary synopsis. Looking awry at the synopsis, interpreting it through the film it represents, we can see that the paratext's displacement of closure from the romantic relationship onto a relationship with the other in fact covers up the Real object of desire in the synopsis. Following the same structure of desire that *Facing Window* shows to motivate Giovanna, the festival's representation of the film, and above all the figure of the other in the film, is motivated by the same desire to fill its inherent lack. While Giovanna as a character is motivated to fill in her lack as a subject, the film's exposition of this highlights attempts made by the synopsis and European A festivals to fill in *their* lack as orders of representation: both are structured in the same way and aim at the disavowal of some fundamental antagonism—the Real split inherent to each. The romantic plot in *Facing Window* can be interpreted as highlighting this logic of fantasy in a way that renders apparent the presence of the same logic structuring the synopsis and, in turn, European A festivals' ideological construction of Italian cinema.

The Radical Antagonism of the Other

To further analyse this structure, I turn to the second point of intersection between *Facing Window* and the Karlovy Vary synopsis: the figure of the other. I examine how *Facing Window* represents Davide as other, considering the extent to which this otherness is shown to be assimilable into the symbolic order (be it of the film, memory or society more broadly). While it could be argued that *Facing Window* follows the logic of the successful sexual relationship in its depiction of Giovanna and Davide's friendship, an alternative reading appears when we view the film from the perspective of its prior depiction of the failure of the sexual relationship and the lack on which it is predicated. From this viewpoint, Giovanna's desire for Davide seems to be subtly represented in its narcissistic dimension. For example, Davide is shown to fill out the lack in Giovanna by teaching her, first, how to become a pastry chef. The two characters are mirrored through their vocation for baking, with Davide, as a renowned pâtissier, standing in as the ego-ideal for Giovanna. This culminates in Giovanna's words to Davide at the end of the film: "I still feel your gestures in mine, your voice in mine," appearing to signal her successful incorporation of him. To what extent, then, does *Facing Window* contrast Giovanna's subjective incorporation of Davide with its representation of marginalised figures' relationships to other orders of meaning, such as Holocaust memory or present-day Italy?

In keeping with the methodology of this book, I highlight the aspects of *Facing Window* that might suggest an unresolvable antagonism between the other and the social order, thus further demonstrating and disrupting the ideology condensed in the Karlovy Vary synopsis. Overall, when read through the notion of otherness, *Facing Window* portrays a social order predicated on exclusion: the present as irreconcilable with the past, Holocaust memory as exclusive of the queer other, and contemporary Italian society as exclusive of the migrant other. This side of the film's representation of otherness counterbalances the sense of wholeness that we could read in the narrative of Giovanna's pursuit of happiness, acting as the "bone in the throat"—the traumatic Real—that permeates and confounds the film's, and the synopsis's, evocation of closure (Žižek, 2003, p. 63). Reading the film in this way highlights the impossibility of a successful relationship with the other: the designation of the other as other means it remains irredeemably open, incomplete, since it can never integrate this element. It is with the aim of demonstrating this that my analysis of *Facing Window* will focus entirely on the film's depiction of a traumatic otherness at the heart of the present, Holocaust memory and contemporary society.

Davide's first appearance in the film signals his status as an othered figure. At first, the camera follows Giovanna and Filippo during a relatively banal exchange as they walk through Rome, the typical trope of the arguing married couple alluding to the status quo (for example, Giovanna's "tired marriage" described in the synopsis). It continues to follow Giovanna as Filippo slips out of view; then, when she realises he is no longer beside her, it cuts to him speaking to an old man. Mystery ensues: the old man is "confused" and cannot remember his name. Filippo's concern and Giovanna's bemused frustration signal Davide's otherness as a stranger to the pair. This sense is visually reinforced and extended to Davide's place in present-day Rome when he is shot on his own after the two have attempted to leave him behind:

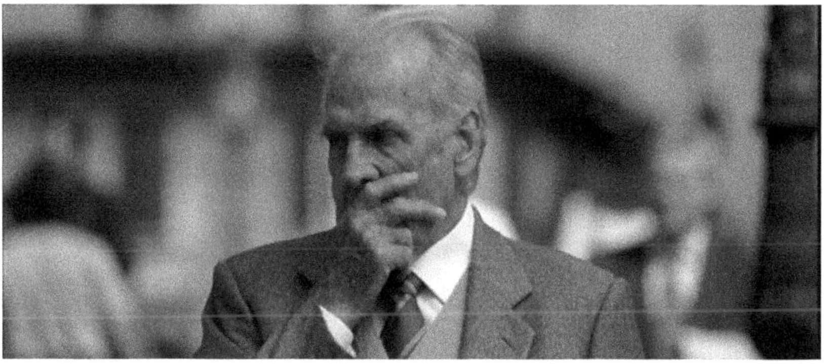

Figure 15: Davide lost in Rome. *Facing Window* (Özpetek, 2003). Sony Pictures Classics.

He appears, confused and distressed, on a busy street. His actions contrast with those of other pedestrians; they walk briskly in a defined direction, while he looks around, stationary. He is shown in shallow focus, which emphasises his wrinkled, pallid skin while placing the colourful buildings and younger Romans out of focus. The film's use of focus here differentiates the two planes, as though Davide and contemporary Rome exist in slightly different dimensions. This visual representation of the character begins his characterisation as someone unable to integrate into the temporality of the present. As the film progresses, we discover that Davide suffers from a kind of psychological disorder, most likely global transient amnesia, a form of temporary memory loss that can cause the sufferer to hallucinate that they are in the past. Davide's depiction as out of joint with the present is reinforced through this condition.

At the beginning of the film, he has no name, and thus no symbolic identity. When he eventually gives his name, he gives the wrong one: that of his lover, Simone, who died during the Holocaust. The past that Davide occupies is thus not only a particularly traumatic one for him as a character, but also on the level of collective memory. This forms the basis of interpretations of the film as one that "works through" Holocaust memory, discussed above.[5] Davide being out of place in the present not only produces a sense

5 See also Dupré (2015), Gordon (2012) and Wood (2005). Scholars do not necessarily agree on whether the film achieves this working through, but all conclude that it gestures towards such

of rupture in the social order as such—the appearance of the past in the present—but does so in a way that foregrounds its traumatic dimension through its evocation of state genocide.

The film often depicts Davide occupying the temporality of the early forties, in contrast with the other characters. This is illustrated most clearly in uncanny scenes in which episodes from Davide's memory are superimposed on the present-day Roman setting:

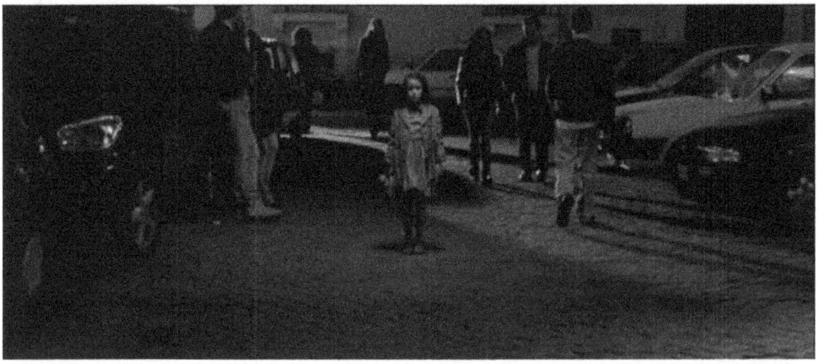

Figure 16: A Shoah girl haunts contemporary Rome. *Facing Window* (Özpetek, 2003). Sony Pictures Classics.

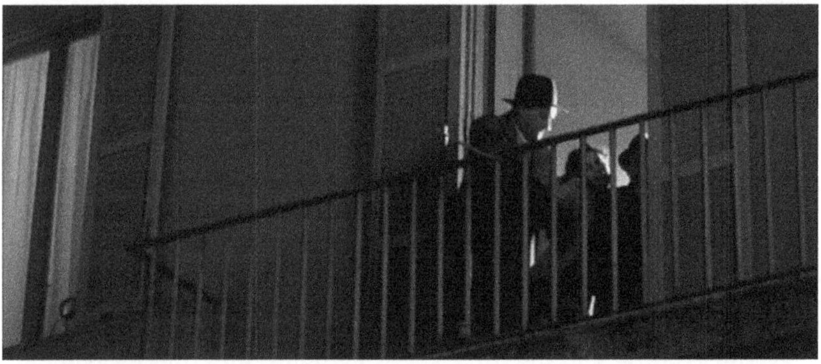

Figure 17: Stasi kidnappings haunt contemporary Rome. *Facing Window* (Özpetek, 2003). Sony Pictures Classics.

This overall produces a sense of the irreconcilability of the past in the present, which results in a kind of haunting of contemporary Rome in the film. Davide's status as other, here signified by his occupying another

a possibility.

temporal reality, makes manifest the presence of a point of trauma (in this case the memory of the Holocaust) in the present.

Arguably, the film provides a gradual integration of temporalities, mirroring Davide and Simone's relationship with that of Giovanna and Lorenzo, and offering a narrative in which Davide's history is eventually explicated. However, by the end of the film it is not clear if Davide's trauma is resolved, and the last image of him depicts him as tired, slumped and somewhat defeated. In explicating the reasons for his condition, the cause of Davide's inability to integrate with the present, the film gestures towards an unresolvable antagonism, this time within the past—within the order of Holocaust memory. This antagonism lies in *Facing Window*'s queer dimension, and potential to foreground queerness as a kind of otherness that resists assimilation into the symbolic order, a "contestational category," as Duncan (2013, p. 259) describes it. As discussed above, scholars have posited that Özpetek's films, including *Facing Window*, are valued for their representation of a "mainstream" or "acceptable" queerness. In this respect, *Facing Window* could evidence a broader trend in which the presentation of an acceptable rather than radical otherness contributes to films' commercial success. However, in contrast with this institutional legitimation, I argue that the film's presentation of a tension between Davide's identity as queer with his identity as a Holocaust survivor suggests a kind of radical otherness that contradicts the notion of an acceptable, assimilable queerness.

In particular, *Facing Window* suggests that the order of Holocaust memory had hitherto been predicated on an exclusion of the queer other. In its complication of Holocaust memory, the film raises a radical antagonism between Davide's identities as queer and Jewish, one that it resolves within the narrative. Through the depiction of Davide's past, Holocaust memory is consistently renegotiated and antagonised through the figure of the queer other. All of Davide's flashbacks and hallucinations revolve around Nazi raids in 1943 and his memories of Simone, and we discover that the crucial moment in this sub-plot is Davide's enforced choice between his lover and his fellow Shoah during one such raid. The trauma of this choice is epitomised in Davide's love letter to Simone, in which he expresses the sense of loss that provoked his hallucinations. Referring to a world liberated from Nazism, but in which Simone is dead, Davide expresses regret: "How can I say that this is a better world. How can that be without you?" Bringing antagonism to the fore, Davide's words imply a kind of heresy: how can a world without Nazism be no better?

The film does not appear to suggest that this should be the case; it is by no means apologetic for the Holocaust. Rather, the film's staging of a choice between Davide's queer and Jewish identities, and his expression of regret at this forced choice present an unresolved tension between the orders of Holocaust memory and queer memory. This is signified by Davide and Simone's relationship being presented as the root cause of Davide's inability to integrate with the symbolic order of present-day Rome. *Facing Window* queers Holocaust memory in a way that does not so much depict the happy integration of the queer other into the social order, but rather presents queer memory as an important and radically antagonistic element.

This reading takes on greater force in relation to the film's representation of exclusion of social others not only in the past, but in contemporary Italy, too. Although a minor aspect of *Facing Window*'s narrative overall (and, as such, one I intend to engage with only briefly), we can read the film's sub-plot of present-day racial exclusion alongside its depiction of historical sexual and racial persecution. Viewing these together, *Facing Window* can be interpreted as a film not about an ideal, closed social order, but one predicated on exclusion. In other words, when read alongside the film's Holocaust narrative, *Facing Window*'s depiction of present-day exclusion of migrant others supports a larger operation in which the radical antagonism between the social order and the other is left unresolved. The film depicts migration and racism through the figures of Turkish migrant Eminè, her family, and undocumented Chinese workers in the abattoir where Giovanna and Eminè also work.

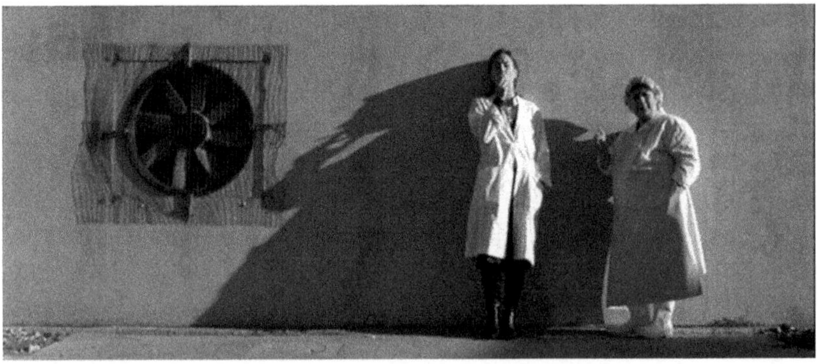

Figure 18: Confidantes: Giovanna and Eminè smoke outside the abattoir where they work. *Facing Window* (Özpetek, 2003). Sony Pictures Classics.

Such figures are absent from Karlovy Vary's presentation of the film, and by focusing on Giovanna's relationship with Davide, the festival synopsis elides an important friendship in *Facing Window*, one that concerns marginalisation in the contemporary social order, the friendship between

Giovanna and Eminè. Eminè arguably supports Giovanna more than Davide: she is a constant presence in the woman's life, acts as her confidante with regards to Lorenzo, and provides a moral compass when Giovanna is about to report another migrant (the unnamed Chinese worker in the abattoir). Meanwhile, racist attitudes are often represented in the contemporary society the film depicts via scenes that allude to Eminè's struggle with them. *Facing Window* includes several moments in which Eminè's marginalisation is foregrounded: when she is called a "dirty immigrant" and threatened with deportation, when she says that the abusive couple in her apartment building were silently calling Giambo a "nigger", and when Giovanna's own daughter says that "non-white" children have to behave better than white children.

In the synopsis, the romantic sexual relationship is substituted for a relationship with the excluded other, and thus romantic desire is replaced with a seemingly more "progressive" desire for the other. This seems to enact a fantasy of closure through individual fulfilment which, as we have seen from the film's representation of Giovanna's desire above, the film shows in its narcissistic dimension. This develops through *Facing Window*'s depiction of the lack in the social order, which takes the form of its structural exclusion of the other. The order of the present is antagonised by the past, while that of Holocaust memory is antagonised by Davide's queer identity. Meanwhile, the social order of contemporary Italian society is antagonised by various characters', but above all Eminè's, racial identities. Far from depicting a fantasy in which these orders of meaning are capable of integrating their constitutive others, on the diegetic level, *Facing Window* leaves antagonism unresolved and traumatic. This highlights the fundamental antagonism that the synopsis (and, by extension, the festival) disavows in its representation of the film. While the synopsis presents Davide as other only to imply that he can be integrated, *Facing Window* makes manifest the paradox in this implication, underlining the radical otherness that precludes such figures' integration and, as such, precludes the possibility of a closed symbolic order.

Conclusion

In this chapter, I have theorised European A festivals' structural preoccupation with difference, and two fundamental manifestations of it. Such festivals represent themselves as institutions capable of integrating that which is other, be that cinemas "othered" by the market or identities marginalised under various regimes of material and/or discursive violence. In so doing, European A festivals position themselves as both platforms for the debate of "topical" social issues and sites of a "harmonious totality" in which the excluded can be integrated into a complete order of meaning. As well as suggesting a form of "elite capture" in which political struggles are appropriated for the benefit of powerful institutions, this ideological procedure enables film festivals to claim universality, disavowing the antagonistic, and often radical, dimension of the other.

We find further evidence for this in its textual instantiation, Karlovy Vary's synopsis of *Facing Window*, particularly when read against the film text. The film makes manifest the Real of the paratext, highlighting the contradictions and ideological procedures that structure it. On one level, the differences between *Facing Window* and the Karlovy Vary synopsis highlight the fundamental ideological procedure of the synopsis as a representation of the film: the synopsis attempts to enclose the film's meaning through a chain of signifiers, while *Facing Window*, as an unstable text, exceeds the meaning ascribed to it. The synopsis is not a closed order of meaning, since its object (the film) continually escapes it.

The particular signifiers with which the synopsis attempts to "fix" meaning are symptomatic of the ideology conditioning the festival's awarding and representation of the film. Reading the paratext through *Facing Window* allows us to observe more fully how the former is structured according to the fantasy of the sexual relationship. The film, particularly through the technique of interface, can be interpreted as making manifest this fantasmatic logic: the desire for another being motived by the more fundamental desire to fill in one's constitutive lack. *Facing Window* suggests that this logic structures Giovanna's subjectivity, guiding her pursuits in the film even after she has refused Lorenzo.

The synopsis, meanwhile, omits the aspects of *Facing Window* that highlight the impossibility of the sexual relationship, and constructs the film in a way that privileges a sense of fulfilment. If the fantasy of closure, particularly romantic closure, is associated with Hollywood cinema, the synopsis subtly fixes *Facing Window*'s meaning in a way that at once renounces and reproduces this structure. It renounces romance as "the fabrication of dreams" while nonetheless reproducing the logic of the sexual relationship through its representation of Giovanna's relationship with the other, Davide. In other words, the enjoyment of fantasy is paid for by the elements that attempt to differentiate *Facing Window* from Hollywood productions (and, in turn, European A festivals from Hollywood).

Above all, this entails a paradoxical representation of the other that foregrounds their difference while positioning them as the second half of the "harmonious totality" fantasised in the sexual relationship. While the synopsis implies that Davide is gradually made legible, assimilable and representable, there are several aspects of *Facing Window* that indicate a radical dimension to otherness—the antagonism between the other and the social order as such. The film represents the past, queer identities and migrant identities as caught in an unresolved antagonistic relationship with the various orders of the present, Holocaust memory, and contemporary "multicultural" society. Interpreting the synopsis through the film, the former's disavowal of this antagonism becomes clearer. In the paratext, otherness is emphasised while its antagonistic dimension is repressed.

European A festivals present themselves as capable of integrating that which is other while disavowing their reproduction of the category of otherness. *Facing Window* is constructed in a way that reproduces a fundamental ideological structure that I have shown to be at work in European A film festivals in general: the fantasy of a closed symbolic order, constructed according to the fantasies of the sexual relationship and suture. As this chapter has demonstrated, these fantasmatic structures appear to support European A festivals' claims to a political-humanist universality organised around the figure of the other.

Bibliography

Bauman, R. (2015). *Divi ambigui*: Ferzan Özpetek's starstruck gaze. *Italian Studies*, *70*(3), 389–401.

Bosma, P. (2015). *Film programming: Curating for cinemas, festivals, archives*. Columbia University Press.

Boutsko, A. (2021). Dieter Kosslick: Berlinale's former head publishes memoir. *Deutsche Welle*. 3 February 2021. Available from: https://www.berlinale.de/en/archive/jahresarchive/2016/01_jahresblatt_2016/01_jahresblatt_2016.html

Cousins, M. (2009). Widescreen on film festivals. In D. Iordanova & R. Rhyne (Eds.), *Festival yearbook 1: The festival circuit* (pp. 155–158). St Andrews Film Studies and College Gate Press.

Damiens, A. (2018). The queer film ecosystem: Symbolic economy, festivals, and queer cinema's legs. *Studies in European Cinema*, *15*(1), 25–40.

De Valck, M. (2007). *Film festivals: From European geopolitics to global cinephilia*. Amsterdam University Press.

Duncan, D. (2013). The geopolitics of spectatorship and screen identification: What's queer about Italian cinema? *The Italianist*, *33*(2), 256–261.

Dupré, N. (2015). La "condivisione" della Shoah: Un confronto tra Perlasca, un eroe italiano e *La finestra di fronte*. In M. Jansen & M. B. Urban (Eds.), *Televisionismo:*

Narrazioni televisive della storia italiana negli anni della seconda Repubblica (pp. 61–68). Edizioni Ca' Foscari.

Elsaesser, T. (2005). *European cinema: Face to face with Hollywood.* Amsterdam University Press.

Frater, P. (2018). Pingyao festival celebrates indie spirit at opening. *Variety.* [Online]. Available from: https://variety.com/2018/film/asia/pingyao-festival-celebrates-indie-spirit-1202976792/

Freud, S. (1917). *Mourning and melancholia.* Vintage.

Gordon, R. (2012). *The Holocaust in Italian culture, 1944–2010.* Stanford University Press.

Halle, R. (2010). Offering tales they want to hear: Transnational European film funding as neo-orientalism. In R. Galt & K. Schoonover (Eds.), *Global art cinema: New theories and histories* (pp. 303–319). Oxford University Press.

Harbord, J. (2002). *Film cultures.* Sage.

Hipkins, D., & Renga, D. (2016). A new canon? Contemporary Italian cinema and television and the role of quality in the anglophone curriculum. *Comunicazioni sociali, 1*(3), 375–397.

Iordanova, D. (2009). The festival circuit. In D. Iordanova & R. Rhyne (Eds.), *Film festival yearbook 1: The festival circuit* (pp. 23–39). St Andrews Film Studies and College Gate Press.

Karlovy Vary International Film Festival. (2003). *Facing Window/La Finestra di Fronte.* [Online]. Available from: http://www.kviff.com/en/programme/film/03383-facing-window/

MacDowell, J. (2013). *Happy endings in Hollywood cinema.* Edinburgh University Press.

Marcus, M. (2007). *Italian film in the shadow of Auschwitz.* University of Toronto Press.

McGowan, T. (2007). *The real gaze: Film theory after Lacan.* State University of New York Press.

Mulvey, L. (1975). Visual pleasure and narrative cinema. *Screen, 16*(3), 6–18.

Shohat, E., & Stam, R. (2014). *Unthinking Eurocentrism: Multiculturalism and the media.* Routledge.

Táíwò, O. O. (2022). *Elite capture: How the powerful took over identity politics (and everything else).* Pluto Press.

Turan, K. (2002). *Sundance to Sarajevo: Film festivals and the world they made.* University of California Press.

Vimercati, G. (2012). Festivals: Karlovy Vary. *Film Comment.* [Online]. Available from: https://www.filmcomment.com/blog/festivals-karlovy-vary/

Wayne, M. (2002). *The politics of contemporary European cinema: Histories, borders, diasporas.* Intellect.

Wong, C. H-Y. (2016). Publics and counterpublics: Rethinking film festivals as public spheres. In M. de Valck, D. B. Kredell, & S. Loist (Eds.), *Film festivals: History, theory, method, practice* (pp. 83–99). Routledge.

Wong, C. H-Y. (2011). *Film festivals: Culture, people, and power on the global screen.* Rutgers University Press.

Wood, M. P. (2005). *Italian cinema.* Bloomsbury Academic.

Zambenedetti, A. (2006). Multiculturalism in New Italian Cinema. *Studies in European Cinema, 3*(2), 105–116.

Žižek, S. (1989). *The sublime object of ideology.* Verso.

Žižek, S. (1992). *Looking awry: An introduction to Jacques Lacan through popular culture.* MIT Press.

Žižek, S. (2001b). *The fright of real tears: Krzysztof Kieślowski between theory and post-theory.* British Film Institute.

Žižek, S. (2002). *Welcome to the desert of the real! Five essays on September 11 and related dates.* Verso.

Žižek, S. (2003). *The puppet and the dwarf: The perverse core of Christianity.* MIT Press.

Žižek, S. (2004a). *Iraq: The borrowed kettle.* Verso.

Filmography

As Far as I Can Walk (*Strahinja Banović*) (2021). Arsenijević, S. dir. Serbia.

Facing Window (*La finestra di fronte*) (2003). Özpetek, F. dir. Italy.

Fahrenheit 9/11 (2004). Moore, M. dir. United States.

Grbavica: The Land of My Dreams (*Grbavica*) (2006). Žbanić, J. dir. Bosnia and Herzegovina.

Hamam: The Turkish Bath (*Hamam Suare*) (1997). Özpetek, F. dir. Italy.

Harem Suare (1999). Özpetek, F. dir. Italy.

Happening (*L'Événement*) (2021). Diwan, A. dir. France.

Ignorant Fairies (*Le fate ignoranti*) (2001). Özpetek, F. dir. Italy.

Still Life (*San xia hao ren*) (2006). Zhangke, J. dir. China.

5. Brutal Humanism: *Fire at Sea* at the Berlinale

Abstract: This chapter analyses European film festivals' construction of a particular "other" that has gained media attention in recent years: the North African migrant. I bring together a short history of European A festivals' cultivation of a specific kind of humanism, a "brutal humanism" founded on the ethics of witnessing the suffering of "others" (Schoonover, 2012), with a detailed analysis of the Berlinale's representation of Italian migration film *Fire at Sea*. Through a consideration of scholarship on neo-colonialism and film festivals, I posit that European A festivals may be underwritten by a brutally humanist conception of the "other" that reproduces not only legacies of Italian neorealism but neo-colonial power.

Keywords: migration cinema, Italian cinema, film festivals, Gianfranco Rosi, neorealism, neo-colonialism

Samuele is twelve and lives on an island in the Mediterranean, far away from the mainland. Like all boys of his age he does not always enjoy going to school. He would much rather climb the rocks by the shore, play with his slingshot or mooch about the port. But his home is not like other islands. For years, it has been the destination of men, women and children trying to make the crossing from Africa in boats that are far too small and decrepit. The island is Lampedusa which has become a metaphor for the flight of refugees to Europe, the hopes, hardship and fate of hundreds of thousands of emigrants. These people long for peace, freedom and happiness and yet so often only their dead bodies are pulled out of the water. Thus, every day the inhabitants of Lampedusa are bearing witness to the greatest humanitarian tragedy of our times.

Gianfranco Rosi's observations of everyday life bring us closer to this place that is as real as it is symbolic, and to the emotional world of some

Johnson, R., Film Festivals, *Ideology and Italian Art Cinema: Politics, Histories and Cultural Value.* Taylor & Francis Group, 2024
DOI 10.5117/9789463720366_CH05

of its inhabitants who are exposed to a permanent state of emergency. At the same time his film, which is commentary-free, describes how, even in the smallest of places, two worlds barely touch.
– *Synopsis of* Fire at Sea *in the Berlinale 2016 print and online programme*

Introduction

Marijke de Valck (2007, p. 74) describes film festival programming as "a political act." Thus far, we have seen that the political dimension of European A festivals and their representations of films can take two directions. Their political dimension can be concealed under the sign of "the art of film," which entails a disavowal of the fundamentally political and contested nature of the term itself. Alternatively, it can be emphasised, provided it operates within certain limits. As was clear from the case study of *Facing Window*, engagement with figures of the other functioned as a marker of distinction from commercial and Hollywood cinema (festivals' constitutive outside) while reproducing the ideological coordinates of otherness, as well as the power relations that such coordinates entail. In a process that may be productively considered as a form of "elite capture" (Táíwò, 2022), festivals achieve the differentiation necessary for their success (securing financial and symbolic capital) through their claim to integrate the other while in fact reproducing the power structures that they claim to challenge. This chapter investigates European A festivals' construction of the figure of the other further, bringing it into relation with the geopolitical dimension of the circuit. The geopolitics I focus on are the legacies of European A festivals' embeddedness in postwar reconstruction through American patrimony, and colonialism. Using this context to frame an analysis of European A festivals' contemporary representations of "Europe" and "Africa," I suggest that these histories continue to condition how such festivals award and represent "politically urgent" filmmaking, taking on new force in the context of the so-called "refugee crisis."[1] This chapter explores further how European A festivals' politics are structured according to the fantasy of the

1 I use the expressions "refugee" and "refugee crisis" following the United Nations report, "The sea route to Europe: The Mediterranean passage in the age of refugees" (UNHCR, 2015), and the UN 1951 Refugee Convention. A refugee is "any person who, owing to a well-founded fear of being persecuted for reasons of race, religion, nationality, membership of a particular social group or political opinion, is outside the country of his/her nationality and is unable, or owing to such fear, is unwilling to avail himself/herself of the protection of that country" (UNHCR, 1951). I do, however, retain some critical distance from the expression "refugee crisis," as the notion of a

sexual relationship, arguing that its actual expression via a politics of liberal humanism may lead to their reproduction of colonial power relations—in particular, a Eurocentric symbolic order that designates Africa, and African migrants, as other.

Migration films have gained increasing visibility across the film festival network, from the almost exponential growth of European migration festivals since 2017 to their continual presence on A festivals' programmes and awards lists since 2011 (Johnson, forthcoming). Both trends are indicative of increased media attention on migration since the "refugee crisis" in Europe began. Meanwhile, migration films' presence at European A festivals suggests migration's status as a "hot topic" that helps to secure the cultural and political relevance of these events. This appears to be a widespread trend, with festivals such as Karlovy Vary awarding the Crystal Globe to *As Far As I Can Walk* (*Strahinja Banović*, Stefan Arsenijević) in 2021, Cannes the Grand Prix to *Atlantics* (*Atlantique*, Mati Diop) in 2019, and San Sebastian its Horizontes Award to *Identifying Features* (*Sin señas particulares*, Fernanda Valadez) in 2020. Even when not winning awards, migration films have been regularly foregrounded in European A festival programmes, for example at Venice in 2017 and 2019, described as "spotlighting migration" (Wallis, 2019; ANSA, 2017).

The 2017 edition of Venice featured not only a large number of migration films, but Italian films too, and this is part of a larger trend of the success of Italian migration cinema on the A circuit. O'Healy (2019, p. 2) argues that there has been "increased attention paid to immigration as a thematic focus" in internationally recognised Italian cinema, and notes several Italian films depicting stories of migration being featured at Venice in 2011. This culminated in *Terraferma* (Emmenuele Crialese, 2011) winning the Pasinetti Award, Special Jury Prize and UNICEF Award at the festival. Similarly, *Mediterranea* (Jonas Carpignano, 2015) was screened during Cannes's Critics' Week to critical acclaim. It then won top prize at another A festival, the Cairo International Film Festival, in the same year. In 2016, *Fire at Sea* won the Golden Bear at an edition of the Berlinale that offered free tickets to refugees. Thus far, *Fire at Sea* has been the most successful Italian film about migration on the European A circuit, in terms of both awards and critical acclaim.

Fire at Sea is not merely the pinnacle of the relationship between Italian migration cinema and European A festivals, however. The 2016 award was

crisis continues to be problematised by scholars and commentators (see, for example, Rajaram [2016]). As such, all instances will be kept in quotation marks.

the first top prize awarded to any film centred on migration since the media began focusing its attention on a so-called "crisis" at the borders of Europe in 2014. This award marks a symbolically significant moment for the European A circuit's engagement with African-European migration at an edition of the Berlinale that defined itself in relation to the phenomenon. Analysing the awarding and representation of *Fire at Sea* by the Berlinale in 2016 thus offers an important starting point for understanding the ideological underpinnings of European A festivals' engagement with migration cinema, migrant others and the Global South more generally. Through this case study, I argue that festivals' representations of migration are marked by legacies of postwar fantasies of not only universal humanism, but a specifically *brutal* humanism theorised by Karl Schoonover (2012), one that reinforces a sense of European agency via the depiction of suffering, racialised bodies of migrants.

European A Festivals' Geopolitically-inflected Humanism

While the artistic universality constructed by European A festivals centres on notions of freedom from commercial constraint, epitomised by the figure of the auteur, the political universality constructed by these festivals is best understood as centring on notions of humanism. In the previous chapter, I suggested humanism's ideological dimension as a fantasy in which all humans can be integrated into the symbolic order. This epitomises the fantasy of sexual relationship. The inherent failure of humanism—its attempt to present a particular symbolic order as universal—has become almost an obligatory point of reference in discussions of the concept. It is well documented that humanism, rather than being universal, "functions within and conditions a predominantly Eurocentric, patriarchal, white, heteronormative, male-dominated global economy and networked society" (Kellner & Lewis, 2007, p. 421). Previous chapters have suggested that European A festivals operate on a similar basis, as evidenced by the othering of queerness in Karlovy Vary's synopsis of *Facing Window*, and the othering of the feminine in Cannes's and Tallinn's synopses of *The Great Beauty*.

The humanist impulse of European A festivals has a long history, one that scholars have argued is intimately bound to the context in which many such festivals were founded. Dorota Ostrowska (2016) apprehends the relationship between A festivals and humanism, and indeed the development of the "humanist film," through Cannes, once again positioned as the trendsetter on the circuit. Cannes, founded in response to the encroaching Fascist influence over the Venice *Mostra Internazionale d'Arte Cinematografica*, held its first edition in 1946, hailing a foundational moment for European film festivals and international film festivals alike. In this first phase of Cannes's development, the festival was oriented primarily towards "a spirit of international collaboration" and pacifist sentiment, underpinned by "the idea of cinema as a vehicle for universal peace" (Ostrowska, 2016, p. 19). Favouring anti-war films from Italy, Poland and the Soviet Union, the festival's early programmes were appraised primarily through the trope of humanism, a critical orientation that "chimed with [...] the festival's utopian and universalising ideal" (Ostrowska, 2016, p. 21). In Cannes's postwar editions, we find an alignment between the ideals of the festival and the film critics who helped to mythologise it, inaugurating a European film culture with universalist and humanist aims.

The most prominent critic whom Ostrowska cites is the editor of *Cahiers* André Bazin, whose writings on cinema and (neo)realist ethics remain foundational to evaluations of film to this day. Schoonover (2012) analyses Bazin's accounts of the French festival in depth, foregrounding the relationship between aesthetic evaluation and humanist ideals that they establish. Bazin's writings on Cannes constituted a crucial part of the "transatlantic refashioning of cinema's medium specificity" (Schoonover, 2012, p. 10), affecting and effected by not only film critics, but, as Ostrowska suggests, cinematic institutions such as festivals. Indeed, Schoonover describes Bazin's writings as "overt attempts to aestheticise a mid-century politics of liberal humanism, to find humanism's aesthetic equivalent in filmic terms, in a popular visual vernacular" (p. 10). At the centre of this vernacular were Italian neorealist films and, in particular, "the revelation of the 1946 festival [...] the anti-fascist *Roma, Città Aperta*" (de Valck, 2007, p. 49). Responding to the exhibition and awarding of *Rome, Open City* (*Roma, Città Aperta*, Roberto Rossellini, 1945), Bazin's writings hailed the film as inaugurating "a new visual politics of liberal compassion" that would come to define notions of cinematic ethics to this day (Schoonover, 2012, p. xiv).

Ostrowska's (2016) delimitation of Cannes "humanist films" such as *Rome, Open City* to those in the war film genre leads her to conclude that this category is "a more historical designation" with only limited resonance today (p. 30). However, when we consider the enduring importance of discourses around Italian neorealism and the visual politics they inaugurated, the legacy of these early cinematic-humanist discourses should be clear. The importance of a certain institutionally recognised Italian neorealism to contemporary notions of cinematic aesthetics and ethics is difficult to understate, and is one of the premises on which this book's study of art cinema through Italian cinema is founded.[2] This is not least due to neorealism's status as one of the perceived cornerstones of European and, later, global art cinema (Galt & Schoonover, 2010; Maule, 2008; Ruberto & Wilson, 2007). As Schoonover (2012) states:

> Neorealism [...] sets the standard for European new wave cinemas, postcolonial cinemas, cinemas of social change and political liberation, the American "new independents" of the 1970s and late twentieth-century explorations of realism by Italian, Danish, Romanian, and Chinese cinemas. (p. 218)

We can thus observe that one of the founding moments of the European festival circuit—Cannes's first edition in 1946—marks, at the same time, the founding moment of Italian neorealism's international prestige, its positioning as a compulsory point of reference for canonical art cinema.

At this point, it becomes crucial to counter the universalising ideals suggested in the accounts of postwar film culture above with the situated approach to film that Aida Vallejo (2020) offers as a remedy to often Eurocentric and (again universalising) histories of cinema. Italian neorealism's legacy is primarily an institutional one, part and parcel of festivals' as well as film critics' and academics' canonisation of a certain kind of cinema (Hipkins & Renga, 2016; O'Rawe, 2008; Guerini Rocco, 2019). Cannes's humanist legacies were, moreover, forged in the specific postwar geopolitical context in which many European A festivals operated, characterised by North American financial and political influence as well as the imperative to counter the perceived threat of Communism from the Soviet Bloc. It is the contingencies of these political realities that led Schoonover to designate the humanism proffered through European film culture a "brutal" one, "more reconciled with than resistant to the geopolitical affinities of large-scale capitalism and its multiple battle zones" (2012, p. xix). In contrast with the seemingly neutral, universal humanism implicit in Cannes's self-representation and appraisal by film critics, we find a partial and geopolitically-inflected humanism, rooted in the requirement for European festivals to act as bastions of a specific set of North-Western values.

2 Recall that "neorealism," like "art cinema," is predominantly an institutional category—a discourse rather than an essence or, as O'Leary and O'Rawe (2011, p. 109) polemically put it, even a perpetrator of "insidious common sense." Throughout this chapter, and indeed this book, I engage with neorealism in its dominant, institutional form. For an important challenge to canonical neorealism and features ascribed to it, see Leavitt (2020) and Fabbri (2015).

Many European countries depended upon North American patrimony for their reconstruction after World War II (a large part of which was the European Recovery Programme, or Marshall Plan). This relationship was also fundamental to the development of the European A festival circuit, since several festivals that gained A accreditation were financed by American organisations in that period. For example, Cannes, although rhetorically claiming to act as a bastion against both Fascism and "America's burgeoning cultural imperialism", was primarily funded by American organisations (Rhyne, 2009, p. 11). Likewise, numerous histories of Berlin demonstrate its conception as a defence against Communism and instrument of Western soft power. The Berlinale, originally named the International Film Festival Berlin, was initiated by American film officer Oscar Martay, and conceived as "an American instrument in the Cold War" (de Valck, 2007, p. 52). As Heidi Fehrenbach (1995, pp. 234–236) argues, the festival was founded as "a celebration of Western values" and "proof of Western economic superiority and cultural dynamism." This West Berlin institution was founded as a "counter-festival" to East Berlin cultural events such as the World Youth Festival (Weltfestspiele der Jugend und Studenten) taking place at the same time. It was also heavily financed by the US military (Harbord, 2002, p. 62). In the postwar period, several European film festivals were created and supported by North American organisations and, as such, were part of geopolitical manoeuvring undertaken with the aim of disseminating their values across the continent.

The hegemony of this North American collaboration had a defining influence on the development of the European A circuit, even beyond the "big three." As Loist notes (2016, p. 55), "[a] clear preference for Western European and North American festivals can be discerned" in FIAPF's accreditation of some, and not other, festivals as A-list. Thus, while Karlovy Vary represents the first Soviet Bloc festival to receive such accreditation, it can be considered an exception rather than the norm. Moreover, the festival's accreditation appears to have come with several conditions. First, just two years after becoming "A-list," Karlovy Vary was required to share its status with Moscow and eventually run only biannually, following FIAPF's 1958 ruling that it could only grant A accreditation to one Eastern Bloc festival (Moine, 2013). Karlovy Vary's acceptance, although embattled, may also have been contingent on its display of relative amenity to the West. A crucial site for economic and cultural exchange between East and West, the festival's programming and awarding has been shown to suggest an openness towards "Hollywood's Eastern European operations," and "the political interests of the US State Department" (Bláhová, 2020,

p. 97; Iordanova, 2006, p. 29). Meanwhile, the case of Locarno highlights how a Western European festival might be seen to overstep its bounds by showing too much sympathy with the Soviet cause: the festival received much criticism for screening Polish and Hungarian films during the Cold War, being seen as "crypto-communist" (Cordoba, 2022). Cases of required openness to North American geopolitical agendas, or enforced exclusion of Eastern ones, demonstrate that the "spirit of international collaboration" that Ostrowska (2016, p. 19) identifies in European film culture at the time operated within strict limits. Less a project of genuine transnational openness, the development of the European A circuit was defined by a deliberately partial, geopolitically-conditioned humanism. To return to Rhyne's contextualisation of Cannes's anti-Fascism within North American patrimony, FIAPF's manoeuvring during the Cold War requires us to ask to what extent European A festivals, both then and today, might either promote a nominal anti-Fascism that nonetheless leaves deep structures of imperialism untouched or advocate for a film culture that rejects not only Fascism, but imperialism in all its forms.[3]

From Universal Humanism to Brutal Vision...

The visual politics of the postwar context were mobilised as part of a transatlantic project in which the US intervened in the economic and ideological reconstruction of Western European countries, including intervention in European film festivals. Central to this cinematic and geopolitical refashioning was the power ascribed to images of brutalised, imperilled bodies, the likes of which we find in many of the "humanist films" to which Ostrowska refers. Such images were thought to trigger concern and sympathy, but also a sense of agency in the spectator—to encourage a kind of transnationally-inflected humanism (Schoonover, 2012, p. 11). Returning to Bazin's writing on Cannes, we discover the founding of "'a phenomenology of death in contemporary cinema'" as a framework for evaluating a film's capacity to "enable experience on a transnational register" (Schoonover, 2012, pp. 11–12). Bazin posited that depictions of death or torture could achieve this aim, involving the spectator in an international, ethical and humanist praxis in which the act of witnessing violence is considered an act of ethical agency (Schoonover, 2012, pp. 12–13).

3 The present context of not only continuing US imperialism, but escalating Russian imperialism, including the war on Ukraine, renders these questions and the requirement that film festivals reject imperialism in all its forms ever more urgent.

In particular, this relationship entails a "politics of pity" that "involves isolating the sufferers as to be seen or to be looked at" and "distancing them from the pitying subject or spectator" (Schoonover, 2012, pp. xiv–xv). Thus, at the heart of the "brutal vision" that instantiates these politics is the relationship between the witness and the figure being looked at. Schoonover (2012, p. xx) argues that a key aspect of neorealist films' address is the way in which "an imperilled body is offered to a bystander's look as an opportunity to exercise ethical judgement." Moreover, while the witness may "exercise ethical judgement," the sufferer is represented as passive, as "offered", and "to be seen or to be looked at." We might say, then, that the witness, either on-screen figure or implied spectator, is positioned as active subject, while the sufferer is positioned as passive object.

Importantly for the relations of power and agency that this entails, the politics of cinematic representation is, Schoonover (2012, pp. 10–11) argues, part of a reconceptualisation of cinema "that emphasises its capacity to broaden the parameters of the Euro-American subject's engagement in the world and authority over it." The relationship between witness and sufferer is not geopolitically neutral but rather asserts a specifically "Euro-American" agency. This impression of agency depends on the fact that sufferers are viewed from a distance, and specifically from "a liberal humanist present" (Schoonover, 2012, p. 148). The "brutal vision" that characterises this postwar regime of representation implies a reciprocal but uneven relation between the "liberal humanist" witness and the sufferer. The elaboration of the former's agency depends upon the subtraction of that of the latter, as well as the performance of a particular kind of distance between the two. Schoonover (2012, p. 66) calls this the "proxied engagement" that defines the spectator's relationship to the imperilled figure. It produces a distance between the sufferer and the witness and situates the powerful witness in the position of liberal, Euro-American subject, implicitly placing the sufferer as other, "isolated" and lacking agency. A crucial manifestation—the "visual vernacular"—of the values of liberal humanism that characterised postwar geopolitics and conceptions of cinema is the representation of a figure in peril as a means of granting the Euro-American subject a sense of ethical agency. This is achieved through the act of looking, the mobilisation of a powerful gaze that the Euro-American subject directs towards the passive, imperilled other. In short, brutal humanism and its cinematic instantiation, "brutal vision," can be defined as a liberal, compassionate stance towards the spectacle of the imperilled figure—a figure defined not only by their suffering but their distance (geographical and temporal but, above all, symbolic) from the Western liberal witness to whom such images are addressed.

To conceptualise these relations of looking and their pertinence to the question of ideology, it is necessary to supplement Schoonover's theory of brutal vision with another theory of perspective. Lacanian theories of the Gaze offer a means of both theorising and challenging the ideological procedures involved in brutal vision insofar as it has the capacity to highlight the disavowals and displacements on which any notion of Euro-American agency may rest. In fact, Schoonover's (2012, p. 183) study contains an undercurrent of the theories elaborated by Metz (1982), Mulvey (1975) and others. This is most apparent in its emphasis on the to-be-looked-at-ness of imperilled bodies: images of suffering others are "offered to a bystander's look" in a way that foregrounds the activity of the witness and passivity of the sufferer (Schoonover, 2012, p. xx). This kind of representation functions in a geopolitical fashion, to bolster the illusion of "the foreign spectator's sovereign gaze" (Schoonover, 2012, p. 183). We might interpret this through Mulvey's (1975) notion of the male gaze as a dominating look that emphasises male agency and female passivity. While Mulvey describes the objectification of the female other, we can extend these insights to consider the colonial gaze, and "othering" more generally (see, for example, Butler [2002], hooks [1992], and Young [1996]). In particular, we might consider how films address an implied liberal, Western spectator as having a sovereign gaze, providing the illusion of mastery over the images they look at and the figures in it, thus (re)producing a sense of "the Euro-American subject's engagement in the world and authority over it" (Schoonover, 2012, p. 11).

The concept of suture outlined in the last chapter also helps explain the ideological procedures involved in the illusion of a "sovereign gaze" as, fundamentally, a form of displacement. The relationship of authoritative onlooker and objectified figure is structured in a similar fashion. As discussed, suture involves displacing the split inherent to the subject—its internal inconsistency or non-totality, which in turn undermines the possibility of total agency—onto an opposition between the subject and an other.[4] This opposition can take two routes. The fantasy of a harmonious totality paradoxically positions the other as outside (that is, "different") *and* assimilable, in an eternal state of to-be-integratedness. Alternatively, it can take the form of antagonistic opposition, in which the other becomes

4 I consider the "Euro-American subject" Schoonover refers to in the sense of the subject implied by a symbolic order of Euro-American identity and its humanist underpinnings. The subject Schoonover describes is an implied spectator and, as such, best conceived of as a part of the symbolic text rather than a real, existing person. Therefore, the inherent split in the subject, in both senses, refers to the inherent split in the symbolic order itself.

perceived as an enemy or threat, the symbolic order's bad object. Crucially, both cases require the other to become the "constitutive Outside" onto whom the symbolic order's internal lack (the Real, as well as various internal conflicts) is displaced, affording the impression of consistency (Žižek, 2004a, p. 102). According to this structure, the Euro-American subject's authority thus depends upon the transformation of an internal split into a relation of difference with the suffering other—for example, the consolidation of a "liberal humanist present" constructed through the distancing and witnessing of imperilled figures.

However, as we know, the other posited through suture necessarily "gives body to an impossibility" (Žižek, 2001a, p. 202). This figure is, in fact, the manifestation of "the impossibility of closure," and bears traces of the ideological operation involved (Copjec, 1994, p. 174). While brutal vision may attempt to address spectators as though they have a sovereign perspective and authority over the world, such efforts are marked by a fundamental impossibility. This is precisely the fundamental impossibility that I have argued films can make manifest through their potential to depict the Gaze, a potential that can challenge the relations of looking that underpin the fantasy of Euro-American agency Schoonover refers to.

... and from Brutal Vision to Colonialism

These relations of power, their manifestation, and the means through which they might be challenged, become crucial to questions of contemporary European A festivals' representations of the other, owing to the implications that the ideology of brutal humanism has for depictions of colonised subjects as well. The fantasy of Euro-American agency has clear implications for relations not only with the Soviet and post-Soviet East but with the Global South as well. This is because the development of the A circuit, and fashioning of a geopolitically-inflected, brutal humanism, also took place in a context of European colonialism. Dovey (2015, p. 29) highlights not only the prevalence of this context, but situates it within "a two-millennia history of practices of collecting, curating, and displaying objects in Europe," conditioning such festivals' participation in "the writing of specific colonial and national histories" and the "universalising of bourgeois views and visions" (Morgan 2013, p. 23). Such festivals' embeddedness in colonialist and "universalising" practices were, moreover, reinforced through the intersections between a European sense of American imperialism and reinforcement of its own imperial power over the subjects whom its states colonised. Dovey (2015) argues that

> [a]ll of the early "A-list" European film festivals [...] were created on a European continent that was not only at war with itself, but that felt the need (partly as a result of these wars, and the sense of threat the US posed) to assert its superiority over other parts of the world, particularly its colonies in "darkest" Africa. (p. 37)

Riven by the effects of two World Wars and North American intervention, Europe intensified its colonial practices: it displaced internal conflict onto a conflict with the African other as a means of regaining a sense of agency. This can be understood precisely as aligning with the ideological project to bolster European authority at a time when that authority may have been perceived as under threat.

What distinguishes this particular displacement is its ultimately antagonistic character, however; unlike the beneficiaries of aid put forward in postwar depictions of brutalised Italians, African figures in the period were still represented as a threatening other. This resulted in their total exclusion from, or stereotypical depiction in, film culture at the time. It is only later, in film festivals' deterritorial phase, that Global Southern subjects, and films, were admitted to festival programmes—and on the basis of a marketable "difference" even then (de Valck, 2007, p. 69). While I discuss this phase of festival development in the next chapter, I turn now to consider the re-inscription of brutal vision in the present day via dominant conceptions of humanism and humanitarianism that define figures from the Global South primarily as beneficiaries of aid.

It would be problematic to assume a direct parallel between the situation and representation of postwar Italians and that of those living under colonial and neo-colonial regimes. Scholars of postcolonialism have alerted us to the dangers of uncritically drawing such comparisons due to Europe's, and in particular Italy's, complex history as both colonial power and site of internal colonialism (Lombardi-Diop & Romeo, 2014). However, provided we remain attentive to this difference, it is possible to consider brutal humanism as structurally similar to the norms of representation that guide depictions of colonised subjects today. Schoonover (2012) repeatedly underlines brutal humanism's ideological persistence in the contemporary, neo-colonial period, as suggested by his claim that "European reconstruction was used as a template for [...] later large-scale humanitarian aid structures" (p. xxiv). If the European A circuit developed in line with the liberal ideology and affective structures that Schoonover identifies, we might wonder the extent to which they reproduce these structures today, above all in relation to the neo-colonial structures that, he argues, have emerged out of the template set out in the postwar period.

In the context of contemporary humanitarianism, staging a figure's helplessness as a means of inciting a sense of agency and pity has become a well-known, and much critiqued, trope of representations of peoples from the Global South. This extends from advertisements for charitable commodities (Wilson, 2016) to direct humanitarian appeals (Bell, 2013; Kessy, 2014; Rumph, 2011). Observing a process highly similar to that involved in brutal vision, Wilson (2016, p. 9) concludes that "the imagined proximity of the helpless and grateful beneficiary is only a prop to sustain his [the consumer's] enjoyment of inequality." As suggested by Schoonover's study, the structures of a humanism that slips into humanitarianism, as well as the structures of representation coextensive with it, developed through the reconstruction of postwar Europe and continue in neo-colonialist projects, such as aid to African states.

This has taken on a new character in the context of the "refugee crisis," in which recent images of refugees circulating in the media have triggered debates regarding the ethics of a compassionate but proxied engagement similar to the one described above. These debates consider images of imperilled refugees in terms of their corporeality and ethical import. Writing of the image of the dead body of the young boy Alain Kurdi, Waldman (2015) argues that

> [t]he assumption is that images are uniquely persuasive in ways that words aren't the impact might turn into some kind of action [...] when confronting a humanitarian crisis. (para. 9)

Waldman's assumption is that showing and witnessing bodies in peril exercises and then stimulates ethical agency and "action." In contrast, cultural theorists such as Žižek (2016) have questioned whether our investment in a compassionate, pitying stance towards the other might fall short of the "global solidarity of the exploited and oppressed" required to combat the conditions giving rise to forced migration (p. 110). Žižek makes an implicit distinction here: on the one hand, the distance between benefactor and other implied in compassion and, alternatively, a more equal relationship achieved through solidarity. However, as the case of *Fire at Sea*'s institutional constructions demonstrates, this solidarity is repeatedly curtailed, owing to the continuing displacement of an internal, European conflict of identity onto figures of the migrant other.

Fire at Sea: Representing the "Refugee Crisis"

Scholars have argued that representations of the "refugee crisis," including by European A festivals, are symptomatic of a broader struggle for a coherent humanist and European identity, echoing the sense of embattlement and displacement discussed above. As Prem Kumar Rajaram (2016, p. 2) has argued, the "crisis" is often considered less one for refugees, and more one for European countries. This can be said of both xenophobic and broadly progressive accounts of the effects of increased rates of migration from Africa to Europe in the new millennium. For example, Cristina Lombardi-Diop and Caterina Romeo (2015, p. 338) identify "what is Europe?" as one of the most pressing questions today due to both the negotiation of the Schengen Agreement and increased rates of migration. They consider Europe's identity in relation to those whom European countries have subjected to colonial oppression. Their study suggests once more the dialectical relationship between European identity and its others, the way in which, perhaps, the notion of "Europe" depends upon the displacement of its inherent split onto a colonised "outside."

O'Healy's (2010) analysis of Italian cinema of migration and abjection raises similar questions about the depiction of migration and migrants in Italian film in a way that clarifies the displacement of a division internal to Italy—and Europe—onto the figure of the other. She argues that Italian representations of migration can be interpreted as expressing an anxiety about Italy's Europeanness. O'Healy's (2010) assessment bears quoting at length:

> The figure of the unwanted immigrant or asylum seeker is deployed in similarly oppositional terms in several other countries of "Fortress Europe" at present [...]. In Italy, however, the national subject or imagined "way of life" is already shot through with the tensions of an internal, Southern "otherness." For generations, the cultural construction of Southern Italy as the "territorial watershed between Italy as Europeanised (or Americanised) and Italy as African" (Pandolfi 1998, 287) undermined any attempt to imagine Italy as a unified political subject. (pp. 7–8)

From this grounding, O'Healy shows that the figure of the "immigrant" was constructed and deployed as part of Italy's more recent "ambition[s] to forge a strong image as a modern, efficient, and progressive European nation" (p. 8). However, this should be read as a displacement: the Italian subject and nation's "tensions of an internal, Southern 'otherness'"—the split between its Southern and European identities—is displaced onto that of the non-Italian (Albanian or African, in O'Healy's account).[5] We find this taken to its xenophobic extreme in present-day Italian politics, characterised by support for far-right politicians such as Matteo Salvini and anti-immigration policies designed to criminalise people crossing the Mediterranean sea as well as those who help them do so safely. That this should be part of a wider European politics towards migration is evidenced in many countries' adoption of similar policies, including Germany's turn from a politics of *Wilkommenskultur* (discussed below) to one of strong borders. Welcoming or xenophobic, Italian and European identity hinges on their relation towards the migrant other.

Meanwhile, O'Healy presents Italian films as counter-narratives, showing that they can problematise "the image of contemporary Italy as a uniformly progressive, affluent nation, with a standard language spoken by all and the shared aspiration of 'European' belonging" (p. 9). O'Healy's analysis raises several questions that demonstrate the importance of Italian films of migration to the notions of European identity and representations of the other: to what extent is Italy and Italian film represented as "European," and on what grounds? To what extent does this "Europeanness" depend upon the displacement of difference onto the figure of the migrant or refugee? And to what extent can films themselves challenge these procedures, undermining the very notion of a coherent Italo-European identity?

Although scholarship on *Fire at Sea* remains relatively limited, a common theme can be traced through the literature, which considers it in relation to the politics of migration and argues that it registers the tension between a relatively privileged European subject position and that of the refugee. The degree to which this is taken to indicate a split internal to Europe, rather than one between Europe and Africa, varies. Sandra Ponzanesi (2016a) compares two films of migration that were recently recognised by European A festivals: *Fire at Sea* and *On the Bride's Side* (*Io sto con la sposa*, 2014, Augugliaro, Del Grande, & Al Nassiry). Ultimately, Ponzanesi (2016a, p. 165) argues for the progressive potential of *Fire at Sea* as a film text, asserting its capacity to "resignify Europe from a location of marginality and hope" (that is, Lampedusa, an island on the periphery between Europe and Africa). In her reading, the film has the potential to produce "new imaginaries for Europe, where a space of solidarity and cosmopolitanism can be regained from new subject positions" (Ponzanesi, 2016a, pp. 151–152).

5 On the racialisation of Southern Italy, see the following chapter.

However, she also considers some of the complexities of the film's reception and portrayal of migrants. Although Ponzanesi (2016a, p. 152) interprets the film as "counter[ing] the EU politics of borders and patrolling," she also acknowledges that the contexts of *Fire at Sea*'s exhibition may signal the possibility of it being utilised as "an easy way to acquit bad consciences by taking part in a drama that is sagely portrayed at a distance." In this analysis, the political potential of *Fire at Sea* risks being undermined precisely by its potential to place European spectators at a distance from the crisis. Given the predication of brutal humanism on a relation of distance between the suffering other and implied spectator, the film's ability to reinforce or undermine this relation of power will be paramount to its relevance to European, and European A festivals', politics towards the refugee other. Before analysing the film and its construction by the Berlinale, suffice to note that Ponzanesi's account highlights a tension that runs through *Fire at Sea*'s status as a film text and its institutionalisation.

Emma Wilson (2018) emphasises the splitting and tension in *Fire at Sea* and does so in a lexicon that might suggest the film's potential to challenge the notion of European agency. She argues that the film powerfully represents a "schism" between the Lampedusan and refugee characters and, with it, between Europe and its others (p. 18). She concludes that the depiction of this schism is part of the film's strategy to make manifest

> the global insanity, the madness of contemporary Europe, where everyday life co-exists, obliviously, with the deathly horror of forced migration, people-trafficking, and flight from war zones. *Fire at Sea* challenges that obliviousness, that disavowal and disconnect. (Wilson, 2018, p. 12)

Although not part of a psychoanalytical interpretation of *Fire at Sea*, we can build on the language of pathology that Wilson deploys. Note that "madness" pertains to Europe, and that the contemporary European condition Wilson claims that the film shows is one of "disavowal and disconnect." This is a disavowal that occurs *within* Europe: within its borders, in the "everyday life" taking place on Lampedusa in the film. That which is disavowed is the European interiority of the "crisis," of the "horror[s]" both Wilson and *Fire at Sea* describe. The film, Wilson argues, challenges notions of a split between Europe and its others, critiquing the "disconnect" that suggests "horror" as something taking place "out there"—in the region of Europe's constitutive outside, Africa. We therefore might question the extent to which the Berlinale's representation of the film reproduces "the madness of contemporary Europe" or underlines *Fire at Sea*'s critique of it, highlighting the disavowal of the interiority of the other on which such madness (or rather, ideology) is predicated.

These analyses of *Fire at Sea* indicate its potential to be assimilated by but also contest the politics that institutions such as European Parliament or the Berlinale promote. Following Ponzanesi (2016a, pp. 151–152), it is ambiguous whether *Fire at Sea*'s contestation of an idea of "Europe" from "new subject positions" has the capacity to fundamentally challenge a sense of European worthiness or agency. Viewed through the lens of brutal humanism, we might argue instead that the film's reception as allowing European viewers to participate in "a drama that is sagely portrayed at a distance" is an important part of its potential to "acquit bad consciences" (Ponzanesi, 2016a, p. 152). However, this is not to say that *Fire at Sea* cannot challenge the ideology of liberal humanism and its attendant power relations. Wilson's emphasis on the film's representation of the unknowability of the other, and the pathology underpinning European responses to the "crisis" provide a ground from which we might analyse *Fire at Sea* in contrast with its institutional construction and the politics that may underpin it. Taking Ponzanesi's and Wilson's interpretations together highlights a productive line of inquiry: an investigation into how *Fire at Sea* might undermine or challenge a European perspective per se, including a compassionate, humanist stance towards the refugee other.

Synopsis Analysis

While the 2016 edition of the Berlinale is a long way from the 1946 edition of Cannes, focusing on broad structures, such as those of Western identity and liberal compassion (or brutal humanism), allows us to see the legacies of certain values across time, including the time of European A festivals. In fact, the awarding of *Fire at Sea*, an Italian film whose title explicitly conjures World War II, is highly evocative of this shared European A festival history and project.[6] Meanwhile, the 2016 edition of the Berlinale took place during what was perceived as the height of the "refugee crisis" and appeared to make explicit political choices as a result of this.[7] Importantly for both Berlin and

6 "Fuocoammare" (fire at sea), as explained in the film, is the title of a World War II song, the "fire at sea" referring to the bombing of the ship *La Maddalena* by the British off the coast of Lampedusa.

7 For a problematisation of discourses which conceptualise migration in relation to time, and above all crisis, see Johnson (forthcoming).

Europe (above all, the EU), in September 2015 Angela Merkel announced Germany's so-called "open-door policy" towards refugees. She committed to settling 800,000 and encouraged other EU countries to make similar pledges. The Berlinale, taking place approximately six months later, seemed to express similar values. In parallel with Merkel's policy, the Berlinale offered them free admission to its film screenings. Organisational decisions as well as those pertaining to the festival's programme and awards therefore appeared to complement the German state politics of humanitarian hospitality or *Willkommenskultur* of the time (Karakayalı 2019). Merkel's words were even mobilised by the Berlinale, the festival's 2016 edition report not only citing her "we can do it" slogan as its inspiration, but explicitly stating that "[i]t is before this particular backdrop that the full power of the International Jury's decision about the winner of the 2016 Golden Bear becomes apparent" (Berlinale, 2016b).

At the awards ceremony, jury president Meryl Streep called *Fire at Sea* "urgent, imaginative and necessary filmmaking" (BBC, 2016, para. 6). Streep's comments allude to the artistic worth of the film but, above all, foreground its political importance—its urgency and necessity. At the award ceremony, Rosi contributed to this impression by stating, "I hope to bring awareness. It's not acceptable that people die crossing the sea to escape from tragedies" (BBC, 2016, para 4). Rosi then dedicated the Golden Bear to the people of Lampedusa, praising their openness to receiving refugees.[8] It is notable here that Rosi's dedication is to Europeans rather than the refugees themselves, suggesting again a European address within the film's presentation at the festival. Complementing these aspects of the representation of *Fire at Sea*, the festival synopsis of the film makes the politics of the Berlinale's engagement with the "crisis" yet more apparent. The text's construction of the film instantiates a brutal vision directed toward the figure of the refugee by: (1) affording only Lampedusan characters the power of looking, defining them as European "witnesses" to a "humanitarian crisis"; (2) characterising the refugee figures as, in contrast, African, and objects of observation and pity; and (3) evoking an ethics based on abstract humanism that allows for the European subject's "proxied engagement" with the other.

As discussed above, an important ideological procedure that structures representations of the other is that of suture: suture displaces the subject's

8 I do not take this as Rosi's ultimate statement on the film. Rather, his comments are themselves conditioned by the context in which he made them—the award ceremony of the Berlinale. The director is as much "spoken by" the festival as they speak at the festival. The contrast between Rosi's speech at the Berlinale and the largely stylistic account of this film he usually gives in interviews underlines this point (Nord, 2016; IDA, 2017).

internal division onto a split between their "inside" and that which appears "outside." For example, the tension inherent to "Europe" (i.e., the impossibility of a coherent "European" ideology or identity) is displaced onto a tension between Europe and Africa; Africa becomes Europe's "constitutive outside." This procedure can be observed in the Berlinale's synopsis of *Fire at Sea*, which posits a coherent European identity and contrasts it with figures of African refugees. The synopsis of *Fire at Sea* is structured around a central point of antagonism, the division between an implied European perspective and that of African refugees. This is exemplified by the text's concluding reference to "two worlds [that] barely touch." The notion of "two worlds" assumes two relatively coherent entities that are then contrasted, separated, one untouchable by the other.

The synopsis continually differentiates between European and African figures, establishing a sense of distance between them. Throughout, the synopsis alternates between the two positions throughout, from Samuele's activities on Lampedusa's port, to "men, women and children trying to make the crossing from Africa" (their contradictory presence emphasised by the "But" that introduces it), to the "inhabitants of Lampedusa" who are "bearing witness" to said crossing. Indeed, through its characterisation of the islanders and the director, the paratext implies a coherent European identity that it associates with agency and the status of witness. While the refugee characters remain nameless throughout the text, the first paragraph introduces the film's protagonist as islander Samuele. As the only named Lampedusan, he is positioned as a representative of the inhabitants of the island in general. The appearance of a named representative implies the status of subject, granted only to the Lampedusans, while the namelessness of the refugees deindividualises them, thus excluding them from the symbolic order posited in the text.[9]

The synopsis gradually moves from Samuele's seeming obliviousness to islanders' witnessing, and then, through a crucial slippage, to the "observations" of the film's director, Rosi.[10] These observations, in turn, "bring us [the implied viewers of the film] closer" to Lampedusa, this site of "metaphor

9 The lack of a refugee character equivalent to Samuele in the film has been criticised by Thomas Austin (2017).

10 Rosi's status as an Italian director should be complicated. He was raised in Eritrea and moved to New York at the age of nineteen, for example. This gives further credence to European A festivals' ideological positioning of "Europe as subject." The festivals ascribe Rosi an Italo-European rather than Eritrean-African, or American, identity. It appears that his status as auteur is bound up with not only the perception of his masculinity (his being male, designated as a man by festivals), but also that of his supposed European identity.

for the flight of refugees to Europe" (italics added). Yet the power to look is afforded only to the European subject position: the Lampedusan islanders, the Italian director and the implied film spectator, who, if we follow to its logical conclusion the slippage from Lampedusa to Italy to "us," is implicitly addressed as European. This slippage in the text subtly elides the potential for a division between, for example, a Lampedusan and European identity, as suggested by Ponzanesi's (2016a) description of Lampedusa as liminal to Europe or O'Healy's (2010) discussion of the tension between Italy's Southern and European identities. Rather, the synopsis downplays these differences and depicts *Fire at Sea* as being about a European tragedy seen, by extension, through a European look.

This sense of a relatively coherent European subjectivity afforded the power of looking underpins the synopsis's distinction between Europe and Africa, and is reaffirmed through the text's depiction of the refugee characters. In contrast with the islander witnesses, the text separates the African figures, positioning them as objects of a brutal humanist look. Refugees are depicted primarily through notions of lack—lacking names, as well as means and agency. In contrast with Samuele's carefree meanderings, his desire to "mooch about the port" of Lampedusa, the refugees are trapped in boats that are "far too small and decrepit" and experience only "hopes, hardship and fate." Rather than bearing witness to their own "fate," the refugees' only activities in the text are "longing for peace" and "trying to make the crossing from Africa."[11] Words such as "longing" and "trying" designate incomplete actions and desire rather than wholeness and agency. This positions Africa as a place of unsatisfied needs—a place from which refugees flee to Europe, a land in which they supposedly might find the "peace, freedom and happiness" they "long" for.

Again, a sense of completeness and power is ascribed to Europe, its lack displaced onto Africa. This is epitomised by the synopsis's final reference to the African characters: "only their dead bodies are pulled out of the water." The representation of dead bodies is, Schoonover (2012, p. xvi) argues, the technique *par excellence* of brutal vision. In this case, the image combines notions of the refugees' peril, lack and passivity. In contrast, agency lies only

11 Note the curtailment of possibilities of refugees' own testimonies here—a curtailment challenged by numerous films made by refugees, as well as film programmes made by and for migrants. A recent example of this I was privileged to attend in Leeds was the T A P E collective's *The Good Immigrant* programme, featuring films such as *I Was Told There's Freedom Here* (Awate Abdalla, 2021). On festivals "by and for" migrants and refugees, see Breyfogle (2020); on the politics of film festivals' programming of migration cinema, see Ostrowska (2019) and Johnson (forthcoming).

with the invisible hands pulling the bodies out of the water. The refugees are, ultimately, depicted as passive objects to be handled or witnessed by the European subject. This again stages the "politics of pity" that underpins brutal vision: the refugees are shown as passive bodies in crisis, lacking subjectivity or agency, while the European subject engages with their suffering from a distance.

This is, perhaps, the interplay of closeness and distance that sustains the brutal sufferer-witness relationship, marked by "proxied engagement whose outreaching hand is assured that it will never actually touch that which it reaches for" (Schoonover, 2012, p. 66). The synopsis thus constructs "Europe" as a coherent entity founded on its humanist and humanitarian ethics: a crucial feature of the film's perspective, as described by the synopsis, is its humanitarianism and the abstract relationship of proximity and distance that it entails. In short, the synopsis depicts *Fire at Sea* as a European film that mobilises a European, humanitarian look towards an imperilled, African other appearing at its borders.

Film Analysis

To demonstrate the ideological procedures at work in the synopsis' representation of *Fire at Sea*, this section focuses on two aspects of both the film and the paratext. First, I analyse the film's representation of its European characters, and how this may present a split internal to Europe similar to that identified by Ponzanesi (2016a)—that is, a split between an official European politics of border policing and a compassionate response to the "crisis." I focus on those characters absent from the synopsis: the island doctor, Dr. Bartolo, and the official rescuers (it is unclear if they are Frontex, the border control agency contracted by the EU, or belong to another organisation). The film's contrasting representations of Dr. Barloto and the officials serve to underline the synopsis displacing an internal division onto an external one between the islanders and the refugees. Second, I engage with the relations of looking made manifest in the film. This final section will contrast *Fire at Sea*'s representation of its own perspective towards refugee characters with the appearance of the neutral, European viewpoint offered by the paratext. I develop the Lacanian theories of the Gaze above through an interpretation of *Fire at Sea*'s metacinematic representation, and problematising, of its own perspective. Considering these issues in relation to brutal humanism, neo-coloniality and European identity not only further highlights the brutal vision mobilised by European A festivals in the context of the "refugee crisis", but opens up a space for them to be challenged via a more self-reflexive acknowledgement of the Eurocentric partiality of liberal humanism.

A Facture Internal to Europe: Frontex and the Doctor

The synopsis evokes the rescue effort taking place on Lampedusa, one of the main narratives of the film, only with the reference to refugees being "pulled out of the water." Here it seems that an invisible hand is intervening in the crisis, which the islanders merely witness. This omission of *who* is pulling the dead out of the Mediterranean Sea effectively obfuscates one of the primary sites of conflict in both *Fire at Sea* and, more broadly, Europe's struggle for identity. In contrast, the film depicts two approaches to engaging with refugees: the official rescue effort, presented as impersonal and dehumanising, and a more personal, compassionate response in Dr. Bartolo. While both are shown to be working towards the same end (rescuing refugees), the way in which they are depicted produces the impression of a division *within* Europe.

In contrast with the notion that the film shows just two worlds that barely touch, *Fire at Sea* portrays fractures within the island community. Significantly, it suggests that it is not the refugees, but the officials running the rescue effort who can be seen as foreign intruders. Throughout the film, the officials have little contact with the lives of the islanders; the rescuers and Lampedusans are never shown together in the same scene. Meanwhile, *Fire at Sea* seems to characterise the official rescuers in a way that critiques their dehumanising approach to refugees, one that emphasises the importance of a strong border to keep the "contagious" "other" out. Ponzanesi (2016) has noted that the contrast between the rescuers' contagion suits and the migrants' barely clothed bodies registers "an encounter that cannot possibly be on an equal footing" (p. 162). Building on this, we can examine the particular way in which this inequality is represented: the rescuers' treatment of refugees as bodies of contagion, a threat from outside that must be repelled with a strong outer layer. This recalls Roberto Esposito's (2011) concept of *immunitas*: the construction of the other as a foreign agent who can make the (social) body sick. This is made most apparent by the fact that we only see the rescuers in contagion suits and masks.

Never shown baring skin, they are characterised as strange, almost inhuman, and dedicated entirely to the containment of the dirt and disease typically associated with the "non-white" other in racist discourses.[12] The extra layer of the contagion suits functions as a border between the healthy rescuer's body and that of the apparently dirty, contagious, threatening African. In the context of the continent-wide debate regarding Europe's borders and the EU's deployment of officials (such as Frontex guards) on such borders, this representation of the rescuers seems to visually register and intervene in an EU politics based on strong borders and keeping "foreign bodies" out.

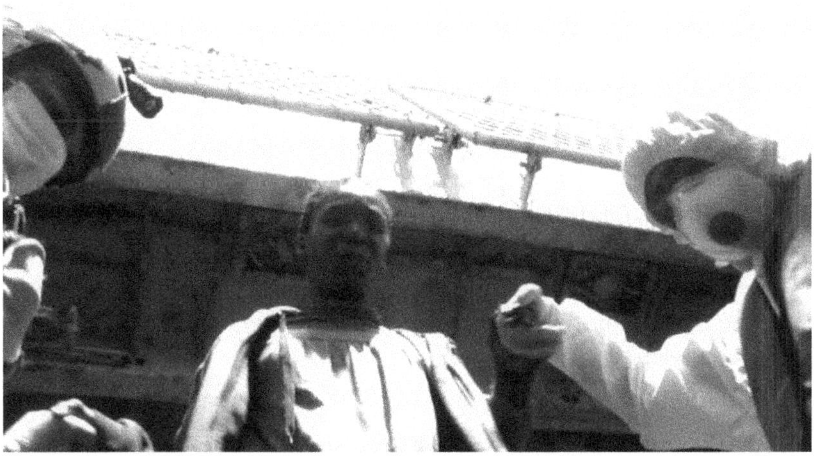

Figure 19: *Immunitas*: contagion suits in *Fire at Sea* (Rosi, 2016). Curzon Artificial Eye.

As well as being faceless, the rescuers also have very little dialogue in the film. Unlike the doctor, none of the officials are shown reflecting on their personal responses to the "crisis." Their speech is usually limited to words that imply a cold pragmatism or disdain towards their mission. Two examples of this stand out. First, a rescuer is heard telling a refugee to "calm down" over the radio. Her pleading for help is met with a coldly pragmatic explanation of the need to remain calm and provide specific information about the boat and its position. This could be taken as nothing more than a sign of efficiency—or perhaps a "small [act] of compassion or practicality" (Wilson, 2018, p. 13)—if it were not complemented by the second instance of the rescuers' speech. The officials in the detention centre are shown complaining about the refugees' smell, again casting them as dirty, contagious bodies. They remain in their contagion suits, roughly handling refugees so that they can be processed in the rescue (read: detention) centre.

12 See Ahmed (2000) and Nicolson et al. (2015). I discuss this in the next chapter, and in relation to of migrant bodies and "Flow" elsewhere (O'Leary & Johnson, 2022).

The lack of empathy suggested by the film's dehumanising representation of the rescuers is thus justified by their dehumanising and unempathetic response to the refugees.

This begins to indicate how *Fire at Sea* may be seen to further complicate the relationship between the inhabitants of the island. In opposition to the representation of the refugees as deindividualised subjects that we read in the synopsis, *Fire at Sea* presents the officials as a deindividualised group. This challenges representations of refugees as a contagious mass typical of the media and official discourse in Europe at the time, an official discourse that we have seen is also represented by the rescuers in the film.[13] This could be a part of an ironic othering of the officials. Instead of refugees, these functionaries and the insular, protectionist politics they represent are shown as strange, faceless—the true inhuman threat to Europe. This portrayal of EU officials seems to be part of a critique of the official European discourse, one downplayed in the Berlinale synopsis.

The everyday clothing and compassionate demeanour of the doctor contrasts with the strangeness of the officials. When shown treating a pregnant and recently rescued refugee, Dr. Bartolo's costume represents an alternative politics of compassion and contact:

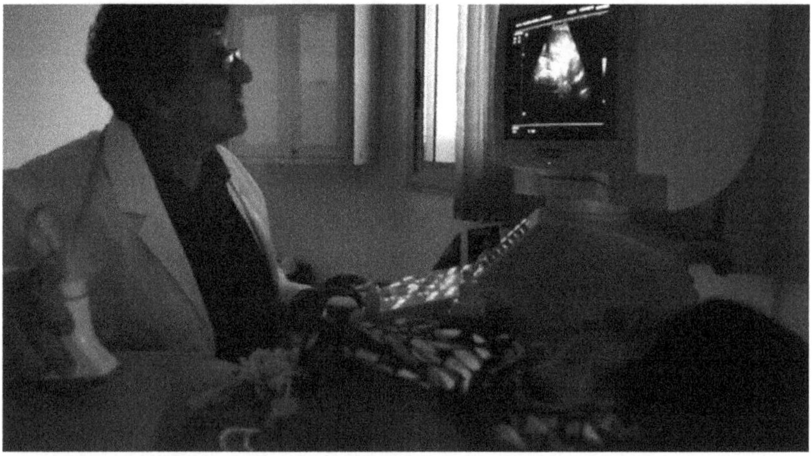

Figure 20: Baring skin: Dr. Bartolo treats a pregnant refugee. *Fire at Sea* (Rosi, 2016). Curzon Artificial Eye.

Aside from his lab coat, which he wears no matter whom he is treating, the doctor wears nothing that would limit contact between himself and

13 Take, for example, David Cameron's (Prime Minister of the UK between 2010 and 2016) description of migrants as a "swarm" (Elgot & Taylor, 2015).

the woman. While it might have been absurd to show a doctor wearing a contagion suit in his practice, Dr. Bartolo does not even wear items of protective clothing that one might expect, such as a mask or latex gloves. The doctor's baring of his skin—that which Sara Ahmed (2000, p. 45) designates a tactile and vulnerable border between a subject and the outside—contrasts with any official protective, insular stance. This seems to represent the humanist response to migration: rather than treating them as a contagious threat, Dr. Bartolo is shown attempting to bridge the border between himself and the refugee.

The film rewards Dr. Bartolo for his compassionate response with a similarly humanising representation. A sense of the doctor as both human and humanist is established through a long interview with him. Unlike the rescuers, the doctor's face is shown and his voice is heard. Such scenes appear to develop him as a character and thus provide a stronger basis for empathy with him than there would be for the faceless officials. Dr. Bartolo's emotional response to the "crisis," registered in the interview, humanises him further, and we might interpret this as part of a cinematic strategy to encourage a humanist politics of compassion. During the interview, he explicitly compares himself with his peers:

> So I have to witness awful things: dead bodies, children... On those occasions I'm forced to do that thing I hate most: examining cadavers [...] Many of my colleagues say, "You've seen so many... You're used to it." It's not true. How can you get used to seeing dead children, pregnant women, women who've given birth on sinking boats, umbilical cords still attached? [...] But it has to be done, so I do it.

Here the doctor's sense of duty is presented as the stoicism of a man deeply affected by the "awful things" he has seen, in contrast with the cold pragmatism of the official rescuers. The film's depiction of the doctor's inner life, his emotions, and sense of duty, encourages identification with this character and, as such, perhaps also the humanist stance that he represents.

However, the doctor's words also foreground the refugees' status as suffering victims, and his own role as their beneficiary. (The film, too, emphasises this role, foregrounding the doctor-patient relationship, itself a relation of power.) As well as treating or helping, Dr. Bartolo also frames his work as *seeing* refugees as a witness to their suffering. His description of their suffering is graphic, evoking the images of "corporeal violence" Schoonover (2012, pp. 12–13) argues are central to the "brutal" aspect of brutal humanism. Moreover, it is compounded with a sense of ethical imperative: "It has to be done, so I do it."[14] While the doctor discusses his activities examining cadavers, the interview is framed by his description of himself as a witness, and the mise-en-scène also alludes to a politics of witnessing:

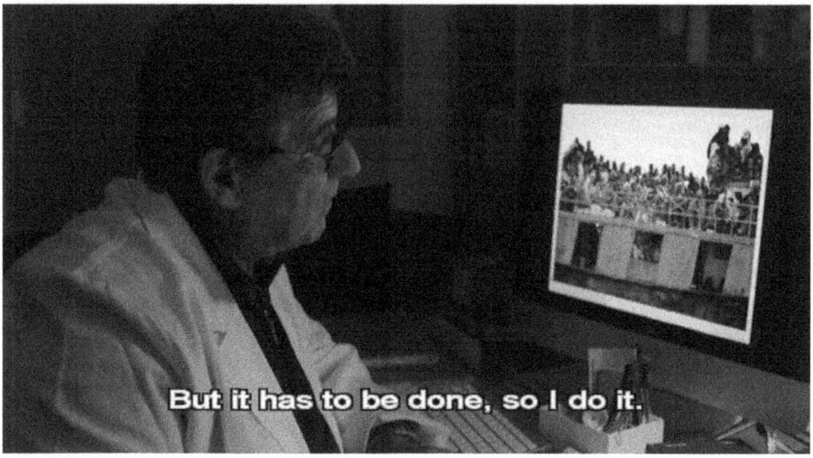

Figure 21: Dr. Bartolo as audience surrogate and ethical witness. *Fire at Sea* (Rosi, 2016).Curzon Artificial Eye.

Here, Dr. Bartolo is sitting in a dark room, illuminated by a screen showing images of refugees and boats, usually in situations of peril. The lighting draws the eye to the screen. In this way, he appears as a shadow, a kind of intermediary between the camera (and spectator) and the images of suffering. The doctor can thus be interpreted as an audience surrogate, a witness whose proximity to the "crisis" stands in for that of the viewer. Paired with his monologue, the scene seems to encourage a "proxied engagement" in which the compassionate spectator is positioned, not unlike the doctor, as an important witness. The viewer is encouraged, likewise, to bear witness to the images of peril on screen. Dr. Bartolo therefore has an ambiguous role in the film when viewed through the framework of brutal humanism. His physical contact with refugee characters implies a challenge to the "culture of transatlantic aid whose outreaching hand is assured that it will never actually touch that which it reaches for" (Schoonover, 2012, p. 66).

14 In light of this, we can better understand the off-screen celebration of Bartolo, who continues to be cast as an ethical witness to the "refugee crisis." The doctor has published a memoir of his experiences, *Lampedusa: Gateway to Europe* (2017). Although actively engaged in treating refugees, Bartolo is valued both on- and off- screen as a compassionate witness.

However, the emphasis on his status as ethical witness, a role that the film may encourage the spectator to similarly assume, also suggests that witnessing the "crisis" is the most urgent imperative.

The impression of the film's compassion and humanism may also fortify European hegemony, inadvertently positing the centrality of a specifically European ideology and perspective. Thus, I would argue that the main difference between the synopsis and the film's representation of a European response to the "crisis" is one of emphasis. Both the film and the paratext in some way appear to be engaged in the struggle for political hegemony—to determine the empty universal "Europe" in line with a politics of liberal (and perhaps brutal) compassion. In the synopsis, this struggle is omitted, perhaps downplaying *Fire at Sea*'s potential to offer a direct critique of an EU politics of border control, undertaken on liberal humanist grounds. In contrast, the film text can be interpreted as taking a clearer stance, suggesting that the official rescuers are, rather than the refugees, strange invaders on the island. Meanwhile, *Fire at Sea* celebrates Dr. Bartolo, casting him as an important witness to the "crisis." The film depicts a division internal to Europe, yet its critique of the official politics of the EU seems to function on the grounds that it has lost its legacy of liberal, humanist compassion, a position that we might consider to neglect the neo-colonial relations of power on which this legacy is founded.

The Irruption of the Gaze in Brutal Vision

This is not to say that *Fire at Sea* can be reduced to these values. Not only does the film represent a fracture *within* Europe, therefore partially signalling the displacement of difference onto the figure of the other; it also contains scenes that challenge our view of the other as such. On several occasions, the film signals the issues and ideological investments involved in its own representation of refugees. It is in this respect that *Fire at Sea* can be interpreted as challenging the politics of brutal compassion most significantly. *Fire at Sea*'s representation of refugees—or rather, its representation of its representation of refugees—demonstrate the risks of objectification involved in screening their suffering, and highlights the partiality of the camera's, the director's, and the viewers' perspectives. In so doing, the film can be interpreted as challenging a sense of mastery over images of refugees (and, more broadly, the other), thus also contesting the agency of the European and/or Western witness.

I have argued that the synopsis's representation of an African other follows the logic of suture: it positions them as an "external" element that may compensate for the split inherent to European identity. As discussed above, this procedure is similar to that theorised by Mulvey gaze theory: looking at an image of an objectified figure reproduces notions of distance and difference from that figure. I have argued that this look can be compared to the "foreign spectator's sovereign gaze" mobilised by brutal vision, since the sovereignty of the spectator suggests a coherent identity, as well as difference from, and mastery over, that which is looked at (i.e., images of the other). As outlined, the Gaze is "on the side of the object" and "gives body to an impossibility"; it can make manifest the ideological and compensatory process of suture that structures the subject's relation to the images they view (Žižek, 2001a, pp. 201–202). Images of the other, when presented in a certain way, can register the lack inherent to the implied subject-onlooker, destabilising a sense of mastery over their image. It is from this basis that the authority of the subject, and the illusion of their dominant viewpoint, can be challenged. When the process of suture is made manifest, the partiality—the ideological nature—of the subject's perspective also appears. The "sovereign gaze" can thus be undermined in moments that allude to the impossibility of a totalising perspective on a scene, moments that signal "the gap within the subject's seemingly omnipotent look" (McGowan, 2007, p. 6). The manifestation of the Gaze in this way "marks a disturbance in the functioning of ideology" (McGowan, 2007, p. 7). This impossibility of self-enclosure that at once constitutes and thwarts suture can be given body through the image being looked at—in this case, an image of the suffering other—particularly when the artificiality of their representation is emphasised.

This process occurs in film through the use of metacinematic elements that reveal that the images on screen have in fact been produced for our witnessing. These irruptions of the Gaze highlight the viewer's implication and ideological investment in the images being screened:

> [T]he existence of the [G]aze as a disruption (or stain) in the picture—an objective [G]aze—means spectators never look on from a safe distance; they are in the picture in the form of this stain, implicated in the text itself. (McGowan, 2007, p. 7).

The image, framed in a metacinematic way, can dismantle the safe distance between spectator and picture by highlighting that the images being screened are projections of the viewer's desires. (I mean this in the sense of the viewer being addressed, implied by the text, rather than any actually existing viewer—the viewer-as-subject.) Rather than being at a "safe distance" that might allow for the illusion of neutrality or mastery required for ethical witnessing, then, the spectator is shown to be "implicated in the text." In the case of brutal humanism, the distance underpinning structures of "proxied engagement" and the power of the witness meets a direct challenge in the form of the "objective gaze" of the suffering other.

Fire at Sea contains several moments in which the refugee is explicitly shown to look back, and the cinematic apparatus registering this figure is alluded to. Together, these manifest the Real; they highlight how "the spectator is accounted for within the film itself" (McGowan, 2007, p. 8). Three shots in *Fire at Sea* epitomise the film's attempt to register and complicate a politics of brutal vision. The first two demonstrate a transition from neutral observation to the representation of the camera's, and viewer's, partial and privileged perspective. The third builds on this interplay of perspectives, highlighting the refugee's subjectivity and our attempt to de-radicalise it by objectifying or taming it.

In contrast with the synopsis, in the film, the refugees look back; they are alive and endowed with the power of vision.[15] Moreover, the second and third images show moments when the film overtly registers the camera's perspective, highlighting its partiality as an artificial representation rather than neutral observation. The first shot (Fig. 22) is of a man who has just been rescued and placed under a blanket on the rescue boat. He is looking into the camera, his facial expression one of suffering. He is one of several such figures filmed in a similar way. The camera usually remains fixed on each person, giving the initial impression of a neutral observer registering the responses of imperilled refugees on film. At first, this seems to confirm the synopsis's description of the film as enacting a "commentary-free" "observation" of refugees with no identity other than as imperilled victims, the passive objects of a one-way, humanist look.

This changes when the boat rocks momentarily, revealing the screen between the camera and the figure (Fig. 23). The outline of the window between them functions as a frame, revealing the artificiality of the film's perspective. This metacinematic aspect highlights that the refugee (and his suffering) is being screened for our look. As discussed in relation to *Facing Window*, the presence of a window/screen can, in this way, be interpreted as making manifest the projection of the viewer's desires onto the image in front of them. If Giovanna projected her desire to find subjective fulfilment onto the screen between her and Lorenzo, we might interpret this window

15 Admittedly, this is a low bar for depictions of refugees. Such is the challenge presented by films such as *Fire at Sea* and the canon they constitute.

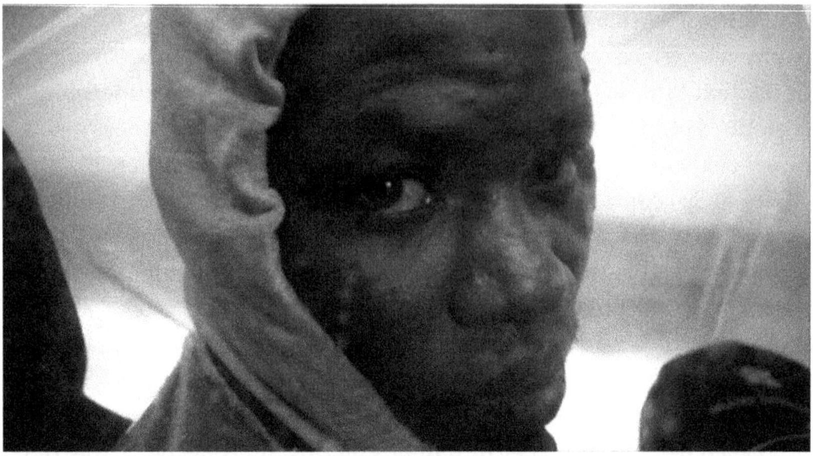

Figure 22: The refugee Gaze (1): man looks into camera on rescue boat. *Fire at Sea* (Rosi, 2016). Curzon Artificial Eye.

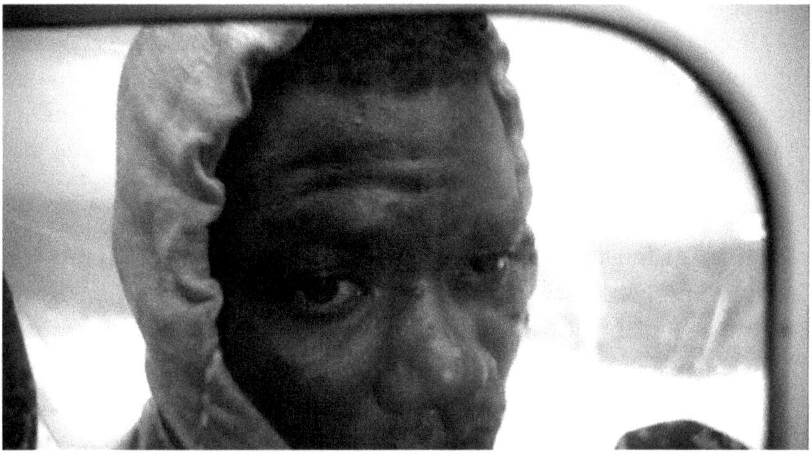

Figure 23: The refugee Gaze (2): boat window as screen. *Fire at Sea* (Rosi, 2016). Curzon Artificial Eye.

as registering the projection of the (implied) viewer's desire for some kind of fulfilment onto the screen between them and the refugee character. Instead of a neutral observation, we are presented with a partial, situated view permeated by desire. In this context, such a desire would be for a coherent, European or Euro-American identity that affords the subject moral agency and authority over both the world and, in particular, the other.

Moreover, this mediation appears predicated on a relation of distance and relative safety, registered by the screen's function as border between the camera/viewer and the refugee. The window manifests the "surrogate proximities" structuring brutal compassion, a relation of imaginary closeness predicated nonetheless on distance (Schoonover, 2012, p. 34). The viewer projects their desires from a distance, from the relative safety across the border of the screen. For a moment, the film demonstrates its, and the viewer's, own implication in the border politics of the official rescuers that I discussed earlier. Through the use of the metacinematic presentation of a screen, *Fire at Sea* suggests that this separation is implied in the relationship of sufferer-witness, problematising its own politics of representation.

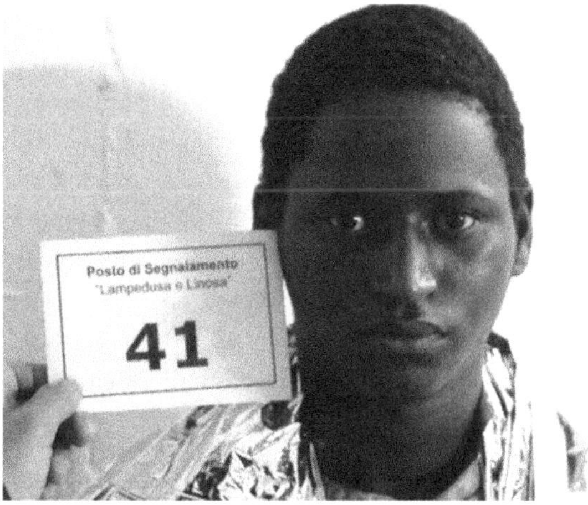

Figure 24: Just a number? The refugee Gaze (3): man looks into official's, and Rosi's, camera. *Fire at Sea* (Rosi, 2016). Curzon Artificial Eye.

Figure 24 is part of a scene that makes these relations more explicit. In this shot, a recently rescued refugee is being photographed next to a number. The number is the only signifier of his individual identity in the frame, and barely fulfils this function. This once again foregrounds the dehumanising procedures at work in how refugees are treated, and represented, by officials. The depiction of photography adds a metacinematic dimension, which continues to signal *Fire at Sea*'s (and, by extension, its audience's) implication in the same procedure of dehumanisation. This becomes especially apparent, since the point of view of the shot is the same as that of the photographer. We, as the audience, are placed in the position of the official photographer, who appears to see the refugee as only a face and a number. There is a palpable tension between the subjectivity of the refugee and the attempt to objectify this subjectivity, signified by the number beside him. This tension takes on a subtle violence as the number repeatedly clashes with the character's face. The tension between the attempt to objectify this figure and his resistant subjectivity—literally, the impermeability of his body—breaks out on screen. This is not a corpse to be pulled out of the water nor an object to be photographed and numbered, but another subject whose power to look back undermines the processes of objectification implicit in the brutal vision of the camera, both that of the photographer and Rosi.

In the Berlinale synopsis, the refugee is offered to the look of the islanders, the director and the implied "foreign spectator." The paratext aligns the film's perspective with, and ascribes agency to, seemingly European characters while rendering the refugee characters as passive and to-be-looked at. This produces a relation of power in which the spectator is implicitly positioned as master of the image, both of the scenes witnessed and the refugees depicted. However, throughout *Fire at Sea*, this relation is challenged in moments when the Gaze is made manifest. Through moments that underline the partiality of the camera's perspective, the film destabilises any notion of a "neutral" or total view of the "crisis." Instead, by associating the cinematic apparatus with fantasmatic screens, distancing borders, and objectifying numbers, *Fire at Sea* highlights the contradictions of a "proxied engagement" that the staging of their suffering entails (Schoonover, 2012, p. 66). In short, these manifestations of the Gaze contain the potential to challenge Europe's liberal compassionate response to the "refugee crisis."

Conclusion

I have argued that this compassion is founded on viewing images of imperilled others from a privileged "liberal humanist present" that characterises brutal vision and its uneven relations of power. Given the ideological persistence of brutal vision in European A festivals' representation of both Italian cinema and the other, Dovey's (2015) contention that European A festivals are engaged in a procedure of "curating Africa" holds true not only for African films and filmmakers, but for festivals' broader politics of representing colonised others, including refugees. Ostrowska (2016), Dovey (2015) and Schoonover (2012) identify the immediate postwar period, the era in which the A circuit had its origins, as the crucial context in which cinematic institutions (from neorealism to film festivals) mobilised a European, or rather broadly North-Western, identity founded on liberal humanism. In Dovey's and Schoonover's accounts, moreover, the coherence of this identity, and the impression of a colonially-inflected agency or mastery, depended upon that which I have theorised as a process of suture: the representation of an imperilled other as a means of displacing the tension internal to a

"European" symbolic order founded on humanism. The case of *Fire at Sea*'s presentation at the Berlinale suggests that this process may continue in the present day, reaching a point of acuity in the context of the "refugee crisis" that has renewed the impression of European identity in crisis.

European A festivals, therefore, may not only ideologically delimit the meaning of "art" (as demonstrated in chapters 2 and 3) but also that of "politics" and, in turn, "Europe." The construction of "art" entails a disavowal of the commerciality of European A festivals—their imbrication in the global third sector as a key component of late capitalism. Meanwhile, the construction of "politics" in its humanist dimension entails a disavowal of the colonialist relations underpinning European A festivals' historical development. The "obscene virtual supplement" to European A festivals' explicit symbolic functioning is their investment in European, or broadly Western, relations of power constituted by the oppression and othering of non-white or non-European subjects (Žižek, 2008, p. 145). The case of *Fire at Sea*, particularly in its status as a migration film, has highlighted a possible connection between the performance of political engagement and European festivals' representation of the other, both of which reproduce the uneven relations of power that such festivals explicitly claim to intervene in. More specifically, it underlines the way in which European A festivals appear to function according to an unacknowledged *brutal* humanism that does not challenge geopolitical regimes of power. This suggests that the European A festivals construct Italian cinema as political, at times even critical, but not in a way that would undermine European hegemony or, perhaps, Western capitalist values. In the next chapter, I bring these two aspects of European A festival ideology together, analysing the confluence of Orientalism and capitalism through the case of Cannes's representation of *Gomorrah*.

Bibliography

Ahmed, S. (2000). *Strange encounters: Embodied others in post-coloniality*. Routledge.

ANSA. (2017). Strong Venice Film Festival line-up heavy on migration. *ANSA Med*. 28 July 2019. Available from: https://www.ansamed.info/ansamed/en/news/nations/italy/2017/07/28/strong-venice-film-festival-line-up-heavy-on-migration_5c87917a-d3f2-48e6-aafc-02b1fbc6ce77.html?idPhoto=2

Austin, T. (2017). *Benefaction, processing, exclusion: Documentary representations of refugees and migrants in Fortress Europ*e. European Cinema: Perspectives on Post-Democracy and the Crisis of the European Project, 19 May 2017, University of Leeds.

Bartolo, P., & Tilotta, L. (2017). *Lampedusa: Gateway to Europe*. MacLehose Press.

BBC News. (2016). *Berlin Film Festival:* Fire at Sea *wins Golden Bear.* [Online]. 20 February. Available from: http://www.bbc.co.uk/news/entertainment-arts-35623412

Bell, K. M. (2013). Raising Africa? Celebrity and the rhetoric of the white saviour. *PORTAL Journal of Multidisciplinary International Studies*, *10*(1), 1–24.

Berlin International Film Festival. (2016a). *Fuocoammare.* [Online]. Available from: https://www.berlinale.de/en/archiv/jahresarchive/2016/02_programm_2016/02_Filmdatenblatt_2016_201614479.php#tab=filmStills

Berlin International Film Festival. (2016b). Yearbook: 66th Berlin International Film Festival, 11–21 February 2016. Available from: https://www.berlinale.de/en/archive/jahresarchive/2016/01_jahresblatt_2016/01_jahresblatt_2016.html

Bláhová, J. (2020). Political significance of a *Butcher in Love*: The 1956 Karlovy Vary International Film Festival, *Marty* and the restoration of contact between Hollywood and Czechoslovakia during the Cold War. *Studies in European Cinema*, *17*(2), 97–112.

Breyfogle, S. (2020). Stories from the margins: The practicality and ethics of refugee film festivals. *Frames Cinema Journal*. Available from: http://framescinemajournal.com/article/stories-from-the-margins-the-practicality-and-ethics-of-refugee-film-festivals/

Butler, J. (2002). *Antigone's claim: Kinship between life and death*. Columbia University Press.

Copjec, J. (1994). *Read my desire: Lacan against the historicists*. Verso Books.

Cordoba, C. (2022). The Locarno Film Festival under the influence? Programming Eastern European movies in anti-communist Switzerland (1946–1962). *Contemporary European History: First View*, *1*(1), 1–19.

De Valck, M. (2007). *Film Festivals: From European geopolitics to global cinephilia*. Amsterdam University Press.

Dovey, L. 2015. *Curating Africa in the age of film festivals*. Palgrave Macmillan.

Elgot, J., & Taylor, M. (2015). Calais Crisis: Cameron condemned for "dehumanising" description of migrants. *The Guardian*. [Online]. 30 July. Available from: https://www.theguardian.com/uk-news/2015/jul/30/david-cameron-migrant-swarm-language-condemned

Esposito, R. (2011). *Immunitas: The protection and negation of life*. Polity Press.

Fabbri, L. (2015). Neorealism as ideology: Bazin, Deleuze, and the avoidance of fascism. *The Italianist*, *35*(2), 182–201.

Fehrenbach, H. (1995). *Cinema in democratizing Germany: Reconstructing of national identity after Hitler*. University of North Carolina Press.

Galt, R., & Schoonover, K. (2010). Introduction: The impurity of art cinema. In R. Galt & K. Schoonover (Eds.), *Global art cinema: New theories and histories* (pp. 3–27). Oxford University Press.

Guerini Rocco, S. (2019). Italian world cinema: Alice Rohrwacher's "Lazzaro Felice" abroad. *International Circulation of Italian Cinema*. [Online]. Available from: https://www.italiancinema.it/italian-world-cinema-alice-rohrwachers-happy-as-lazzaro-abroad/

Harbord, J. (2002). *Film cultures*. Sage.

Hipkins, D., & Renga, D. (2016). A new canon? Contemporary Italian cinema and television and the role of quality in the anglophone curriculum. *Comunicazioni sociali, 1*(3), 375–397.

hooks, b. (1992). *Black looks: Race and representation*. South End Press.

International Documentary Association (IDA). (2017). Gianfranco Rosi on "Fire at Sea." Video interview. Available from: https://www.youtube.com/watch?v=xzNVTUziT8k

Iordanova, D. (2006). Showdown of the festivals: Clashing entrepreneurships and post-communist management of culture. *Film International, 4*(5), 25–37.

Johnson, R. (forthcoming). On studying film festivals and migration: Borderlands and beginnings. In D. Ostrowska & T. Falicov (Eds.), *Contours of film festival research and methodologies*. Amsterdam University Press.

Karakayalı, S. (2019). Solidarity with refugees. In J. Bock & S. Macdonald (Eds.), *Refugees welcome? Difference and diversity in a changing Germany* (pp. 191–214). Berghahn Books.

Kellner, D., & Lewis, T. (2007). Liberal humanism and the European critical tradition. In W. Outhwaite & S. P. Turner (Eds.), *The SAGE handbook of social science methodology* (pp. 405–422). SAGE.

Kessy, R. (2014). *Decoding the donor gaze: Documentary, aid and AIDS in Africa* [PhD thesis]. University of Huddersfield.

Leavitt, C. (2020). *Italian neorealism: A cultural history*. University of Toronto Press.

Lombardi-Diop, C., & Romeo, C. (2015). State of the union: Survival blankets and falling stars. *Postcolonial Studies, 18*(4), 337–352.

Loist, S. (2016). The film festival circuit: Networks, hierarchies and circulation. In M. de Valck, D. B. Kredell, & S. Loist (Eds.), *Film festivals: History, theory, method, practice* (pp. 49–64). Routledge.

McGowan, T. (2007). *The real gaze: Film theory after Lacan*. State University of New York Press.

Maule, R. (2008). *Beyond auteurism: New directions in authorial film practices in France, Italy and Spain since the 1980s*. Intellect.

Metz, C. (1982). *The imaginary signifier: Psychoanalysis and the cinema*. Indiana University Press.

Moine, C. (2013). La Fédération internationale des associations de producteurs de films: un acteur controversé de la promotion du cinéma après 1945. *Le movement social, 243*, 91–103.

Mulvey, L. (1975). Visual pleasure and narrative cinema. *Screen, 16*(3), 6–18.

Nicolson, M., de Oliveira Andreotti, V., & Mafi, B. F. (2015). The unstated politics of stranger making in Europe: A brutal kindness. *European Journal of Cultural Studies, 19*(4), 335–351.

Nord, L. (2016). "Fire at Sea": How Gianfranco Rosi made an anti-documentary. *No Film School*. [Online]. Available from: https://nofilmschool.com/2016/09/fire-at-sea-gianfranco-rosi-interview

O'Healy, Á. (2010). Mediterranean passages: Abjection and belonging in contemporary Italian cinema. *California Italian Studies, 1*(1), 1–19.

O'Healy, Á. (2019). *Migrant anxieties: Italian cinema in a transnational frame*. Indiana University Press.

O'Leary, A., & Johnson, R. (2022). Flow. In D. Duncan & J. Burns (Eds.), *Transnational modern languages: A handbook* (pp. 123–131). Liverpool University Press.

O'Leary, A., & O'Rawe, C. (2011). Against realism: On a "certain tendency" in Italian film criticism. *Journal of Modern Italian Studies, 16*(1), 107–128.

O'Rawe, C. (2008). "I padri e i maestri": Genre, auteurs, and absences in Italian film studies. *Italian Studies, 63*(2), 173–194.

Ostrowska, D. (2016). Making film history at the Cannes film festival. In M. de Valck, B. D. Kredell, & S. Loist (Eds.), *Film festivals: History, theory, method, practice* (pp. 18–33). Routledge.

Ostrowska, D. (2019). "The migrant gaze" and "the migrant festive chronotope" – Programming the refugee crisis at the European human rights and documentary film festivals. The case of the One World International Human Rights Documentary Film Festival. *Studies in European Cinema, 16*(3), 266–281.

Ponzanesi, S. (2016a). Of shipwrecks and weddings: Borders and mobilities in Europe. *Transnational Cinemas, 7*(2), 151–167.

Rajaram, P. K. (2016). Europe's "Hungarian Solution." *Radical Philosophy, 197*, 2–7.

Rhyne, R. (2009). Film festivals circuits and stakeholders. In D. Iordanova & R. Rhyne (Eds.), *Film festival yearbook 1: The festival circuit* (pp. 9–22). St. Andrews Film Studies & College Gate Press.

Ruberto, L. E., & Wilson, K. M. (Eds.). (2007). *Italian neorealism and global cinema*. Wayne State University Press.

Rumph, R. S. (2011). *I am African: Branding Africa through the gaze of philanthropy* [PhD thesis]. New York University.

Schoonover, K. (2012). *Brutal vision: The neorealist body in postwar Italian cinema*. University of Minnesota Press.

Scott, A. O. (2016). "Fire at Sea" is not the documentary you'd expect about the migrant crisis. It's better. *New York Times*. [Online]. Available from: https://www.nytimes.com/2016/10/21/movies/fire-at-sea-review.html

Táíwò, O. O. (2022). *Elite capture: How the powerful took over identity politics (and everything else)*. Pluto Press.
UNHCR. (1951). *Protocol relating to the status of refugees*. The United Nations Refugee Agency.
UNHCR. (2015). *The sea route to Europe: The Mediterranean passage in the age of refugees*. The United Nations Refugee Agency.
Vallejo, A. (2020). Rethinking the canon: The role of film festivals in shaping film history. *Studies in European Cinema, 17*(2), 155–169.
Waldman, P. (2015). Aylan Kurdi, and the ethics of an image that shocked the world. *The Week*. 4 September 2015. [Online]. Available from: https://theweek.com/articles/575415/aylan-kurdi-ethics-image-that-shocked-world
Wallis, E. (2019). "Beyond the Beach": Venice Film Festival spotlights migration. *InfoMigrants*. 5 September 2019. Available from: https://www.infomigrants.net/en/post/19328/beyond-the-beach-venice-film-festival-spotlights-migration
Wilson, E. (2018). From Lampedusa to the California desert: Gianfranco Rosi's scenes of living and dying. *Film Quarterly, 71*(3), 10–20.
Wilson, J. (2016). The joy of inequality: The libidinal economy of compassionate consumerism. *International Journal of Žižek Studies, 9*(2), 1–26.
Young, L. (1996). *Fear of the dark: "Race," gender and sexuality in the cinema*. Routledge.
Žižek, S. (2001a). *Enjoy your symptom! Jacques Lacan in Hollywood and out* (2nd ed.). Routledge.
Žižek, S. (2004a). *Iraq: The borrowed kettle*. Verso.
Žižek, S. (2008). *Violence: Six sideways reflections*. Profile Books.
Žižek, S. (2016). *Against the double blackmail: Refugees, terror and other troubles with the neighbours*. Penguin.

Filmography

As Far as I Can Walk (Strahinja Banović) (2021). Arsenijević, S. dir. Serbia.
Atlantics (Atlantique) (2019). Diop, M. dir. Sengeal, France.
Fire at Sea (Fuocoammare) (2016). Rosi, G. dir. Italy.
I Was Told There's Freedom Here (2021). Abdalla, A. dir. UK.
Identifying Features (Sin señas particulares) (2020). Valadez, F. dir. Mexico.
Mediterranea (2015). Carpignano, J. dir. Italy/USA.
On the Bride's Side (Io sto con la sposa) (2014). Augugliaro, A., Del Grande, G., & Al Nassiry, K. S. dirs. Italy.
Rome, Open City (Roma, città aperta) (1945). Rossellini, R. dir. Italy.
Terraferma (2011). Crialese, E. dir. Italy.

Section III

Capital

6. Capitalism and Orientalism: *Gomorrah* at Cannes

Abstract: Through the case study of *Gomorrah*'s (Matteo Garrone, 2008) presentation at Cannes, this chapter re-assesses film festivals' claims to both artistic and political universality through the lenses of capitalism and Orientalism. I argue that European A festivals disavow their reproduction of oppressive power structures by displacing the excesses of global capitalism onto a fantasmatic, orientalised South. I investigate the dynamics of transnationalism and "uneven development" in competitive film festivals' programming of films produced and/or set "outside" the North Atlantic. I show that, while Cannes' presentation of *Gomorrah* effectively localises its critique to Southern Italy, the film itself makes manifest the imbrication of the Global North—and even European film festivals—in the ecological and commercial corruption it depicts.

Keywords: globalisation, Eurocentrism, film festivals, Italian cinema, Matteo Garrone, eco-cinema

Power, money and blood: these are the "values" that the residents of the Province of Naples and Caserta, have to face every day. They hardly ever have a choice, and are almost always forced to obey the rules of the "system", the Camorra. Only a lucky few can even think of leading a "normal" life.

Five stories are woven together in this violent scenario, set in a cruel and apparently imaginary world, but one which is deeply rooted in reality.
– *Synopsis of* Gomorrah *in the Cannes 2008 print and online programme*

Introduction

In this book I have analysed the ideological effects of European A festivals' position within, dependence upon, and reproduction of, global capitalism.

Johnson, R., Film Festivals, *Ideology and Italian Art Cinema: Politics, Histories and Cultural Value.* Taylor & Francis Group, 2024
DOI 10.5117/9789463720366_CH06

I have considered how the figure of the auteur, as a *sinthome* of "universal" cinematic art, both conceals and reveals the contradictions of art cinema as a commodity and European A festivals as commercially constrained institutions. Building on this, I have analysed the gendered dimension of this figure to show that the festivals' ideological dependence on the auteur entails the reproduction of masculine dominance or patriarchy. I have also considered how European A festivals' claim to represent the other functions to differentiate them and the films they award from their constitutive outside, Hollywood, while nonetheless reproducing coordinates that make the totality of representation that festivals claim structurally impossible. From this perspective, I have argued that the specific way in which European A festivals represent the other is, when shown as a subject of humanitarian aid, characterised by a "brutal humanism" that is "more reconciled with than resistant to the geopolitical affinities of large-scale capitalism and its multiple battle zones" (Schoonover, 2012, p. xix). In each case, the ideological operation and its effects appear to have a basis in European A festivals' commercial aspect, their need to perform within and ultimately maintain the power structures of a dominant, globalised, capitalist economic system.

Moreover, the effects of this ideological structure—an othering of the queer, the feminine, the migratory—highlight some of the inadmissible or excessive consequences of this economic system, festivals' adherence to it, and the ideological operations required for its upkeep. Such consequences are not solely inadmissible from, say, my perspective as a critic, but appear to be inadmissible to European A festivals themselves. Chapters 3 and 5 have demonstrated some of the specific contortions that these festivals perform in order to both maintain and disavow these excesses: sublimating the masculine auteur as a universal figure of "art" rather than a gendered signifier of patriarchal oppression, or framing the other as a beneficiary of humanitarian aid while disavowing their collusion in the structures that created (for example) refugees' need for aid. In this chapter, I approach the question of European A festivals' relationship to capitalism and its excesses directly. I aim to show one of the ways in which European A festivals might disavow this excess precisely as a necessary consequence of the global dominance of capitalism and the uneven power relations that it entails. European A festivals appear to disavow their reproduction of oppressive power structures not only through claims to artistic universality and humanitarian politics, but also through a displacement of the excesses of global capitalism onto the other constructed by that system—the Global South.

One method of tracing this structure is to analyse how European A festivals construct space, such as the way they represent certain territories within a global capitalist system. I use the term "territory" to designate these large, delimited areas of the globe, profiting from the fluidity of the term as well as its connotations of sovereignty and power (to be territorial is to defend one's territory). I theorise European A festivals' construction of territories through Said's (2003 [1978]) theory of Orientalism, which I put into dialogue with Iain Chambers's (2015) discussion of Orientalism as a constitutive part of Northern, capitalist hegemony. I follow both Chambers and Said in their use of the Gramscian term "hegemony" to designate the intersection between material and symbolic or ideological dominance. Furthermore, on the basis of Chambers's argument, I use the terms "South" or "Global South" over Said's "Orient," as this seems to more accurately reflect the contemporary geopolitical situation, including the well-established "orientalisation" of Southern Italy, a pertinent consideration for this chapter.[1]

Using theories of capitalism as an economic system marked by an "inherent structural imbalance" and "permanent production of an excess" that is ideologically displaced onto the figure of the other, we characterise Orientalism as yet another ideological process of displacement. This leads me to categorise European A festivals' differentiation between North and South as orientalist, as effecting a displacement of global capitalism's antagonisms onto the South as other. I investigate this orientalist dimension of festival ideology through the case of *Gomorrah*'s (*Gomorra*, Garrone, 2008) presentation at Cannes, where it won the Grand Prix in 2008. This marks an exception in the book's methodology, since the film has not won Best Picture (e.g., the Palme d'Or) but a secondary prize. My exclusion of such prizes was largely pragmatic, undertaken on the basis that it would not have been possible to offer the necessary depth of engagement if I included every Italian film that won first and second prizes at a European A festival. Yet, secondary prizes awarded by the "big three," such as the Silver Lion, Silver Bear and Grand Prix, do significantly increase the number of countries in which a film is distributed (Mezias et al., 2011, p. 179).

I have made a specific exception for *Gomorrah*, and not other Italian Grand Prix winners, for several reasons. First, it is, alongside *The Great Beauty*, an Italian film that has had exceptional critical and financial success in the new millennium, becoming a *cause célèbre* of Italian cinema. This

1 See Chambers (2008, 2015), Schneider (1998) and Verdicchio (1997), discussed below. The state of the field regarding Orientalism and Southern Italy is usefully summarised in Ponzanesi (2016b).

can be observed through the film's box office takings and the number of countries in which it was distributed: overall it has made $33,282,383 worldwide and achieved theatrical distribution in 33 countries (Box Office Mojo, 2018a). The film's box office takings are even higher than those of *The Great Beauty* ($24.6 million worldwide between 2013 and 2014) (Box Office Mojo, 2018b). Having secured international attention for Garrone and consecrated him as an auteur, *Gomorrah*'s Grand Prix thus contributed to an institutional and auteurist construction of Italian cinema through the director, alongside Sorrentino and Moretti. Since 2008, the discourse of a "rebirth" promoted by critics, scholars and festivals has focused on these three auteurs (Zagarrio, 2016, p. 7). Cannes in particular has contributed strongly, for example by selecting films directed by the three directors for its main competition in 2015—an unusually strong presence of Italian cinema at the festival.[2] Aside from the significance of films directed by all three being included in the same Cannes programme, the framing of the auteurs' inclusion by key cinema and festival publications also suggests their centrality to discourses of Italian film. CineEuropa photographed Sorrentino, Garrone and Moretti and reported that they were "in it together for Italian film" (De Marco, 2015). The piece promoted the trio as emblematic of the Italian film industry, as embodying Italian cinema (see chapters 2 and 3). From his breakthrough with *Gomorrah* to the time of writing (having won a further Grand Prix for *Reality* [2012]), Garrone has become a key figure in the international construction of Italian cinema. Since this book is concerned with the films that best exemplify European A festivals' construction of Italian cinema, this *cause célèbre* is a crucial case study.

Moreover, *Gomorrah*'s institutional legitimation and representation exemplifies the intersection between global capitalism and the North's construction of the other. The idea of *Gomorrah* as a realist depiction of a violent, distant locality of Southern Italy permeates both scholars' and film festivals' paratextual constructions of the film, indicating the prevalence of an orientalist "radical realism" that structures representations of othered cultures, representations that "can create not only knowledge but also the very reality they appear to describe" (Said, 2003 [1978], p. 72). I demonstrate and critique the ideological process at work in the Cannes synopsis through

2 We might note the same level of participation by Italian films was reproduced in 2018, now with two female directors: Garrone's *Dogman* and Alice Rohrwacher's *Happy as Lazzaro* were both screened in competition and won awards, while Valeria Golino's *Euphoria* was screened as part of the Un Certain Regard programme. Neither Rohrwacher nor Golino have been afforded the status of "representative" of Italian cinema in the way Garrone has, signalling the persistence of patriarchal biases in European film culture and criticism.

an analysis of scenes and narratives that are not only omitted by the Cannes text, but directly contradict its depiction of the film as being set in a distant territory characterised by otherness and excess. Through its eco-Mafia and fashion narratives, *Gomorrah* makes manifest the North's exportation and displacement of its most inadmissible aspects onto an exploited, orientalised South. The latter fashion narrative contains real footage from the Venice film festival, implicating the film, the viewer, and the European A festival apparatus in this process of displacing and disavowing the othering of the South, a process that underpins the uneven circulation of products and power in the global capitalist system.

European A Festivals' Construction of Space

Transnational or Territorial?

European A festivals' transnationality paradoxically requires an ideological investment in notions of national or territorial difference. These festivals can be thought to construct a world—and one that largely reproduces existing power relations. This involves not only the performance of European hegemony, but the representation of certain areas as "outside" that hegemony, often through the characterisation of them as homogenous, distant or inferior. The world that European A festivals construct aligns with the interests of a global capitalism that requires the unfettered transnational flow of goods and services, and non-(re)distribution of power.[3] Several studies of film festivals demonstrate or, at least suggest, a contradiction between these institutions' relationship to the transnational and territorial. On the one hand, film festivals are the "driving force of the global circulation of cinema" and "international flow of culture and capital" (Iordanova & Rhyne, 2009, p. 1; Andrews, 2010, p. 10). They are "transnational spaces," or "post-national," and even embedded in a global economic system that emphasises "deterritorialisation" (Mazdon, 2006, p. 23; de Valck, 2007, p. 69). On the other hand, their promotion of the transnational and facilitation of global trade to an extent depends on their differentiation of films and cultures along national and territorial lines. This entails a symbolic reconstruction of those very borders that would limit the transnational flow of goods.

3 This is one of the ways in which European A festivals participate in one of the fundamental paradoxes of our times: the contradiction between globalised, "free" trade and heavily policed borders. See Amin (2018), Jabri (2013), Rose (2007), Bauman (2000) and Appadurai (1990).

De Valck (2007, p. 68) argues that major film festivals (including, but not only, European A festivals) are embedded within a global system invested in the reproduction of difference—that which she designates the "postmodern" capitalist system. She describes the "new power relations on the international film festival circuit" through Michael Hardt and Antonio Negri's (2000) theory of "Empire" in postmodernity (defined as the 1980s and '90s, although de Valck implies that it extends to the present):

> [T]he ideology of the world market comes into full bloom when matched with postmodern and post-colonial convictions, because postmodernity's pet subjects such as circulation, mobility, diversity, and mixture are profitable to global trade. The world market embraces the deconstruction of nation-states and promotes open global markets and product differentiation. The differences between people, in their turn, are seen as market opportunities. (de Valck, 2007, pp. 69–70)

In the postmodern period, film festivals are embedded in the "ideology of the world market," which requires them to sell difference, in turn reproducing neo-colonial power relations. De Valck thus argues that, despite major festivals' claims to post-nationalism, the national reappears on the festival agenda in a way that reproduces the uneven development and power relations that characterise the film industry in the current global economic system.

De Valck's assessment implies that festivals' means of securing economic and symbolic capital through a process that differentiates cinemas on the basis of where they were produced may also entail the reproduction of colonial power structures. Likewise, writing on the spatial and power dynamics of film festivals, Stringer (2001, p. 137) argues that the construction of space across the festival network is "a metaphor for the geographically uneven development that characterises the world of international film culture." This entails the reproduction of the "core" via larger, more successful festivals (for example, the concentration of A festivals in Europe) and the "periphery" to which smaller festivals are relegated (social interest festivals, major un-accredited festivals outside Europe) (Stringer, 2001, p. 138).[4] Moreover, this results in an uneven distribution of power over which films, and from which territories, receive legitimation: Stringer (2001, p. 135) identifies the assumption across institutional representations of film that "non-Western cinemas do not count historically until they have

4 One might similarly theorise the peripheral status of "women's festivals"; see Chapter 3.

been recognised by the apex of international media power, the center of which is located, by implication, at Western film festivals." Such an analysis epitomises the relationship between the spatial politics and economic system that European A festivals reproduce. Uneven development, the economic impoverishment of some territories and not others, is reflected through cultural unevenness, for example the ghettoisation of films from some territories and legitimation of those from others.

While the differentiation of films on the basis of their main country of production may still occur in film festivals' representations of all sorts of films, the power relations implied vary depending on how that site of production is framed. Here we might productively consider the distinction between production fetishism (defining a product through its relation to its perceived site of production) and cultural essentialism (defining a location or territory in a way that ascribes it an intrinsic truth or homogenous meaning).[5] When the two intersect, a product is defined in relation to an essentialised culture, as an artefact representing the "truth" of that culture. While cultural essentialism and production fetishism are not mutually exclusive, identifying when and how each is deployed assists an understanding of the power dynamics involved in European A festivals' construction of certain territories.

This distinction is most apparent in the way that A festivals construct borders through their programming, the most obvious case of their symbolic reconstruction of space within the event. Using the examples of the Toronto International Film Festival's "Planet Africa" or "Discover Canada" sections, Liz Czach (2004, p. 83) argues that the differentiation between films shown in these territorially-defined fringes and those that enter the main competition constructs a "hierarchy," with fringe sections "perceived as ghettos for underperforming work." However, in taking both "Planet Africa" and "Discover Canada" as examples of the same kind of differentiation or ghettoisation of filmmaking from countries not yet perceived as canonical in world cinema, she misses a crucial distinction between the two sections. Toronto's "Discover Canada" fringe affords Canada national specificity and can best be understood as a typical example of a festival promoting the cinema of the country in which it takes place. On the European A circuit, for example, the Berlinale has its "Perspektive Deutsches Kino" section, Karlovy Vary, its "Czech Films" section and so on. This is part of a process

5 For an extended discussion of production fetishism and its role in obscuring the contradictions of global capitalism, see Appadurai (1990). I take cultural essentialism in its basic sense for now but develop it later through the theory of Orientalism.

of production fetishism in which a festival differentiates and therefore markets itself and its host country's films on the basis of their association with a particular national culture.

The politics implied by Toronto's "Planet Africa" section are, by contrast, expressive of a wider trend in A-list festivals, in which "difference" is included "within token sidebar programmes [in a way that] protects the structures absences and margins of the festivals" (Rastegar, 2012, p. 312). Presenting "other" cultures, particularly those from the Global South, within fringe programmes is an extension of the "anglo-western impulses to construct representations of third-world and developing countries" that Rastegar (2012, p. 312) argues is characteristic of many festivals' practices, encompassing not only their programming but also discursive construction of nations (Chan, 2011) and aid-inflected funding schemes (Ross, 2011). Such practices do not entail only production fetishism, but a cultural essentialism that homogenises and differentiates filmmaking from the entire Southern Hemisphere.

Manthia Diawara's (2010) study of African cinema underlines a further level of cultural essentialism: African filmmaking is often not even afforded specificity as a regional cinema but is rather subsumed into notions of "world cinema." Anticipating recent challenges to the term as a cipher for peripheral (read: non-Western) films (Jeong, 2021), Diawara argues that this is a category "by which festivals understand everything that is neither American nor European [...] a new invention of films from the non-Western world that comfort Europeans in their paternalistic supremacy vis-à-vis the Third World and in their struggle against Hollywood" (p. 86). Dovey (2015, p. 53) resumes Diawara's criticism of the treatment of African cinema by European A festivals, particularly Cannes, demonstrating their relative homogenisation under notions of world cinema vis-à-vis "the same, uniform, worldly language" and an exoticist exhibitionism with roots in the world fairs of colonial times. She grounds this in A festivals' "sporadic and isolated" programming of African films, further noting their particular absence from main competitions and award lists.[6] That such films remain

6 Dovey (2015, p. 51) notes, for example, that *Chroniques des années de braise* (Mohammed Lakhdar-Hamina, 1975) was, in 2015, the only "film by and African and set in Africa to be awarded the Palme d'Or." While other African films have won awards at other A festivals, they remain few and far between, with the top prize continuously elusive. For example, although Dovey suggests that *Camp de Thiaroye* (Ousmane Sembene, 1989) won the prize for "best film" at Venice, it actually won the Special Jury Prize. While still an important prize, this does not counter African filmmakers' exclusion from the "gold" category of awards, and even if it did, this would remain an exception rather than the rule.

under-represented at European A festivals overall and, when programmed, often find themselves out of competition or winning minor, specialised prizes, suggests a further "ghettoisation" of the type suggested by Czach and Rastegar. That such practices appear to result in vague apprehension of African films under that geopolitically-complex category of world cinema suggests a mode of deterritorialisation that not only essentialises the African continent, but the entire Global South.

While Dovey's focus is primarily on Cannes and African cinema, her argument has implications for programming practices towards "non-European" filmmaking across the European A circuit. Such practices are commonplace, and so, for the sake of brevity, I offer just one here: Karlovy Vary's "East of the West" section, which groups together films from "Central and Eastern Europe, the Balkans, Greece, the countries of the former Soviet Union and the Middle East" (Karlovy Vary, 2019). In an intriguing case of self-orientalisation, Karlovy Vary differentiates the films produced in these areas of the world through their status as "Eastern" in relation to a "West" positioned as core: the East is "*of*" the West, not vice versa (italics added). The contrast between A festivals' sections indicates one way in which they might construct filmmaking from outside North America and Europe—more precisely, *Western* Europe—on the basis of its difference from a hegemonic centre. In such cases, the film product is fetishised as not from a particular nation, or even a vaguely coherent region, but a large, homogenised territory that includes, with ever-diminishing specificity, Greece, the Balkans, former Soviet countries and the Middle East. Such instances, while they may appear innocent or even playfully ironic on the surface, reproduce the spatial dynamics that characterise globally uneven development and geopolitical regimes of power, affording the Global North the status of subject and everywhere else that of other.

Moving the discussion towards how films and filmmakers are represented within the main competition, Elsaesser (2016, p. 27) has considered how films and auteurs from all territories are caught up in the process of "performing nationalism" required by the film festival apparatus. Appearing to apply a post-colonial framework to the construction of films from both colonial and colonising countries, he highlights the centrality of this power dynamic at work in film festivals' apparent internationalism: "this openness can be a trap: it is an open invitation to self-conscious ethnicity and re-tribalisation, it quickly shows its affinity or even collusion [...] with a post-colonial [or neo-colonial] and subaltern sign-economy" (p. 25). Reminiscent of the critiques of world cinema above, Elsaesser locates this sign-economy along-side the broad structures of capitalist globalisation that gave us "cultural tourism, [and] fusion-food-world-music-ethnic-cuisine Third Worldism in the capitals of the first world" (p. 25). From world music to world cinema, this performed cosmopolitanism produces "a tendency of films within the festival circuit—whether from Asia, Africa, or Europe—to respond and to comply, by gestures that amount to a kind of 'self-exoticising' or 'auto-orientalism'" (p. 26). Elsaesser identifies a power dynamic similar to those involved in the negotiation of production fetishism and cultural essentialism in film culture. Moreover, this leads to a performance of identity that prompts the kinds of "self-exoticising" or "auto-Orientalism" we saw in cases such as Karlovy Vary's "East of the West."

Elsaesser applies this dynamic to European cinema, including Italian cinema. *Gomorrah*, for example, "performatively enacts" a "national cinematic lineage" of "neorealism, spaghetti Western, and Pasolini" (p. 27). Again, while Elsaesser's assessment is not incorrect, it misses the distinction between the performance of nationalism that assists the production fetishism required to market films from any part of the world and the auto-Orientalism that assists the cultural essentialisation of films and territories in the Global South. There is an important qualitative difference here: performing a national heritage, if that heritage is not discursively defined as "oriental" or other, is distinct from Orientalism. Therefore, one must analyse how films associated with the Global North are represented in an aspect that may be nationalist but still maintains their place within the dominant centre, while those associated with the Global South are positioned as outside this centre.

Building on Elsaesser's assessment, I would like to pose three counter-questions: (1) beyond a cinematic lineage, what other kinds of territorial or national identity are films required to perform? (2) How does this relate not only to where a film is made, but where it is set? And (3) how and when does this take on a specifically orientalist character, and in relation to which spaces? I hope to begin answering these questions by picking up Elsaesser's reference to Orientalism and showing its relevance as a framework for understanding both how cinematic institutions such as European A festivals construct the Global South, and how this is, in fact, a procedure intimately bound up with such festivals' dependence on and maintenance of global capitalism. I argue that these festivals' embeddedness in a postmodern capitalist system requires their marketing of difference, and also necessitates that this difference take on an orientalist dimension in representations of the Global South. In the latter case, this is because the global capitalist system in which festivals are imbricated also depends upon the construction of a subordinate other that it can exploit economically and onto which it can displace its internal antagonisms.

Orientalism and Capitalism

Randal Halle (2010) approaches the questions I have asked above using a similar lens. The crucial feature of Orientalism, he argues, is "an elaborate set of textual references [that] had developed in Europe by which that which was fundamentally proximate is kept distant" (Halle, 2010, p. 314). This arises "through the intervention and mediation of a set of cultural texts that speak the truth of the other on behalf of that other" (p. 314). Halle demonstrates the prevalence of these tropes of distance and of cultural texts that speak the truth for the other in a way that intervenes in the intersection between production fetishism and cultural essentialism. Using the case study of the German Federal Agency for Civic Education's educational pamphlets about films, he argues that co-productions funded through the EUROMED programme (an EU programme that offers financial support for co-productions involving countries along "Mediterranean trade routes") are institutionally framed in a way that essentialises both their supposed country of origin and their setting (p. 305).[7] First, the pamphlets present these films as national productions, focusing on the non-European production partner. Developing Halle's claim, we can note that this is a particular case of production fetishism that lays the foundation for cultural essentialism: the catalogues present these films as originating solely in a conceptually distant and other culture.

The texts also describe the films as "revealing a truth" about the culture they depict, a tendency unseen in respective representations of films wholly produced by and set in European countries (Halle, 2010, p. 316). This, Halle argues, reproduces a cultural essentialisation of the Global South in which films made and set there are constructed as intrinsically culturally distant from Europe. To return to a quotation from Chapter 4:

> Something happens in films and in the institutions of promotion and criticism to establish a (cultural) distance between the viewer and viewed, to establish a differential on one side of which the story is about another culture through which I learn. (Halle, 2010, p. 315)

Central to this is the idea that such films can "offer insight into a type of person, if not an entire people," which, in turn, implies that these people have an essential quality that can be represented and pinned down for

7 On the ambivalences of film funding schemes offered to Global Southern filmmakers, particularly via film festivals, see Falicov (2010) and Ross (2011).

the European viewer. Production fetishism is complemented by cultural essentialism in which a film is framed as being both from and about a non-European culture in a way that distances and essentialises this culture.

To specify further how the Global South might be represented, and whose interests this might serve, I turn to the source underpinning Halle's analysis: Said's *Orientalism*. For the purposes of this chapter, the most useful definition of Orientalism that Said (2003 [1978] offers is his third "more historically and materially defined" one, as it concerns the institutional construction of the "Orient" (taken as fluid, its borders changing over history) as a means of consolidating European, capitalist hegemony since the Enlightenment (p. 3). Orientalism is, in this sense,

> the corporate institution for dealing with the Orient—dealing with it by making statements about it, authorising views of it, describing it, by teaching it settling it, ruling over it: in short, Orientalism as a Western style for dominating, restructuring, and having authority over the Orient (Said, 2003 [1978], p. 3).

Said's definition here aims at Orientalism in its corporate, institutional manifestation in which certain authorised ways of representing the "Orient" (or Global South) assist in its domination. This domination is economic, but also reproduced "politically, sociologically, militarily, ideologically, scientifically, and imaginatively" (p. 3). In relation to the European A festival apparatus outlined above, this form of Orientalism is best understood, therefore, as at the intersection of economic, political and ideological-cultural reproduction of the North's hegemony.

In its corporate-institutional aspect, Orientalism is tightly bound up with capitalist expansion. Orientalism in this sense originated and continues to be mobilised as a means of reinforcing a particular definition of "civilisation" that would later benefit Northern Atlantic states' pursuit of capitalist economic development (from industrial to post-industrial), colonial expansion (including neo-colonial interventions in the Middle East) and a liberal democracy suited to supporting these values.[8] Building on Said's work, Chambers (2015) has noted how the differentiation of the Global South is crucial for the maintenance of a capitalist hegemony that originated in and still favours European and American territories. Viewed from metropolitan centres such as Los Angeles, Berlin or Paris (and, perhaps, Cannes), the South is symbolically framed as "inadequate," "rendered subordinate and

8 Said develops this argument himself in *Culture and Imperialism* (1993).

subaltern to other forces, and [...] exploited, not only economically, but also politically and culturally, in order for that subalternity to be reproduced and reinforced" (p. 13). In fact, the North's hegemony depends upon its construction of a subaltern other:

> the South, of Italy, of Europe, of the Mediterranean, of the world, is rendered both marginal but paradoxically central to the reproduction of that [Northern, capitalist] economy. If the whole world were equally modern, then modernity as we know it would collapse. (Chambers, 2015, p. 13)

Global capitalism depends upon "subordinate" places for its economic sustenance (for example, cheap labour) as well as its symbolic authority (exemplified by the relation of power implied in terms such as "subordinate" and "inadequate"). Taking Chambers's analysis together with the scholarship on film festivals reviewed above, we can hypothesise that the Global South continues to fulfil the role of constitutive other not only in literary and academic texts, but also in those produced by European A film festivals.

As we saw from Chambers's description of the metropolitan North's construction of the South, Orientalism is central to an economic and ideological order that relies upon the construction of subordinate places—on the reproduction of inequality. To delve more deeply into the ideological aspect of this, I return to Said's (2003 [1978]) original theory:

> [T]he imaginative examination of things Oriental was based more or less exclusively upon a sovereign Western consciousness out of whose unchallenged centrality the Oriental world emerged [...] according to a detailed logic governed not simply by empirical reality but by a battery of *desires, repressions, investments and projections*. (p. 8; italics added)

Such "projections" and "repressions" can be best understood in relation to psychoanalytical theory, as this is where the terms originated. The orientalised South is represented as Europe's "contrasting image, idea, personality, experience" and, more pointedly, its "surrogate or underground self" (Said, 2003 [1978], p. 3). This culminates in a catalogue of stereotypes, according to which "European superiority"—as rational, modern and humanist—depends upon its construction of ideas of "Oriental backwardness," as irrational, uncivilised and autocratic (Said, 2003 [1978], p. 7; Macfie, 2000, p. 8). Since the foundation of Said's theory is the claim that the tropes through which orientalist discourses characterise the South are generated in the North, these stereotypes can generally be understood as the excessive, obscene underside of the colonisers' community, each being the binary opposite, the "underground" version, of Europe's self-image (Said, 2003 [1978], p. 3). These discourses involve the displacement of the North's negative, inadmissible aspects onto an other. Developing the implicit psychoanalytical reasoning in Said's theory (which functions alongside and in tension with its Foucauldian foundations), Homi K. Bhabha (1983, p. 31) summarises how this works: the colonised figure is an "alienating other, (or mirror) which crucially returns its image to the subject." Understanding Orientalism through the framework of psychoanalysis, we can therefore describe it as the process by which the hegemonic system constructs its own positive image by displacing its excessive aspects onto its constitutive outside.

We can elucidate this process's ideological character and its function within global capitalism further by using Žižek's theory of capitalism as excess, and fantasy as a means of managing this excess (a sort of waste management, as we will see later). Žižek argues that capitalism is defined by "inherent structural imbalance," a "permanent production of an excess" (Žižek, 1993, p. 208). This excess is, however, not only economic, as in the classical Marxist notion of surplus value, but also symbolic, as in the Lacanian notion of the Real—the unrepresentable "excess" of the symbolic order. The only way to manage such imbalance, to give the impression of capitalism as a coherent, viable economic system, is to displace it onto an "alienating other." This is observable in that which Žižek designates the "fascist dream [...] to have capitalism without its 'excess,' without its structural imbalance" (p. 210). This "fascist dream" requires the figure of an "alien intruder" who is constructed as the "cause [of] the antagonistic imbalance" (p. 210). This results in a typical procedure of othering, with its corollary stereotypes of dirt, irrationality and greed (p. 210). As such, this ideological process may be operative beyond fascist ideology per se, understandable in relation to Orientalism or even, as I suggested in the previous chapter, liberal humanism. Žižek uses Lacan's theory of the mirror stage in a similar way to Bhabha, concluding that "the fascinating image of the Other gives a body to our own innermost split [...]. The hatred of the Other is the hatred of our own excess of enjoyment" (p. 206).

Through this displacement, the Southern other becomes representative of the "excessive" aspects of capitalism: violence, corruption, poverty and filth. As I have argued throughout this book, a Lacanian framework allows us to understand the other as a destabilising, rather than securing, figure. Their image can be mobilised to critique the social order, revealing the excess and antagonism internal to it. Beyond the structural level—the social order's inherent split—a psychoanalytical reading of Orientalism allows us to consider the way in which the particular characteristics of the other make manifest the inadmissible characteristics of the social order in global capitalism, as well as European A festival ideology (itself embedded within global capitalism). The violence and corruption associated with the Global South can be interpreted as the Global North's own displaced violence and corruption. To interrogate the excessive other in this way (as I will argue *Gomorrah* does) opens the possibility for a radical critique of the hegemonic social order from which this excess originates.

Overall, European A festivals appear to invest in a territorial distinction between a hegemonic North and an othered South that can be understood as Orientalism in its corporate-institutional form. I have shown this, in part, through a discussion of film festivals' construction of space in a way that produces the Global South as a homogenous and culturally distant territory, defined in opposition to the North. Film festivals' perceived status as "the driving force of the global circulation of cinema" and their ability to "facilitate international flows of culture and capital" via their main competitions may depend on their categorisation of cinema in terms of territories, with part of their prestige coming from their claim to offer "encounters with unfamiliar cultures" (de Valck, 2007, p. 71). European A festivals invest in an ideological differentiation between the Global South and the Global North, the former being ascribed particularity and the latter universality—and this is crucial to the festivals' status as institutions that facilitate (and depend on) the circulation of financial and symbolic capital. However, there is still much work to be done to comprehend the extent to which European A festivals' construction of the South may also translate into a representation of this territory as not only distant but other in the sense of corrupted, excessive; it is a figure representing, in short, the inadmissible "underground" aspects of the North. Moreover, there has to my knowledge not yet been a study of how these festivals represent culture and territory *within* their descriptions of certain films. Film festivals' depictions of films as being about, and perhaps set solely within, a certain territory is an important aspect of their overall construction of that territory that goes beyond their promotion of certain "new" cinemas (or new waves) via, for example, fringe sections or competition selections and awards. The remainder of this chapter will therefore focus on how European A festivals construct the countries or territories a film is framed as being *produced* in but also *set* in. To provide a foundation for analysing European A festivals' orientalist representation of the South as not only an effect of but also a means of reinforcing a system of global capitalism that favours the North while exploiting the South, I turn now to the case study of *Gomorrah*'s presentation at Cannes.

Gomorrah: An Orientalist Realism?

The categorisation of South as other also recurs in both scholarly and various paratextual interpretations of the film. These use notions of realism to imply that *Gomorrah* represents the "truth" of Naples as a violent, Southern (orientalised) place. *Gomorrah*'s setting in Southern Italy appears to have been the basis for the reproduction of orientalist representations of the film by critics, scholars and, as we will see later, Cannes. I ground this interpretation of institutional representations of *Gomorrah* and its setting in theories of Southern Italy's complex post-colonial condition often interpreted through theories of Orientalism. This tradition of thought begins with Antonio Gramsci's (1994 [1926]) analysis of the "Southern Question" and has since been developed by scholars such as Paolo Verdicchio (1997), who raises the question of internal colonisation in Italy, and Jane Schneider, whose introduction to a collection of essays entitled *Italy's "Southern Question": Orientalism in One Country* moves from a framework of internal colonisation to internal orientalisation.

Schneider (1998) observes that the "Southern Question" evokes an opposition between provinces south of Rome and those in the North (Italian and European). This opposition generates a "tenacious catalogue of stereotypes" that casts Southerners as "unable to build the rational, orderly, civic cultures that, in the North, underwrote the emergence of industrial capitalist society" (p. 1). Regions south of Rome are continuously opposed to an image of the North as rational, democratic, prosperous and orderly through tropes of Southerners as "passionate, undisciplined, [and] rebellious" (p. 1). Similarly, the South is cast as a site solely of "poverty and underdevelopment [...] a clientalistic style of politics [...] patriarchal gender relations and various manifestations of organised crime" (p. 1). These stereotypes are imbricated with the material subordination of the Italian South. Scholars have repeatedly shown that the area's continuing "economic underdevelopment" (for want of a less loaded term) was caused by successive, North-based Italian governments' forceful integration of the South into its economy and political structure, treating the South as "a *terra dimissione*" (Tarrow, 1996, p. 394). This process has resulted in regions such as Sicily occupying a subordinate position in relation not only to Italy, but to global capitalism.

Being both within and outside this system, the South occupies a liminal space between European modernity and Global Southern post-coloniality, and appears most clearly as the site of both Italy's and Europe's projected anxieties—again, its inadmissible underside, as argued by O'Healy (2010). Chambers (2008, p. 32) describes the Mediterranean as "an intricate site of encounters and currents" between North and South, which reveals the former's "repressed rhythms and reasons." Building on this assessment, Ponzanesi (2016b, p. 152) argues that "the Italian South can be a place from where a critique of Western developmental teleologies can be sustained [...] from within, demonstrating modernity's incompleteness and interruptions." Viewing Southern Italy through theories of Orientalism not only corresponds with its symbolic and material construction as European capitalist modernity's other, but shows its important position as a liminal space from which a critique of this centre can be mounted.

Critical constructions of *Gomorrah* often appear to reproduce Orientalism in their characterisation of the film as operating in the realist mode. Such descriptions of the film manifest a latent investment in an orientalist "radical realism" that affords access to the "truth" of the South from the vantage point of the relationally superior North (Said, 2003 [1978], p. 72). Significantly, this permeates reviews of *Gomorrah* in the festival press. The *Screen Daily* review that accompanied the film's presentation at Cannes described it as "[p]robably the most authentic and unsentimental mafia movie ever to come out of Italy" (Marshall, 2008, para. 1). Likewise, the *Variety* review praises the film's blending of fiction with a "dispassionate docu style" to "show how the Camorra's vice-like grip on the region infects everyone, creating a permanent miasma of fear that terrorises some while proving impossibly seductive to others" (Weissberg, 2008, para. 3). *Gomorrah* may be fictional in some respects, but Weissberg ascribes its style and content a revelatory function. The article implies that the film offers audiences access to the truth about a despotically controlled region whose inhabitants are subjects of violence or seduction. The focus on the film's Southern Italian setting is accompanied by the same orientalist stereotypes of autocracy (as opposed to humanism and democracy) and irrationality (violent or sexual impulses, as opposed to rationality) discussed above. Key articles in the festival press already indicate the festival apparatus's potential to construct the film as a realist depiction of a distant, Southern territory defined by its oriental character, a character determined by its opposition to the supposed norms of the democratic, rational North.

Ideas of *Gomorrah*'s objective representation of Southern Italy are also ubiquitous in scholarly discussions of the film. They might be considered, therefore, in relation to Orientalism as a discourse engaged in "authorising views," producing norms for "describing" or "teaching" about the South. In the institutions of film criticism and scholarship, realism and objectivity seem to constitute the authorised views of *Gomorrah* as a film about Southern Italy. For example, Flavia Cavaliere (2010) argues that

> [i]n contrast to Hollywood's appropriation and glamorisation of the gang culture of Italy, "*Gomorra(h)*" stands in the Italian neorealist tradition, preferring actual locations to elaborate film sets and ordinary people to movie stars in order to expose the rest of the world to the actuality of the contemporary violence of the Camorra and the extent to which its tentacles reach. (p. 176)

This assessment reproduces several of the tropes discussed in previous chapters, pertaining to the ideological construction of Italian cinema: opposition to Hollywood, a neorealist, perhaps brutal address, and representation of the other. Such tropes, as with the other case studies I have analysed, may be key to *Gomorrah*'s success at Cannes.

However, Cavaliere's evaluation of *Gomorrah* alerts us to another important value: the representation of othered cultures in relation to a film's claim to realism and ethics. She asserts that *Gomorrah*'s

> bleak portrayal of what is represented to be present reality can be compared to a film such as Fernando Meirelles's *City of God* (2002), the Brazilian movie which portrayed ferocious teenage drug gangs in one of Rio de Janeiro's slums. (Cavaliere, 2010, p. 176)

This comparison implies a shared project of realistically depicting and critiquing the violence of a place in the Global South and on the peripheries of global capitalism (gang-controlled slums in Brazil or suburbs in Naples). Given the comparable success of *City of God* and *Gomorrah*, they might be productively understood in relation to a global ideology of cinema in which films are valued for their depiction of Southern places in a realist mode. (*City of God* earned $30,641,770 in box office takings worldwide, a similar figure to *Gomorrah* [Box Office Mojo, 2019].) Notably, however, realism is more a claim than inherent aspect of a film. *Gomorrah*'s realism, like that of *City of God*, lies in tautology: "what is represented to be present reality" (Cavaliere, 2010, p. 176). Therefore, one ought to be vigilant when this claim is made and consider what ideology it may serve. Such questions will become crucial to understanding the orientalist-capitalist ideology condensed in Cannes's representation of *Gomorrah* as a realist, critical and territorially-circumscribed film.

The relationship between realism, critique and othered places continues, but is complicated, in Fabrizio Ciliento's (2011) analysis of the film. Ciliento argues that *Gomorrah* can be read within the heritage of Roberto Rossellini's war trilogy, *Rome, Open City, Paisan* (*Paisà*, 1948) and *Germany*

Year Zero (*Germania anno zero*, 1949), and Gillo Pontecorvo's *The Battle of Algiers* (*La battaglia di Algeri*, 1966)—above all, through the film's use of techniques such as long takes, natural lighting, use of dialogue in dialect or local languages, and its cast mixing professional and non-professional actors. For Ciliento, the film's engagement with what he describes as an Italian neorealist heritage is integral for the film's representation of Le Vele as "the Neapolitan junkspace [...] a symbol of the country's different economic synchronies and of the permanence of the Third World within the First World" (para. 23). This realist depiction of Naples is crucial to the film's critique, which re-inserts the imagined space of the "Third World" back into that of the "First World." This association of Naples with the "Third World", and celebration of a realist aesthetic as that which is best suited to represent it, echo Cavaliere's comparison of *Gomorrah* with *City of God*. Again, the notion of a realist depiction of an othered place (i.e., the "Third World") contains orientalist overtones, implying as it does an essential reality that *Gomorrah* is able to "realistically" represent. The celebration of *Gomorrah* and its realist style, while taken as a marker of its national heritage, at once obscures and reproduces the power dynamics involved in these notions of the film's representation of Southern Italy.[9]

Ciliento does not restrict the film to an Italian political and/or realist tradition, however, arguing that "*Gomorrah* is an ambitious film that overcomes the present impasses of Italian neorealist heritage by blending it with noir moral ambiguity and visual culture" (para. 7). He argues that *noir* is crucial to *Gomorrah*'s political commentary insofar as it cites *noir* and science fiction films such as *Double Indemnity* (Billy Wilder, 1944) and *Blade Runner* (Ridley Scott, 1982), and invokes a similar critique of global capitalism. This, he continues, complements *Gomorrah*'s depiction of Nigerian and Chinese Mafia, and the superimposed text that appears at the end of the film (which states that the Camorra has invested in the rebuilding of the Twin Towers site) to facilitate the film's critique of global capitalism. Thus, style and content give *Gomorrah* a transnational dimension adapted to depicting the unlocalisable power that characterises relations in and beyond Naples (para. 26). It is significant here that Ciliento associates the film's Italian and realist dimension with its representation of a locality—Naples as "Third World"—in contrast to its transnational and generic dimension (*noir*, science fiction), here associated with the film's critique of global power structures. This is not to say that Ciliento creates a stable binary; his article overall can be read as a synthesis that, perhaps like the film, complicates binary notions

9 On the relationship between post-colonial representation and neorealism, see Chapter 5.

of local/global or realist/generic. However, the piece also responds to, and thus highlights, a trope we should be aware of when we approach Cannes's representation of *Gomorrah*: the association of realism with the critical depiction of localised themes, in contrast with that of supposedly more transnational styles (such as science-fiction) with the critical depiction of global themes and unlocalisable power. Therefore, it seems pertinent to ask how far Cannes's representation of the film foregrounds the film's local or global location, and the relations of power condensed in such a representation.

We can begin to find a basis from which to answer these questions in other paratexts accompanying its presentation at Cannes. Focusing on interviews and press packs, Holdaway (2014, p. 202) analyses a "realist rhetoric" that he argues is not only present in the film but, above all, in its paratexts.[10] Most significant for our purposes is Holdaway's analyses of the descriptions Garrone and scriptwriter Roberto Saviano offer of the film in press packs and in interviews at Cannes. He takes these descriptions as rhetorical—not objective statements of the filmmakers' intentions, but part of a highly mediated strategy. These representations of the film *perform* realism, and are "symptoms" of a critical discourse about realism and its ethical import. In this way, the paratexts Holdaway analyses can and should be read alongside the synopsis of the film in the Cannes programme, here taken as symptomatic in the same sense. Both are surface-level indications of a similar overarching "rhetoric" or, more pointedly, ideology.

The texts Holdaway highlights merit reproduction here, since they are pertinent to the Cannes synopsis of *Gomorrah* analysed below:

> The events you are about to witness are inspired by real events and ones that continue to occur in areas of Naples such as Scampia and Caserta. There, as in other places, the lives of thousands of men and women, many youths among them, are conditioned by the power and violence of criminals. (Saviano, 2008, p. 6; cited in Holdaway, 2014, p. 201)

Holdaway reads Saviano's introduction to the film, written to accompany its Cannes premiere, as an appeal, addressed to the audience (the Cannes-accredited film critics and professionals), to take the film as a "testimony of the real Scampia" (p. 201). Saviano frames the film as a realist depiction of a specific place—Scampia, the suburbs of Naples. The writer invokes the trope of a film "inspired by real events," which he locates first in Naples, but also in "other places." The term "other" is overdetermined; it has a variety of

10 All translations of Holdaway's article and its sources are my own.

meanings, some of which may appear more pertinent in certain contexts. If we consider the limitations to meaning effected by the European A festival apparatus (its actual construction of the other and of territory), Saviano's reference to other places can (and is likely to) be interpreted as signifying a generalised notion of the Global South, of which Naples is a signifier. These "other places" likely refer to, in this context, the othered places of the Global South, homogenised and associated with "criminal power and violence," represented through a realist lens that claims to speak the truth of these places on their behalf.

A rhetoric of realism continues in Garrone's "director's note" included in the Cannes press pack:

> The material that I started from when filming *Gomorrah* was so visually powerful that I limited myself to shooting it in an extremely simple manner, as though I were a spectator who had happened upon the place by chance. This seemed to me to be the most effective way of reproducing the emotional experience that I'd had during the course of working on the film. (Garrone, 2008, p. 4; cited in Holdaway, 2014, p. 203)

These comments, Holdaway argues, imply that *Gomorrah* should be understood as "objective, like a form of video surveillance," attested to by the expression "an extremely simple manner, as though I were a spectator" (p. 204). Holdaway (2014, p. 204) continues that Garrone has also emphasised "verisimilitude" and his use of "war reportage" techniques in interviews held at Cannes. Garrone's comments promote a reading of *Gomorrah* as a film whose political status is bound up with its documentary value, its "ability to be informative and objective" (p. 204). Again, we find the tropes of realism as objectivity, an objectivity with an ethical charge, informing viewers of the violence (war) taking place in Naples. We might intuit another dimension in terms such as "surveillance" and "informative and objective," a kind of surveillance that claims objectivity and produces knowledge about its subjects. This realism, when framed as providing an objective depiction of a place associated with violence and corruption—as surveilling the place, no less—takes on a powerfully orientalist dimension.

Synopsis Analysis

Gomorrah's institutional construction, from scholarship to festival paratexts, is underpinned by several orientalist characteristics: producing a cultural distance between the South and the site of its construction and reception; claiming to represent the South on its behalf, revealing an essential truth about it; and constructing this truth in line with a catalogue of stereotypes such as irrationality, despotism and backwardness. We find yet further evidence of this in the central construction of the film in the European A festival context: Cannes's representation of *Gomorrah* in its official programme. The synopsis accompanying the film's exhibition at the festival condenses many of the tropes I have identified above, suggesting the institution's ideological investment in the construction and differentiation of the South underpinned by an orientalist framework. Moreover, as will become clear when I analyse the film against the synopsis, the text not only produces the South as other, but does so in a way that suppresses *Gomorrah*'s potential to critique the structures of global capitalism from the perspective of Naples. Overall, the synopsis effects a displacement of the excesses of global capitalism onto the image of a strange, distant and irrationally violent Southern Italy.

As with Cannes synopses in general, this text contains little explicit description of the film's style or genre. However, the synopsis of *Gomorrah* does represent the film as fictional but realistic, and strongly emphasises its authenticity. According to the text, *Gomorrah* contains several imaginative elements: "stories" and a "scenario," each of which implies a fictional narrative. However, the imaginary nature of this construction is brought into question in the conclusion, a rhetorical construction that retroactively determines the meaning of the text. In fact, the stories that the film depicts are only "apparently imaginary," being, rather, "deeply rooted in reality," implying a profound grounding in the "reality" of that which the film depicts. We might contrast this with Ciliento's (2011) and Holdaway's (2014) arguments that the film's aesthetics are surreal, stylish or spectacular, related to science fiction or Hollywood gangster movies. Following Holdaway's argument in particular, we can interpret the synopsis as a paratext that also participates in the film's rhetoric of realism, emphasising objectivity and eliding style or artifice.

When we examine the "scenario" that *Gomorrah* is described as depicting, the presence of the orientalist trope of a realist text objectively showing a strange and irrational—an other—place becomes apparent. The "world" of *Gomorrah* is "cruel," "violent" and "rooted in reality." It appears marked by an inadmissible excess. But to what extent is this "world" global or circumscribed to a particular territory? The opening words of the synopsis, "Power, money and blood" (organised into a rhetorical triad of nouns and given emphasis by the brevity of the clause), provide a powerful frame for the world of *Gomorrah*. They designate the "values that the people of

Naples and Caserta have to face every day." Power and money are implicitly shown in their negative, excessive aspect. That such values have to be faced or struggled with implies an unregulated, excessive control of power and money. While this can be thought of in global terms, the text both implicitly and explicitly locates this struggle in the South. The effect is initially produced by the presence of the word "blood" as the final term in the triad. Blood, here, creates a subtle distance between the circulation of money and power in the world and its excessive "mis"-use in the Global South. It retroactively frames the excess of the first two terms in relation to a word heavy with connotations of "backwards" political practices (as in nepotism), irrationality (as in passion), violence (as in the spilling of blood through war), and contagion (as in the unregulated flow of infected blood). Together, the first three of these connotations evoke the orientalist stereotype of Southern Italy as "unable to build the rational, orderly, civic cultures that, in the North, underwrote the emergence of industrial capitalist society" due to the "passionate, undisciplined, rebellious character of its inhabitants" (Schneider, 1998, p. 1). In contrast with the humanist, democratic North, where power and money supposedly circulate freely, the South's subjection to blood values cause it to be constrained to a despotic "underdeveloped" political life and thus a concentration of power and money in the wrong hands. On the subtler level of the fourth connotation, that of contagion, the word "blood" may also reproduce ideas of the other as excessive, dirty and threatening.

Blood, as a potential carrier of infection is a threatening substance—its flow must be regulated as a means of protecting the social body. This is imagery most commonly used in racist discourses that cast the non-white other as a threatening presence who must be kept out of the "clean" Northern social body—for example, Enoch Powell's (1968) notorious "Rivers of Blood" speech. The Cannes synopsis *contains* this fluid and the excesses it is perceived to carry: the social body of the South may be contaminated but, by localising contagion there, the text could be read as preserving a sense of the Northern social body as clean. The synopsis is fixated on Naples and Caserta, circumscribing the "world" of *Gomorrah* to this region. The text refers solely to Naples and Caserta as the setting of the film, eliding any sense of its place within a world system.

It distinguishes this place further by constructing an impression of distance between the region and the place from which the text speaks (and the implied viewer/reader looks). It establishes "a (cultural) distance between the viewer and viewed" that follows an orientalist logic (Halle, 2010, p. 315). This distance is achieved primarily through that which we might describe, following Said (1993, p. 198), as "narrating [...] strangeness." The synopsis explicitly underlines the abnormality of life in the South, in the short sentence used to conclude the first paragraph: "Only a lucky few can even think of leading a 'normal' life." In this region, normality is a distant concept, barely conceivable to its residents. From this concluding sentence, rhetorically powerful due to its position at the end of the section, a hierarchy is produced between life in Caserta and an implicit "normal" condition. As we saw in chapters 4 and 5, another technique that renders a figure strange is that of deindividualisation. Here, in contrast with the full identity of the (Northern) subject, the (Southern) figure is depicted as identity-less, almost as an object, and certainly as other. These figures are referred to in generic terms: "people," "inhabitants" or the impersonal "they." As discussed both in the previous chapter in relation to brutal humanism and above in relation to festivals' homogenisation of cultures outside the Global North, this participates in a hierarchy of power in which the hegemonic North is afforded specificity and the South is constructed as an indistinct mass, defined only by its difference.

Overall, the text's portrayal of the characters recalls many orientalist descriptions of Southern Italy—for example, Pasquale Villari's *Southern Letter on the Camorra* (1885), in which

> both the bodies of the city and of its inhabitants become a homogenous and undistinguished mass of dirt and "filth." The insalubrious slums reflect the amorality of the "brutes," the Neapolitan masses coerced to live in poverty and become criminals. (in Ridda, 2017, p. 471)

The Cannes synopsis of *Gomorrah* reproduces centuries-old tropes that cast Neapolitans as a homogenous, criminal and/or impoverished mass, tropes commonly mobilised in the frameworks of Orientalism and othering. When the Cannes synopsis claims that *Gomorrah* will represent a reality located specifically in Naples and Caserta, a region associated with the Global South, it reproduces the orientalist creation of knowledge about, and fetishisation of, that place. Moreover, if the orientalist stereotype registers an attempt to displace the inadmissable underside of the hegemonic North onto an other, the Cannes synopsis can be read as constructing the South (via *Gomorrah*) in a way that instantiates this process.

Focusing on the film, and using it to "speak back" to the synopsis, I aim to further demonstrate and intervene in this procedure. I use *Gomorrah* to consider Naples as that "alienating other, (or mirror) which crucially returns its image to the subject" and, in turn, reveal "the hatred of the

Other" (Bhabha, 1983, p. 31) as the European A festival apparatuses' and global capitalism's "hatred of [its] own enjoyment" (Žižek, 1993, p. 203). In the next section, then, I offer an interpretation of *Gomorrah* that focuses on the way in which its depiction of the South might offer a critique of capitalist hegemony. I argue that the film can be read as "returning the image of the North," framing excess as constituent of the Northern capitalist system rather than a feature of some unregulated outside (the orientalised South).

Film analysis

Much has been written about *Gomorrah* in relation to realism, and I do not wish to add to an already saturated debate. What concerns me below is not so much the extent to which *Gomorrah* is or is not "deeply rooted in reality"; instead, I consider the nature of the "reality" it depicts. We have seen the Cannes synopsis describe this reality as violent and hopeless, located in a precise locality. According to the synopsis, Naples and Caserta are part of a region outside of normality and the global order of things; they are sites of excess and antagonism inassimilable to the symbolic order of the capitalist, hegemonic North. However, *Gomorrah* contains elements that destabilise the binary between the North and its other that structures the Cannes synopsis. There are several moments in the film at which corruption, pollution and violence are shown as irruptions of an excess constitutive of global capitalism rather than features of its "outside." Rather than the South's excesses exploding onto Northern screens, in *Gomorrah* the excesses of the North contaminate the social and ecological orders of the South, and the film grapples with Southern Italy's forced assimilation into a globalised, extractive and capitalist reality.

This appears most clearly in the three narrative threads with an explicitly global aspect: (1) the *Scarface* (De Palma, 1983) narrative, which focuses on two young men, Ciro and Marco, whose idealisation of Hollywood mobsters eventually results in their assassination by local Camorra bosses; (2) the eco-Mafia narrative, which centres on Franco and Roberto, two businessmen in the Camorra-run waste disposal business; and (3) the high fashion narrative about a *camorrista* tailor, Pasquale, who makes "designer" dresses that appear on the red carpet at glamorous film events, including film festivals. These three narratives can be understood in relation to three corresponding themes: (1) Hollywood and the impossibility of unmediated identity under globalisation; (2) abjection and waste, the unassimilable excess of capitalism; and (3) exploitation: the hidden underside of fashion and film (associated with the Made in Italy brand).[11]

As with the question of realism and *Gomorrah*, scholarship on the *Scarface* narrative in relation to the Mafia movie, Hollywood and mediation has saturated the debate. This is perhaps due to its implications for the debate on realism: as Pierpaolo Antonello (2011) points out, traditional notions of realism are complicated by the way in which *Gomorrah* shows the mediation of today's "reality." Both Antonello (2011) and Renga (2013) analyse the striking mises-en-abyme in the film that contribute to this impression, such as the scenes in which Marco and Ciro act out *Scarface*, shot on location in Camorra boss Walter Schiavone's mansion. This mansion was modelled on the same film. Thus, *Gomorrah*'s on-location shooting actually, in some respects, takes place on a set, a simulacrum of Tony Montana's house in *Scarface*. Any authentic, even Italian, realism (on-location shooting is a much-celebrated trope of Italian neorealism) that could be ascribed to the film is complicated by contemporary Italian reality's mediation through Hollywood movies. Both realism and nationality collapse in such moments.

Since I do not wish to rehearse work already done on the film, I will not undertake a detailed analysis of this same narrative and its relation to the themes of transnational cinema and mediation. I would like to note, however, its significance for my argument. The cyclic relationship between the really existing and fictional Mafia depicted on screen, along with the relationship between Southern Italy, the US and Hollywood, destabilises the boundary between centre and periphery, North and South. If the Mafia once provided inspiration for highly lucrative Hollywood gangster movies such as *Scarface* (see Renga, 2014), and these now provide inspiration for the really-existing Mafia in Italy and around the world, one might question precisely how Southern the "reality" *Gomorrah* supposedly depicts is. *Gomorrah* not only cannot be realist in the sense of unmediated, but it also cannot be set solely in Southern Italy, given the permeation of North American culture in the region and vice versa. Therefore, the Cannes synopsis attempting to designate *Gomorrah* as a Mafia movie about just Naples and Caserta obscures the impossibility of any Mafia movie—in the new millennium, at least—being set in just one place. While this narrative functions solely on a cultural

11 Made in Italy is a brand used to sell goods on the basis of their Italian origin and connotations of quality and luxury. It is traditionally thought of as being comprised of three types of product: fashion, furniture and food.

level, being about the image of the Mafia, we can find representations of continuities between the South and North on economic levels in the other two narratives I have identified above: the eco-Mafia and high fashion narratives.

Eco-Mafia, Disposing of Capitalism's Abject Excess

Renga (2013) argues that *Gomorrah*'s eco-Mafia narrative "shed[s] light onto the eco-Mafia and its ties to international politics and big business" (p. 136), referring to transnational waste management, the import and export of companies' excess. Building on Saviano's (2007, p. 310) description of dumps as "the most concrete emblem of every economic cycle," Simona Bondavalli (2011) analyses how *Gomorrah* depicts the centrality of waste management to global capitalism in a way that "renders all viewers complicit in the criminal acts performed on the screen" (p. 1). Rather than simply abject—repugnant matter to be expelled from the system or (social) body—waste has been assimilated into the structures of capitalism, since the waste management industry now makes money from waste; waste produces value (Bondavalli, 2011, p. 8).

Although Bondavalli does not make this connection explicit, we might notice a corollary in *Gomorrah*'s depiction of Camorra-controlled waste management, which also shows an "excessive" element (the Mafia) as a constitutive part of the structures of value production and circulation. Indeed, "[w]hile a socially defined, localised and dirty-handed *camorra* would relate to most viewers [...] a network of businessmen circumventing the ever-increasing EU regulations to realise a profit may situate most viewers differently" (p. 9). When we read this analysis alongside the Cannes synopsis, its significance becomes clear. The Camorra are typically represented as "socially defined" (other), "localised" (Southern), and "dirty-handed" (abject), as reproduced in the Cannes text. However, the film's portrayal of a network of businessmen exploiting EU regulations for profit undermines the demarcation between crime and capitalism, abjection and value.

Viewing the cycle of production and this pollutant excess through *Gomorrah*'s depiction of waste dumping in Southern Italy, it becomes clear that this excess can also be thought of as a metonym: the environmentally-destructive toxic waste as a side-effect of production symbolises the excessive production of an othered and exploited South. *Gomorrah*'s eco-Mafia narrative brings these two kinds of abjection together, depicting the exploitation and poisoning of the South as an effect of global capitalism's displacement of its excesses onto the region.[12] *Gomorrah* manifests these effects through the figure of a dying father whose family, having had their land and bodies contaminated by toxic waste, plead for yet more to be dumped near them. If the abject can be understood as "death infecting life," the man's poisoned body makes the abject waste visible—capitalism's toxic excess, death, infecting Neapolitan people's lives (Kristeva, 1982, p. 4).

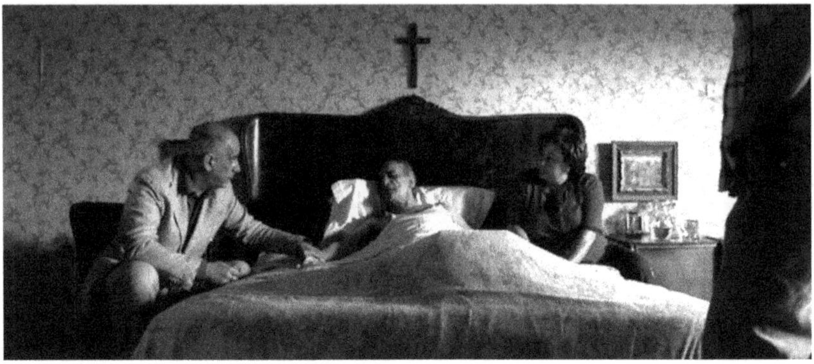

Figure 25: Toxicity and abjection: poisoned Neapolitan man asks for euros in *Gomorrah* (Garrone, 2008). Optimum Releasing.

The economic situation of Naples is presented in microcosm here: the contaminated body (the land); the desperate family that one would expect to care for both the land and the father, but instead is coerced by poverty into contaminating them further; the opportunistic businessman who mediate between the land, its people, and the uneven circulation of capital. The father's status as sacrificial figure is made apparent by religious symbolism that characterises the scene. He is shot, centre-frame, lying beneath a crucifix with no shirt on and one arm outstretched, in an almost Christ-like position. However, this figure is being sacrificed for a different religious order, as implied by his ritualistic repetition of the word "Euro." His son reveals the mechanism by which this sacrifice is to take place: despite having just described the refuse being dumped on their land as "poison," the family bargain with Franco, pleading for more, since "everything

12 I am struck here by the resonance with Kenneth Harrow's (2013) description of "trash" in African cinema as a signifier of the same world system. This is picked up later by Ella Shohat and Robert Stam in their *Unthinking Eurocentrism* (2014, p. 394): "All this trash, for Harrow, points to the insidiously complementary processes by which the "Global North" forms the locus of commodity capitalism, while the 'Global South Africa' becomes the site where consumerist waste is dumped. While raw materials—agricultural products, oil, human labor—sustain the 'Global North,' the 'slag' created by producing goods for consumption, fouls and bedevils the 'Global South.'"

costs double in Euro." The affective power of this scene, in providing an embodiment of the polluted Neapolitan land, and thus making visible an otherwise invisible excess, marks a departure from the "cold gaze" and "brutality" usually ascribed to *Gomorrah* in the festival press. This is one of several moments in the film where its supposed "objectivity" contrasts with emotional direction employed to symbolise, dramatise and condemn the pollution of Naples and Caserta, a pollution on which global capital (signified here by the Euro) depends. The periphery becomes a wasteland, the site of capitalism's excremental excess, filtered away from the centre in order to maintain the façade of efficiency and cleanliness. Naples as a site of the abject, an othered place—embodied by the sick man, the sick land—is dramatised, and the origin of this abjection, its necessitation by the metropolitan centre's production of a polluting excess (literally, toxic waste), is made explicit.

In fact, this is one of the few scenes followed by some kind of consequence and comment. In a rare moment in which the film could be described as approaching the didactic, the apprentice waste manager Roberto resigns from his position, initiating a dialogue that confronts the relationship between poverty in the region and the politics of the Eurozone. The relationship between the two scenes is reinforced by the contaminated peaches carried over from the former to the latter. These objects, further manifestations of the polluted land, appear to provoke Roberto's resignation from his role and the following exchange:

> F: Think this job sucks? You know that guys like me put this shit country in Europe? Know how many workers I've helped by saving their companies money? Stop and look! What do you see? What do you see? Debts! All these people have been saved only thanks to us.
> R: I saw how you helped them live. You save a worker in Mestre and kill a family in Mondragone.
> F: That's how it works, but I didn't decide it. We solved problems created by others. I didn't create chromium and asbestos. I didn't dig up the mountain. That's how it works.

Throughout this scene, the handheld camera moves around the faces of the two men, uncomfortably close to each face at any given time. As Franco asks, "What do you see?" the camera follows his gesture, panning across the Neapolitan countryside.

The camerawork immerses the viewer in the exchange, placing us in line with Roberto's perspective as he looks at the field that Franco has

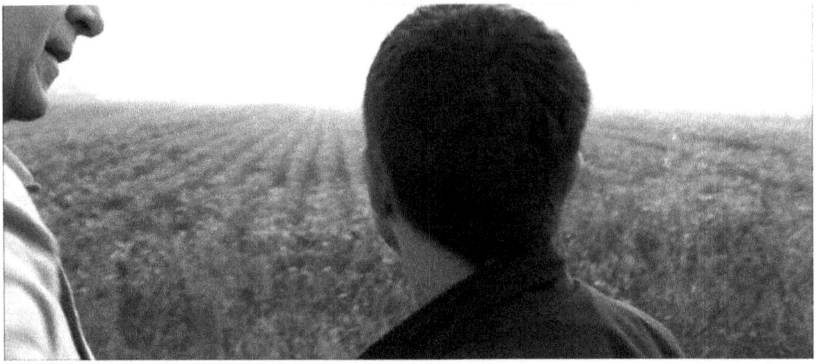

Figure 26: The Real of debt beneath a Neapolitan pastoral. *Gomorrah* (Garrone, 2008). Optimum Releasing.

indicated. The shot of the countryside invites us to contemplate the Real of the region and its place in global capitalism. Nothing particularly out of the ordinary is visible, even if the low saturation might contrast with the luscious greens usually featured in films and advertisements depicting the Italian countryside. However, the image is then defined through a bizarre signifier: "Debts!" The image's immediate visual meaning is confronted with its "symbolic real" meaning, its abstract underpinning in a system of debt (Žižek 2004b).

Franco's position throughout this dialogue manifests a cynical acceptance of the symbolic real: rather than an obstacle, or something traumatic, Franco accepts the land's transformation into debt as a sign of capitalism's proper functioning: "That's how it works." His cynical description, and Roberto's response to it, outline the global nature of capitalism's production of excess and displacement of it onto exploited Southern territories. Franco's attempt to designate these economic processes as capitalism's proper, even successful, functioning is repeatedly met by negation from Roberto. Franco argues that businessmen like him "put this shit country in Europe," securing its place as part of a Northern territory and saving workers. This characterisation of his work simultaneously reproduces and disavows the anxieties caused by Italy's duality as at once Northern and Southern: Italy was once a "shit" country, perennially "backwards" in comparison with Northern Europe, but this has been overcome thanks to its successful assimilation into both Europe and the capitalist system.

However, his attempt to disavow the North/South divide—both within Italy and between Europe and its "outside"—is countered by Roberto's re-instatement of it: "you save a worker in Mestre and kill a family in Mondragone." This exchange emphasises that Italy's status as European depends upon the reinforcement of the North's hegemony (saving workers in Venice) through the exploitation of the South (killing families in Caserta). Moreover, Roberto's evocation of death highlights the cost of this assimilation, recalling the dying father and thus re-evoking its potential to affectively critique an economic system that depends upon the exploitation of the South as a means of securing the relative wealth and health of the North. Through its depiction of the exportation of capitalism's excesses—waste and debt—into Southern Italy, *Gomorrah* can therefore be interpreted as positioning the South as constitutive part of global capitalism. Rather than a distant site of irrational, criminal violence, Naples and Caserta are depicted as sites onto which Northern hegemonic capitalism displaces its inadmissible excess, its abjection carefully managed by the regulation of the flow of abjection towards the South.

Camorra Couture: Mediating Made in Italy

The place of the South in global capitalism, and the need for such a system to export its excesses away from the North, also appear in *Gomorrah*'s narrative of a Camorra tailor who produces high fashion dresses to be sold on the global market. This narrative implies that Naples, the Camorra, and even Chinese underground workers in the region, are the criminal centre of Italy's fashion industry and, by extension, Italy's image abroad. The centrality of Italian fashion to the Made in Italy brand is well-known as one of the "F's of Made in Italy: fashion, food, furniture and film (La Porta, 2013; Balicco, 2013). *Gomorrah* moves Italian fashion from its imagined centre, Milan, and shows the industry's underground, its "underground self," in Naples. The narrative opens with an auction set in a school gym. A beautiful cream designer dress fills the opening shot; all we see is decontextualised luxury. This moment quickly passes as the camera moves round the dress to reveal Pasquale's bald head and, behind him, a basketball hoop, all shot in low saturation, emphasising the unglamorous surroundings that contradict typical representations of Italian high fashion.

The camera continues its movement, showing more couture dresses alongside props that highlight the school gym setting. Thus, we are presented with a contrast between the products and the site of their production, a locality starkly at odds with the usual image used to market them. This contrast is the basis of a disconnect that rends the fashion narrative throughout the film. The luxurious appearance of the dresses and the connotations of quality that underpin the Made in Italy brand are confronted with the film's portrayal of their site of production. While the Southern, unglamourous setting may reproduce Cannes's depiction of Naples and Caserta as an othered place—far from the "modernity being triumphantly pursued elsewhere" (Chambers, 2015, p. 13) —the designer goods shown in this same setting place an entire system of capitalist production in a far more continuous relationship with the Global South than the synopsis implies. *Gomorrah* defamiliarises the common image of Italian high fashion by placing it in a run-down, criminal setting. In so doing, it reproduces the traumatic materiality beneath the symbolic brand of Made in Italy.

Maria Tulante (2013) analyses this as a part of *Gomorrah*'s "revelatory" function, the manifestation of Garrone's "consistent interest in finding the truth of a matter," even when deploying a "liberal interpretation of realism" (p. 256). Although the analysis above supports such a reading, Tulante's argument misses the importance of mediation in both the construction of the Made in Italy brand and the film. *Gomorrah* complicates the idea of film as straightforwardly revelatory, and perhaps signals its own complicity in the system it purports to critique, through the theme of mediation, a theme mentioned above in relation to Marco and Ciro, the *Scarface*-inspired would-be *mafiosi*. *Gomorrah* screens the disconnect between Italian designer dresses' conditions of production and their brand image, explicitly implicating the film industry (especially film festivals) in this contradictory reality. The fashion narrative ends with Pasquale having, like Roberto, quit the Mafia-controlled industry and become a truck driver. On the television screen in a rest stop, Pasquale sees one of his creations on Scarlett Johansson on the red carpet at Venice:

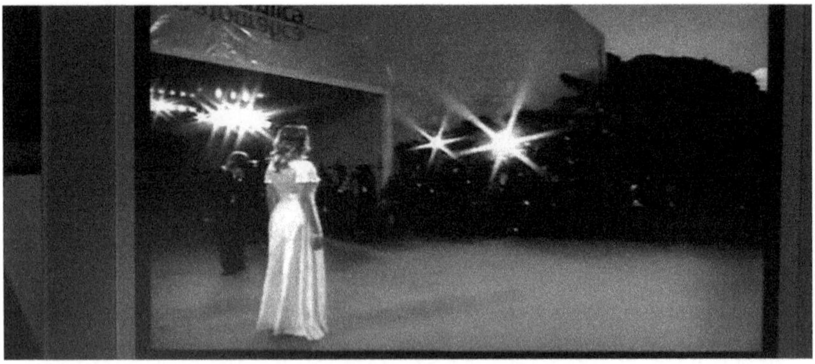

Figure 27: Screening the Venice film festival in *Gomorrah* (Garrone, 2008). Optimum Releasing.

This is the cream dress featured in the opening scenes of this narrative arc and that the film shows on several occasions subsequently, making it a central prop within this plotline. Pasquale draws attention to the dress: in the first scenes, he remarks on its complexity, and he is shown working on the dress throughout. In a later scene, he caresses the fabric as it hangs on a dummy. In this arresting mise-en-abyme, the dress from the film is transported into "real" life through the employment of footage of the Venice film festival. Fashion meets film, offering a glimpse into the interconnectedness of different industries.

It is telling that this moment combines two industries related to the Made in Italy brand: designer clothing and cinema (specifically the kind of cinema associated with European A festivals such as Venice). As such, *Gomorrah* can be interpreted as alluding to the mediation of Italy's image abroad, including through the film festival apparatus. The film's use of interface, the redoubling of an image on screen, is crucial here. In projecting the dress onto a television screen, *Gomorrah* highlights the mediation of Italy's image and, in some respects, the film's own complicity with this process. Here, Johansson and the festival red carpet appear on the interface-screen (the television), showing the "absent cause" of both the diegetic events of the high fashion narrative and, on a metacinematic level, the film to be the film festival apparatus and its place in a global circulation of goods and images.

As previously discussed, interface reveals the viewer's perspective on screen, making manifest the Gaze—the partiality of this perspective and the ideological investments on which it is founded. The use of this technique in *Gomorrah* holds a particular power given the context of the film being premiered at Cannes. It seems to anticipate that film's audience is likely to have watched the same kinds of red carpet displays, either live or on screens around the festival. Seeing the same image appear in the midst of a competition premiere, in a film about the Mafia, no less, would have an uncanny familiarity. In screening such images, *Gomorrah* can be read as highlighting its own status as a product involved in the mediation of Italy's "brand." Rather than having a straightforwardly revelatory function, as Tulante argues, the film performs its own contradiction. This scene highlights *Gomorrah* as a film whose depiction of Southern Italy at once critiques the area's exploitation in Northern, capitalist hegemony, yet nonetheless depends upon an apparatus in which it is embedded and that actively reproduces this exploitation. The appearance of Scarlett Johansson on the red carpet at Venice, dressed in an outfit that the film has (in a kind of temporal short circuit) retroactively determined as Camorra couture, suddenly brings into relief the structures of labour, migration and oppression on which festivals such as Cannes depend for their pomp and glamour. It makes manifest the film's, the viewers', and the festival apparatus's complicity in the excesses of exploitation, pollution and violence depicted in *Gomorrah*'s earlier scenes. Moreover, in screening this via the glitz and glamour of the festival red carpet, the film depicts the enjoyment—the senseless ideological complicity—that maintains the South's construction as the constitutive other of Northern capitalist hegemony.

Conclusion

Once more, the stakes of the synopsis's representation of the film as a realist, regional tale become clear. It would seem from the above that several of *Gomorrah*'s narratives contain global dimensions in a way that undermines the ideas of Northern, capitalist modernity and Southern, criminal otherness that characterise the logic according to which the Cannes synopsis constructs the film. The festival synopsis represents *Gomorrah* as a solely Neapolitan affair, founded on the displacement of criminality, excess and otherness, onto a location presented as "outside" the hegemonic system. Naples becomes the culturally essentialised other, effecting a disavowal of the antagonisms underpinning global capitalism. Thus, the Cannes synopsis reproduces "the political economy of location," best summarised in Chambers's (2015) analysis of the "Southern Question":

> [The South] is maintained at a distance, transformed in to a separable "other" and then rendered subaltern and subordinate within the institutions and practices of "advanced" capitalist culture [...] at the same time structurally integral to the very production and reproduction of dominance and subordination. (p. 20)

Reading *Gomorrah* against the Cannes synopsis suggests the presence of this orientalist logic on the European A circuit: while the text constructs the South as other, displacing its inadmissible excesses onto this territory, the South depicted in *Gomorrah* holds up a mirror to the North, revealing precisely these excesses as its own. Taken together with the previous chapter, it should become clear that European A festivals are invested in the "politics of location" that Chambers describes, not only in the politics of where they take place, nor the way they represent films' territories of production, but also in their representations of films' settings.

Finally, *Gomorrah*'s depiction of a criminality that is not the excess, but the constitutive feature of global capitalism—from waste management to the fashion industry, to film festivals themselves—highlights the ideological process through which a European A festival's representation of a film may effect a containment of its radical potential. *Gomorrah*'s status as an emblem of Italian cinema and culture has allowed us to explicitly consider one of the crucial themes underlying this book: the influence of capital on A festivals' awarding and construction of Italian cinema. One of the aspects of the ideology of Italian festival cinema that has become apparent throughout this chapter is the way in which festivals appear to localise, to contain or co-opt, the political critiques a film might pursue—and to do so in such a way that attenuates the threat that such critiques may pose to global capitalism. With the final case study, this book thus comes full circle: while Chapter 2 showed that European A festivals' construction of the universal of "the art of film" via the auteur was at once a symptom and disavowal of their dependence upon capital, this chapter has demonstrated how festivals' claim to (geo)political universality, entrenched in a politics of the other, is, too, a crucial component of their reproduction of capitalism as both an economic and ideological system. All that remains, therefore, is to tie together the threads that have run through the book so far, and summarise the relevance of this relationship between European A festivals' embeddedness in, and maintenance of, global capitalism and their ideological construction of Italian art cinema in the new millennium.

Bibliography

Amin, S. (2018). Globalisation and its alternative. *Political Notebook #1*. Tricontinental Institute for Social Research. Available from: https://www.thetricontinental.org/wp-content/uploads/2018/10/181029_Political_Notebook_1_EN_Final_Web.pdf

Andrews, D. (2010). Art cinema as institution, redux: Art houses, film festivals, and film studies. *Scope: An Online Journal of Film and Television Studies, 18*, 1–21.

Antonello, P. (2011). Dispatches from hell: Matteo Garrone's *Gomorrah*. In D. Renga (Ed.), *Mafia movies: A reader* (pp. 377–385). University of Toronto Press.

Appadurai, A. (1990). Disjuncture and difference in the global cultural economy. *Theory, Culture & Society, 7*(2–3), 295–310.

Balicco, D. (Ed.). (2013). Conoscere l'Italia contemporanea. Indagine sul Made in Italy. *Allegoria, 68*.

Bauman, Z. (2000). *Liquid modernity*. Polity.

Bhabha, H. K. (1983). The other question. *Screen, 24*(6), 18–36.

Bondavalli, S. (2011). Waste management: Garbage displacement and the ethics of Mafia representation in Matteo Garrone's *Gomorra*. *California Italian Studies, 2*(1), 1–17.

Box Office Mojo. (2018a). *Gomorrah: International box office results*. [Online]. Available from: https://www.boxofficemojo.com/movies/?page=intl&id=gomorrah.htm

Box Office Mojo. (2018b). *The Great Beauty: International box office results.* [Online]. Available from: http://www.boxofficemojo.com/movies/?id=greatbeauty.htm

Box Office Mojo. (2019). *City of God: International box office results.* [Online]. Available from: https://www.boxofficemojo.com/movies/?id=cityofgod.htm

Cavaliere, F. (2010). *Gomorrah*: Crime goes global, language stays local. *European Journal of English Studies, 14*(2), 173–188.

Chambers, I. (2008). *Mediterranean crossings: The politics of an interrupted modernity.* Duke University Press.

Chambers, I. (2015). The "Southern Question"... again. In A. Mammone, E. G. Parini, & G. A. Veltri (Eds.), *The Routledge handbook of contemporary Italy: History, politics, society* (pp. 25–34). Routledge.

Chan, F. (2011). The international film festival and the making of a national cinema. *Screen, 52*(2), 253–260.

Ciliento, F. (2011). Saviano, Garrone, *Gomorrah*: Neorealism and noir in the land of the Camorra. *Fast Capitalism, 8*(1). [Online]. Available from: https://www.uta.edu/huma/agger/fastcapitalism/8_1/ciliento8_1.html

Czach, L. (2004). Film festivals, programming, and the building of a national cinema. *The Moving Image, 4*(1), 76–88.

De Marco, C. (2015). Moretti, Sorrentino, Garrone: "In it together for Italian film." *Cineuropa*. [Online]. Available from: http://cineuropa.org/nw.aspx?t=newsdetail&l=en&did=289826

De Valck, M. (2007). *Film festivals: From European geopolitics to global cinephilia.* Amsterdam University Press.

Diawara, M. (2010). *African film: New forms of aesthetics and politics.* Prestel Verlag.

Dovey, L. 2015. *Curating Africa in the age of film festivals.* Palgrave Macmillan.

Elsaesser, T. (2016). The global author: Control, creative constraints, and performative self-contradiction. In S. Jeong & J. Szaniawski (Eds.), *The global auteur: The politics of authorship in 21st century cinema* (pp. 21–41). Bloomsbury.

Falicov, T. (2010). Migrating from south to north: The role of film festivals in funding and shaping global south film and video. In T. Falicov et al. (Eds.), *Locating migrating media* (pp. 3–22). Lexington Books.

Festival de Cannes. (2008). *Gomorra (Gomorrah).* [Online]. Available from: https://www.festival-cannes.com/en/films/gomorra

Garrone, M. (2008). *Nota di regia, Gomorra.* Press pack. [Online]. Available from: http://www.archimedefilm.it/docs/gomorra_pressbook_ita.doc

Gramsci, A. (1994 [1926]). Some aspects of the Southern Question. In R. Bellamy (Ed.), *Antonio Gramsci: Pre-prison writings* (pp. 313–337). Cambridge University Press.

Halle, R. (2010). Offering tales they want to hear: Transnational European film funding as neo-orientalism. In R. Galt & K. Schoonover (Eds.), *Global art cinema: New theories and histories* (pp. 303–319). Oxford University Press.

Hardt, M., & Negri, A. (2000). *Empire*. Harvard University Press.
Harrow, K. (2013). *Trash: African cinema from below*. Indiana University Press.
Holdaway, D. (2014). Osservazioni sulla retorica di *Gomorra*. In W. Hope, S. Serra, & L. D'Arcangeli (Eds.), *Un nuovo cinema politico italiano? Il passato sociopolitica o, il potere istituzionale, la marginalizzazione* (pp. 198–210). Troubador.
Iordanova, D., & Rhyne, R. (Eds.). (2009). *Film festival yearbook 1: The festival circuit*. St Andrews Film Studies and College Gate Press.
Jabri, V. (2013). *The postcolonial subject: Claiming politics/governing others in late modernity*. Routledge.
Jeong, S. (2021). World cinema in a global frame. *Studies in World Cinema, 1*(1), 29–38.
Karlovy Vary International Film Festival. 2019. *Programme Sections*. [Online]. Available from: https://www.kviff.com/en/about-the-festival/programe-sections
Kristeva, J. (1982). *Powers of horror: An essay on abjection*. Columbia University Press.
La Porta, F. (2013). Il film in questione: *La grande bellezza* (2013). *Allegoria, 68*, 213–216.
Macfie, A. L. (Ed.). (2000). *Orientalism: A reader*. New York University Press.
Marshall, L. (2008). Gomorrah (Gomorra). *Screen Daily*. [Online]. Available from: https://www.screendaily.com/gomorrah-gomorra/4038782.article
Mazdon, L. (2006). The Cannes Film Festival as transnational space. *Post Script, 25*(2), 19–30.
Mezias, S. et al. (2011). Transforming film product identities: The status effects of European premier film festivals, 1996–2005. In B. Moeran & J. S. Pedersen (Eds.), *Negotiating values in the creative industries: Fairs, festivals and competitive events* (pp. 169–196). Cambridge University Press.
O'Healy, Á. (2010). Mediterranean passages: Abjection and belonging in contemporary Italian cinema. *California Italian Studies, 1*(1), 1–19.
Ponzanesi, S. (2016b). Does Italy need postcolonial theory? Intersections in Italian postcolonial studies. *English Literature, 3*, 145–161.
Powell, E. (1968). Rivers of Blood (also known as The Birmingham Speech). Address to the Conservative Political Centre, Birmingham, 20 April 1968. Transcript. *The Telegraph*. [Online]. Available from: http://www.telegraph.co.uk/comment/3643823/Enoch-Powells-Rivers-of-Blood-speech.html
Rastegar, R. (2012). Difference, aesthetics and the curatorial crisis of film festivals. *Screen, 53*(3), 310–317.
Renga, D. (2013). *Unfinished business: Screening the Italian Mafia in the new millennium*. University of Toronto Press.
Renga, D. (2014). *Mafia movies: A reader*. University of Toronto Press.
Ridda, M. (2017). The siren's children: Rethinking postcolonial Naples. *Interventions, 19*(4), 467–486.
Rose, J. (2007). *The last resistance*. Verso.

Ross, M. (2011). The film festival as producer: Latin American films and Rotterdam's Hubert Bals Fund. *Screen*, *52*(2), 261–267.

Said, E. (1993). *Culture and imperialism*. Vintage.

Said, E. (2003 [1978]). *Orientalism: Western conceptions of the Orient*. Penguin.

Saviano, R. (2008). *L'impero criminale, Gomorra*. Press pack. [Online]. Available from: http://www.archimedefilm.it/docs/gomorra_pressbook_ita.doc

Saviano, R., & Jewiss, V. (2007). *Gomorrah: A personal journey into the violent international empire of Naples' organised crime system*. Farrar, Straus and Giroux.

Schoonover, K. (2012). *Brutal Vision: The neorealist body in postwar Italian cinema*. University of Minnesota Press.

Schneider, J. (1998). *Italy's "Southern Question": Orientalism in one country*. Berg.

Shohat, E., & Stam, R. (2014). *Unthinking Eurocentrism: Multiculturalism and the media*. Routledge.

Stringer, J. (2001). Global cities and the international film festival economy. In T. Shiel & T. Fitzmaurice (Eds.), *Cinema and the city: Film and urban societies in a global context* (pp. 134–144). Blackwell.

Tarrow, S. (1996). Making social science work across space and time: A critical reflection on Robert Putnam's *Making Democracy Work*. *American Political Science Review*, *90*, 389–397.

Tulante, M. (2013). High fashion in film: Italian identity and global anxiety in *Valentino: The Last Emperor* and *Gomorrah*. *Journal of Italian Cinema & Media Studies*, *1*(3), 245–262.

Verdicchio, P. (1997). The preclusion of postcolonial discourse in Southern Italy. In B. Allen & M. Russo (Eds.), *Revisioning Italy. National culture and global culture* (pp. 191–212). University of Minnesota Press.

Weissberg, J. (2008). Gomorrah. *Variety*. [Online]. Available from: https://variety.com/2008/film/markets-festivals/gomorrah-1200522327/

Zagarrio, V. (2016). Una certa tendenza del cinema italiano. *Flinders University Languages Group Online Review*, *5*(1), 1–8.

Žižek, S. (1993). *Tarrying with the negative: Kant, Hegel, and the critique of ideology*. Duke University Press.

Žižek, S. (2004b). *The reality of the virtual* [lecture]. Recorded 11 December 2003. Ben Wright Film Productions.

Filmography

The Battle of Algiers (*La battaglia di Algeri*) (1966). Pontecorvo, G. dir. Italy/Algeria.

Blade Runner (1982). Scott, R. dir. United States.

Camp de Thiaroye (1989). Sembene, O. Senegal.

Chroniques des années de braise (1975). Lakhdar-Hamina, M. Algeria.
City of God (*Cidade de Deus*) (2003). Lund, K., & Meirelles. F. dirs. Brazil.
Dogman (2018). Garrone, M. dir. Italy.
Double Indemnity (1944). Wilder, B. dir. United States.
Euphoria (*Euforia*) (2018). Golino, V. dir. Italy.
The Great Beauty (*La grande bellezza*) (2013). Sorrentino, P. dir. Italy.
Gomorrah (*Gomorra*) (2008a). Garrone, M. dir. Italy.
Happy as Lazzaro (*Lazzaro felice*) (2018). Rohrwacher, A. dir. Italy.
Paisan (*Paisà*) (1948). Rossellini, R. dir. Italy.
Reality (2012). Garrone, M. dir. UK.
Rome, Open City (*Roma, città aperta*) (1945). Rossellini, R. dir. Italy.
Germany Year Zero (*Germania anno zero*) (1949). Rossellini, R. dir. Italy.
Scarface (1983). De Palma, B. dir. USA.

Conclusion: Da capo senza fine

Abstract: The Conclusion discusses the two universals that European A festivals construct, and on which they stake claims to legitimacy as canon-makers: artistic universality and political universality. Bringing the book's five main case studies into dialogue with a wider corpus of Italian prize-winning films, this chapter summarises and expands prior analyses of the figures of the auteur and the "other," as well as regimes of taste and difference. Responding to Žižek's (2000, p. 223) claim that "today's Real which sets a limit to resignification is capital," I argue for a discursive-materialist approach to not only studying film festivals, but seeking just models of film culture and cinephilia.

Keywords: cinephilia, film festivals, decolonization, ideology, discourse, film culture

European A festivals are in the business of creating art cinema. This can take many forms, from festivals' role in the funding and production of films, through their cultivation of filmmakers via film education programmes and labs, to their facilitation of international film distribution through markets and networking events. I have been concerned with European A festivals' production of art cinema as a discursive regime, one founded on the imperative (economic as much as representational) to fix the meaning of certain films within a common framework. Through their programming, paratexts, pronouncements and prizes, festivals bring art cinema tentatively into being. This process always fails, giving rise to the cycle of repetition and reproduction that characterises festivals as annual film events—not just festivals, but a series of festival editions, pursuing the same impossible object. It is within the space of this failure and repetition, the space of desire, that ideology emerges. Each repetition brings with it a moment of undecidability, the moment opened up by failure, which is then captured, tamed and taken back up into a dominant system of signification. European A festivals' construction of art cinema is underpinned by a series

Johnson, R., Film Festivals, *Ideology and Italian Art Cinema: Politics, Histories and Cultural Value.* Taylor & Francis Group, 2024
DOI 10.5117/9789463720366_CON

of ideological structures, or fantasies, that secure not only the meaning of the films they represent but the power of these institutions themselves—their claims to universality.

The claim to universality is, in its most fundamental sense, part and parcel of festivals' struggle for hegemony—hegemony over art cinema's meanings—as well as hegemony over the field of film festivals (the hierarchies that structure the festival "network"). As discussed in Chapter 2, for a meaning to appear hegemonic, – universal rather than particular, the very processes of struggle through which such meaning is constituted must be retroactively erased; "a minimum of 'naturalisation' is a condition of effectiveness of the hegemonic operation" (Žižek, 2004a, p. 96). Thus, European A festivals' hegemony is dependent upon the naturalisation of the highly contingent practices in which they engage, as well as both the discursive and material regimes that underpin them. This gives rise to a series of displacements that tend to support festivals' claims of artistic and political universality, while nonetheless effecting the simultaneous disavowal and reinforcement of the power structures of Global Northern capitalism that enmesh these institutions.

Universal Art

European A festivals are best known for operating under the sign of "art," founded on their claims to privilege aesthetic brilliance above all else. While this claim has repeatedly been complicated by studies that show the influence of commercial concerns on festivals' programming and awarding of films (Peranson, 2009; de Valck, 2014; Ostrowska, 2016), or the entanglement of their very operation with the workings of neoliberal "third sector" funding models (Rhyne, 2009), it is one that persists stubbornly. The effect of European A festivals' conjuring of a purified notion of "Art" to which they are beholden is to naturalise the very definition of art in which festivals participate—to obscure the continuous struggle for meaning in which festivals are engaged, one which is cut through by contingent interests, histories, economic pressures and so on. This process finds its most potent expression in European A festivals' continuing obsession with the figure of the auteur as a privileged representative of an unconstrained artistic expression. The auteur functions as a *sinthome* of the festivals' claims to operate under the universal sign of "art"; the figure of the auteur is the crucial representative of European A festivals' "professed commitment to artistic excellence and nothing else" (Elsaesser, 2005, p. 95).

The auteur appears and re-appears in synopses of films across this book's corpus. *Facing Window* is "Özpetek's new film" (Karlovy Vary, 2003). *The Great Beauty* is Sorrentino's "finest film," and one made in the tradition of that arch-auteur, Fellini (Tallinn, 2013). Meanwhile, *Fire at Sea* is constituted by "Gianfranco Rosi's observations of everyday life" (Berlinale, 2016). In the extended corpus of Italian award-winners, the trend continues. Another film directed by Rosi, *Sacro GRA* (2013), is framed by Venice in relation to the auteur's oeuvre and autobiography:

> After the India of Varanasi's boatmen, the American desert of the dropouts, and the Mexico of the killers of drug trade, Gianfranco Rosi has decided to tell the tale of a part of his own country, roaming and filming for over two years in a minivan on Rome's giant ring road—the Grande Raccordo Anulare, or GRA. (Venice International Film Festival, 2013)

Just as *Sacro GRA* is described as the product of Rosi's "roaming and filming for over two years in a minivan," *Caesar Must Die* (*Cesare deve morire*, Paolo and Vittorio Taviani, 2012) is the result of the directors' having "spent six months following rehearsals for this stage production" (Berlinale, 2012). The production in question is itself a symbol of "artistic excellence," this time taken from the world of English literature—the William Shakespeare play *Julius Caesar* (1599). *Caesar Must Die* is legitimised as the work of both literary and cinematic authors, evoking a long tradition of authorship and art.

Such notions of artistry and auteurism function to disavow European A festivals' character as sites of struggle. Yet, in its contradictory dimension as a particular, contingent representative of a universal, the auteur-as-*sinthome* also highlights this disavowal. The exceptional case of *The Son's Room* shows the contradictions that beset auteurism: the way in which notions of the auteur at once signify and limit artistic freedom. Cannes's synopsis of *The Son's Room* attempts to represent the film as free from constraint, as a neutral artwork, while disavowing the fact that the film's meaning, exhibition and awarding at the festival was contingent upon Moretti's persona and reputation. The paradoxical constraint of the meaning of *The Son's Room* through its relation to the *sinthome* of its very freedom—its universal ideality as "art"—erupts in moments in which the film performs its contradiction as an a-Morettian Moretti text. Through a metacinematic hysteria grounded in Moretti's appearance on screen as both character and auteur, *The Son's Room* foregrounds its own internal split as an ambivalent artwork. This, in turn, reveals the fundamental ideological structure of European A festivals' construction of Italian and art cinema: the presentation of "art" as universal through the deployment of contingent signifiers that in fact delimit art to a particular meaning.

The auteur's privileged position as *sinthome* at once manifests and contradicts European A festivals' claim to function under the sign of the universal of the "art of film" while in fact being engaged in a hegemonic struggle for the contingent meaning of this universal. I showed that this struggle is, furthermore, marked by contingency: such festivals' embeddedness in global capitalism. Since the auteur has traditionally been conceived as at once a guarantor of artistic freedom and a "brand name" to "sell" art films, this figure is *sintho-matic* of the economic necessity that European A festivals cultivate their own brand identity, paradoxically under the sign of art unconstrained by commercial concerns. Constructing this image under the sign of a universal (art) disavows both festivals' own constraint by economic necessity and the constraint to which their construction of certain notions of art is subject.

Just as the universal of "the art of film" is constrained by its construction via the auteur (a constraint necessitated by films' and festivals' commercial aspects), so the auteur, as a human figure, is constrained to another kind of particularity. As the case studies in this book suggest—indeed, as every top prize-winning Italian film since 1946 suggests—the "art of film," in its constraint via the auteur, is subject to a gendered particularity. This occurs not only through the practice of prize-giving, but on a symbolic level too, through festival paratexts. As we saw in Chapter 3, Cannes's and Tallinn's representations of *The Great Beauty* are structured around an "art" characterised by the expression of a masculine creative look towards a feminine object. The *sinthome* constructed by European A festivals renders the universal of "the art of film" particular through its investment not only in the auteur as such but in the *male* auteur and the masculine artistic vision his presence connotes. The unwritten law of European A festivals' construction of "the art of film" via the auteur is not only the (disavowed) law of capital, but the law of sexual difference—the investment in a masculine/feminine gender binary that, as is so often the case, results in the privileging of the masculine and exclusion of the feminine. Developing this idea, we might observe that the ideological procedure of disavowing contingency through the *sinthome* of the auteur may give rise to a whole host of particularities that colour the content of the universal under which European A festivals claim to operate, resulting in fetishisation of both art and identity.

Political Universality

While the sign of "art" may be the ultimate guarantor of European A festivals' hegemony as purveyors of art cinema, these institutions also reinforce their cultural relevance through engagement with the political and social issues of the time. Underpinning this engagement is a binarised, structural preoccupation with difference: European A festivals' construction of the "other." On the fundamental level, the artistic and political mix here, as that which is "other" initially stands in as a signifier for alternative, niche, even "world" cinema, as well as for figures and places "othered" by dominant regimes of power. This entails a performative opposition to Hollywood, festivals' "bad object," which at once secures their claim to a more inclusive artistic and social alterity, and obscures the internal hierarchies and exclusions through which the European A circuit operates.

Such hierarchies come into relief when we consider the second key figure in these festivals' representations of art cinema: the social other. While the figure of the auteur stands in for the artistic universality European A festivals posit, the figure of the social other signifies humanist universality, the fantasy of a socio-symbolic order that can integrate every element.[1] In this ideological formation, the "other" is presented as at once inside the social order, filling its lack, and as a "constitutive Outside" perpetually marked out by difference (Žižek, 2004a, p. 102). European A festivals' construction of a series of "others" instantiates this fantasy as well as the tension that undercuts it. The presence of these figures in the symbolic order of European A festivals is contingent upon their legibility as others-to-be-integrated, caught in a perpetual state of limbo between difference and inclusion. Yet, when we examine the precise means through which festivals construct them, the implications of this paradoxical representation become clear.

Visibility is the key word in European A festivals' construction of art cinema through figures of the "other": art cinema is defined by these institutions as a cinema that makes "othered" subjects visible, and legible. Karlovy Vary's synopsis of *Facing Window*, for example, enacts a gradual revelation of the "strange" Davide, culminating in the promise of fulfilment for both the film's protagonist and its audience. This presentation of the film, which clearly offers the hope of a "harmonious totality" through the integration of the "other," obscures aspects of *Facing Window* that confront us with irruptions of radical alterity that produce a rift in European Holocaust

1 At times these figures are condensed into one, as we saw in the case of Ferzan Özpetek's presentation as the acceptable face of a queer, multicultural Italy.

memory via queer counter-history, or in anaemic multiculturalism via the film's explorations of race and migration.

This negation of radical alterity also entails a negation of agency and, with it, the possibility for European A festivals' "others" to disrupt the material and discursive regimes of power in which such institutions operate. The visibility of the "other" is underpinned by unequal relations of looking in which an implied European subject is afforded the agency to observe or witness, while the "other" is positioned as the object of such observations. In the Berlinale's presentation of *Fire at Sea*, we find the re-emergence of a legacy of brutal witnessing, a kind of pitying humanitarian look with roots in postwar, "humanist" cinema, particularly Italian neorealism. The Berlinale's celebration of the film makes the stakes of neorealism's enduring influence on conceptions of art cinema clear. In the context of the so-called "refugee crisis," we find the reappearance of a brutal humanist legacy that reinforces Euro-American agency via the ethical witnessing of dead or dying "others." When applied to refugees, this becomes a legacy of not only European postwar reconstruction, but European colonialism as well. This case shows how European A festivals' engagement with migration, and perhaps crises more generally, is figured in line with a visual politics of neo-colonial, humanitarian aid, a form of humanism "more reconciled with than resistant to the geopolitical affinities of large-scale capitalism and its multiple battle zones" (Schoonover, 2012, p. xix).

Such geopolitical affinities are, too, the affinities of Global Northern power, and the othering of refugees is part of a larger ideological procedure in which the Global South is figured as a site of lack, excess or, in the paradox proper to Orientalism, both. As we saw in Chapter 6, Cannes's representation of *Gomorrah* exemplifies European festivals' construction of Southern spaces as distant, strange and simultaneously immoderate and inadequate. The setting of the film, observed through the lens of an orientalist "radical realism," was construed as a distant site marked by violence, tyranny, irrationality, and dehumanised, victimised or corrupt masses. As my discussion of the film shows, the Global South thus becomes abject: the dumping ground for the toxic waste of the North's excessive and unassimilable aspects.

We find similar tropes in other Italian award-winners such as *Certi bambini* (Andrea and Antonio Frazzi, 2004). Karlovy Vary's descriptions of the film instantiate ideas of Southern Italy as a Mafia-ridden, impoverished and irrational territory, while foregrounding the film's realist depiction of the place. This is best summarised in the concluding statement: "This fascinating film bears cruel witness to how easy it is for a troubled child to get mixed up in the Naples camorra" (Karlovy Vary, 2004). The sentence combines a brutally humanist conception of ethical witnessing and a fetishisation of Southern Italy as a "fascinating" site of Mafia violence and the corruption of innocence. Karlovy Vary's summary *Certi bambini* exemplifies European A festivals' ideological designation of the South as fascinating "other" space paired with a fantasy of integrating the "other" through a pitying look.

European A festivals' construction of "others" to-be-looked-at or to-be-integrated is the mechanism by which they assert a claim to humanist universality, and by which these institutions assert hegemony not only over art, but over the acceptable horizons of politics, a horizon that stops just short of destabilising the Global North's power. This ideological procedure affords that which Edward Said (2003 [1978], p. 7) has called a "flexible positional superiority" over the "other," in this case ensuring that their integration is conditional upon the maintenance of hegemony for European A festivals and the geopolitical regimes in which they are imbricated. We might wonder, then, to what extent these institutions' performance of political engagement can be considered a form of "elite capture," theorised by Olúfemi O. Táíwò (2022) as a procedure in which political and cultural institutions mobilise discourses and practices taken from grassroots struggles for equality in order to further their own ends. As I have discussed throughout this book, as long as the representation of "others" at European A festivals leaves the fundamental ideological structures through which they operate untouched, the risk of elite capture will remain, even while these institutions perform an ever-greater concern with inclusion and diversity.

Yet the films such festivals exhibit offer a ground from which to challenge such hegemony. We find figures, and sometimes objects, gazing back, making manifest the antagonisms at the heart of the socio-symbolic order. These figures (and the occasional lighthouse) are screened in a way that foregrounds the failure of the look that European A festivals proffer. This perspective is shown not to be coherent, nor objective in any sense, but rather entangled in the scenes it would otherwise witness at a distance. *Fire at Sea* highlights the presence of the cinematic apparatus, the fact of refugee figures being presented for a European look (including at the Berlinale), and the ideological investments that come with it. *Gomorrah* takes this further and actually screens the film festival, with Scarlett Johansson appearing on the Venice red carpet in a disquieting mise-en-abyme that targets not only the representational politics of these events, but their participation in an exploitative, and extractive, economic regime.

The Real of Capital

While European A festivals' embeddedness in certain geopolitical histories and economic arrangements is well-known, the effects of this mutual dependency have rarely been questioned outside of a handful of academic studies, most often in relation to Eurocentrism. Much more needs to be done to understand these effects, although work is emerging that considers the environmental impact of festivals (de Valck & Zielinski, 2022) and their labour practices (Leão, 2022; Vogel, 2022). I have sought to offer an account of the role that the European A festival apparatus has played in constituting, and naturalising, a certain representative regime, the regime of art cinema, conditioned by the power structures just alluded to.

The impact of these factors on the reproduction of a canon of art cinema, and the tropes that underpin it, is rarely studied, much less theorised through the lens of ideology. Yet, it is precisely the study of intersections between material ("apparatic") and representational structures, as well as regimes of institutional power and legitimation, to which ideology critique lends itself so well. I have aimed to demonstrate this by putting forward a methodology that analyses the apparatus of European A festivals in relation to, and sometimes in productive tension with, the paratextual representations of the films they award, as well as the unruly or excessive aspects of the films themselves.

Conceptualising European A festivals' re/production of art cinema through notions of ideology allows us to apprehend the effects of global capital not only on the material level (for example, funding), but on the level of signification, or rather resignification. In the essay from which this chapter takes its name, Žižek (2000a) deploys a notion of the Real as the limit to resignification, the repressed law that constitutes today's dominant ideology:

> In so far as we conceive of the politico-ideological resignification in terms of the struggle for hegemony, today's Real which sets a limit to resignification is Capital: the smooth functioning of Capital is that which remains the same, that which "always returns to its place," in the unconstrained struggle for hegemony (p. 223).

The repressed element that "always returns to its place" in the order of European A festivals, the repressed Real "which sets a limit to resignification," is, *alla fine* (in the end), capital. Italian cinema and indeed art cinema may be signified and resignified in myriad ways: as a decadent tour through Rome in the tradition of Fellini or an ethical witnessing of a humanitarian tragedy in the tradition of neorealism. Yet the guiding principle, the "unwritten rule" that sets the limit to signification, is European A festivals' need to maintain "the smooth functioning of Capital." Such festivals' construction of films may celebrate "art" and attempt to perform an integration of the other, but only do so provided that the Real of capital is left in place, and the symbolic coordinates of the global capitalist system (e.g., North/South) remain intact. It is not only that European A festivals are "business festivals" or enterprises caught between "art" and "commerce," as scholars such as Peranson (2008), Chan (2011), de Valck (2014) and many others have argued; rather, their character as such actively delimits the meanings they ascribe to art cinema. This, in turn, delimits the canons of films that audiences, critics and academics have access to and implicitly invest in.

Futures of Cinephilia

European A festivals' awarding and representation of Italian cinema in the new millennium is a relatively limited phenomenon but, as I have shown, a significant one for our understanding of the ideological underpinnings of dominant canons of art cinema. The framework of discursive materialist ideology critique, the investigation into the relationship between an institutional apparatus and its representation of both itself and its object, offers a means through which to interpret film culture beyond the case studies I have shared here. The other traditional pillars of European art cinema—French, German and Spanish—are likely to have been constructed in similar ways (it is hard not to think of these as another list of male auteurs, for example), but their study might bring to light new tropes that further nuance the account of institutional art cinema above. Such a study offers the possibility to comprehend the conditions under which not only European films, but films from around the world are permitted to "speak," via exhibition, attention, awards, and the opportunity to gain international circulation. For many films, festivals remain the gateway to international circulation, whether that be further exhibition within the festival network or through distribution deals that take such films to cinemas and streaming platforms. Understanding the ideological coordinates of this system, from festivals through to cinemas and platforms, is crucial if we are to understand the kind of reproduction of certain categories of art cinema and the values that underpin them.

The role of digital film circulation, above all platforms such as Netflix and Mubi, will become increasingly important in the reproduction of art cinema canons in future. The COVID-19 pandemic accelerated an already fast-moving shift to digital, with several festivals moving online (although Cannes staunchly resisted this move), and the exclusive window for both a film's premiere at a festival and, later in the distribution cycle, exhibition in film theatres being dropped. It remains to be seen if and how this might shape taxonomies of cinema to come. At present, platforms still appear to be somewhat dependent on festivals for the discovery of new films and new talent. This goes beyond Thierry Fremaux's triumphant assertion that Netflix is yet to discover "one great director" in 2021 (Fremaux cited in Yossman, 2021), and is borne out by academic studies of the phenomenon so far. Roderick Smits's and E. W. Nikdel's (2019) analysis of Mubi—by far the most relevant Global Northern online platform for art cinema—showed that their selections remain dependent on festival exhibition and awards.[2] Although in the context of their now much larger catalogue (they dropped the "film a day" model for a more expansive offering during COVID), Mubi aggregates films from a variety of festivals and many of the platform's spotlighted film strands showcase films from the European A list, reinforcing these institutions' dominant position in online and offline film culture.

In tracing the broad structures and historical legacies operative across European A festivals and their representation of films, this book may have given the impression that both the institutions of film festivals, and the institution of art cinema, are monolithic. However, the radical and destabilising potential of the films shown at festivals offers one avenue through which this sense can be challenged. In not only producing paratexts about and giving awards to films, but exhibiting them to audiences, film festivals offer a means through which even their own claims about cinematic value might be challenged. That such challenges are repeatedly contained by elements of the festival apparatus and festivals' paratextual representation of films has been a source of continuous tension within both European A festivals' attempts to delimit the meaning of art cinema, and this book's attempt to grapple with the phenomenon. However, in choosing to end each chapter on the moments of resistance that each film offers, I have tried to open up a utopic space in which these dominant ideological formations might be refuted. This is, I argue, a necessary project for all those involved in the legitimation of films and thus regimes of meaning, from academics to film critics, film programmers to fans.

In today's climate, our appraisals of art cinema can no longer afford to adhere to the old horizons of aesthetic and political value. Considerations of

2 For an extensive analysis of Mubi, curation and online streaming, see Frey (2021).

a film's merit must go beyond a vague apprehension of "technical achievement" rooted in legacies of that which Girish Shambu (2019) has designated the "old cinephilia," a cinephilia of white, male, straight auteurs and a very limited number of "exceptional" directors who might be afforded entry into the canon. European A festivals have been among the purveyors *par excellence* of the old cinephilia, setting standards of cinematic value that, as I have shown, continue to permeate the legitimation of art cinema today. Shambu (2020), among others (Vetter, 2022; Iyer, 2022), has proposed alternative modes of evaluating cinema that look beyond the film text, offering holistic assessment of not only its style but the relations of care, production, pedagogy and identity that underpin it. The insistence on the "art of film" as the singular sign under which European A festivals operate (an insistence I have deconstructed throughout this book) should thus be expanded to include the art of constructing decolonial relations of co-authorship and collaboration, or developing narratives that are "creative" not only in their utilisation of some technical conceit, but in their practical responses to and perspectives on a human society wrought by the effects of climate breakdown, colonisation, displacement, and numerous forms of inequality.

Yet, throughout this book, I have argued against self-congratulatory narratives of inclusion that do not touch the structures that gave rise to these exclusive notions of cinema in the first place. If my starting premise was that art cinema does not exist, I do not seek to argue now for the construction of a new "universal" secured only by greater diversity. Art cinema's non-existence must be asserted with ever greater force, our relationship to it organised by an apprehension of the impossibility of meaning. The crucial ideological procedure is not the flawed attempt at representation, but the act of concealing such flaws through disavowals and displacements. On the purely structural level, this means that European A festivals' representation of art cinema must somehow do away with their claims to universality: they must no longer claim a film's meaning on behalf of the festival but foreground the impossibility of ever doing so—the instability of film canons, notions of quality and even meaning. Such a move would be radical, challenging the very function of the film festival as an institution that produces meanings for films, as well as the historical imbalance of power accorded European film festivals the primary producers of such meanings. This would offer the ground for a "radical rearticulation" of the festival framework as well as the hierarchies through which the festival network has been constituted.

Abstract structures of representation and universality are not all that is at stake, however; as I discuss above, the Real that cuts through these festivals' representation of cinemas is capital. Thus, while the disruption of European

A festivals' representational hegemony remains an important step, it cannot be severed from a project that seeks to destabilise the material conditions on which they are founded and in the reproduction of which they participate. Rather than a retreat into a series of language games, then, it is necessary to assert the imperative to intervene at the material-discursive level. I do not think it is unfair to say that European A festivals, along with several other major festivals, hold a monopoly on film culture outside Hollywood. In its ideological form, this entails the universalisation of ultimately partial discourses about aesthetic value, progressive politics, and identities and geographies. While the film interpretations in this book have sought to counter the universality on which European A festivals stake their power, much more work is needed to undo the monopoly of a few festivals at the "top" of an artificially-constructed hierarchy.

In contrast with the continued centring of these institutions and their ideals—a centring in which this book participates—what is now required is the creation of a horizontal, multiplicitous "pluriverse" of film festivals and their study (Mignolo & Walsh, 2018, p. 3). As Lewis Gordon and Jane Anna Gordon (2006, p. ix) argue, the aim can no longer be to dismantle the master's house, but to build more houses such that not only one master's hegemony, but mastery itself becomes insignificant. With over 11,000 festivals now operating around the world, that work is surely underway, but the imbalances of power that have led us to this point remain. Such imbalances are, as I hope this book has made clear, a product of capital as at once a material and representative regime. To ignite the radical potential of the films, and festivals, film culture must be transformed by anti-capitalist, decolonial and environmental struggle. The stakes are too high for any lesser solution.

Bibliography

Berlin International Film Festival. (2012). *Cesare deve morire.* [Online]. Available from: https://www.berlinale.de/en/archiv/jahresarchive/2012/02_programm_2012/02_Filmdatenblatt_2012_20125150.html#tab=boulevard

Berlin International Film Festival. (2016a). *Fuocoammare.* [Online]. Available from: https://www.berlinale.de/en/archiv/jahresarchive/2016/02_programm_2016/02_Filmdatenblatt_2016_201614479.php#tab=filmStills

Chan, F. (2011). The international film festival and the making of a national cinema. *Screen*, *52*(2), 253–260.

De Valck, M. (2014). Film festivals, Bourdieu, and the economization of culture. *Canadian Journal of Film Studies*, *23*(1), 74–89.

De Valck, M., & Zielinski G. (2022). Greening film festivals. In M. de Valck & A. Damiens (Eds.), *Rethinking film festivals in the pandemic era and after* (pp. 307–328). Palgrave MacMillan.

Elsaesser, T. (2005). *European cinema: Face to face with Hollywood*. Amsterdam University Press.

Festival de Cannes. (2001). *La Stanza del Figlio (The Son's Room)*. [Online]. Available from: http://www.festival-cannes.com/en/films/la-stanza-del-figlio

Festival de Cannes. (2008). *Gomorra (Gomorrah)*. [Online]. Available from: https://www.festival-cannes.com/en/films/gomorra

Festival de Cannes. (2013). *La Grande Bellezza (The Great Beauty)*. [Online]. Available from: http://www.festival-cannes.com/en/films/la-grande-bellezza

Frey, M. (2021). *MUBI and the curation model of video on demand*. Palgrave MacMillan.

Gordon, L., & Gordon, J. (2006). Introduction: Not only the master's tools. In L. Gordon & J. A. Gordon (Eds.), *Not only the master's tools: African-American studies in theory and practice* (pp. i–xi). Paradigm.

Iyer, U. (2022). A pedagogy of reparations: Notes toward repairing the film and media studies curriculum. *Feminist Media Histories*, *8*(1), 181–193.

Karlovy Vary International Film Festival. (2003). *Facing Window/La Finestra di Fronte*. [Online]. Available from: http://www.kviff.com/en/programme/film/03383-facing-window/

Karlovy Vary International Film Festival. (2004). *A Children's Story/Certi bambini*. [Online]. Available from: https://www.kviff.com/en/programme/film/04996-a-childrens-story/

Leão, T. (2022). *Can we openly talk about precarious and voluntary work at film festivals? Reflections on the Portuguese case*. NECS annual conference, Epistemic Media: Atlas, Archive, Network, 22–26 June 2022. Politechnica University of Bucharest.

Mignolo, W. D., & Walsh, C. E. (2018). *On decoloniality: Concepts, analytics, praxis*. Duke University Press.

Ostrowska, D. (2016). Making film history at the Cannes film festival. In M. de Valck, B. D. Kredell, & S. Loist (Eds.), *Film festivals: History, theory, method, practice* (pp. 18–33). Routledge.

Peranson, M. (2008). First you get the power, then you get the money: Two models of film festivals. *Cineaste*, *33*(3), 37–43.

Priimägi, T. (2013). *The Great Beauty*. Tallinn Black Nights Film Festival. [Online]. Available from: http://2013.poff.ee/eng/films/programmes.p/official-competition-eurasia-1/the-great-beauty

Said, E. (2003 [1978]). *Orientalism: Western conceptions of the Orient*. Penguin

Schoonover, K. (2012). *Brutal vision: The neorealist body in postwar Italian cinema*. University of Minnesota Press.

Shambu, G. (2019). For a new cinephilia. *Film Quarterly*, *72*(3), 32–34.
Shambu, G. (2020). Rethinking film evaluation. *Quorum*. Available from: https://filmquarterly.org/2020/03/11/rethinking-film-evaluation/
Smits, R., & Nikdel, E. W. (2019). Beyond Netflix and Amazon: MUBI and the curation of on-demand film. *Studies in European Cinema*, *16*(1), 22–37.
Táíwò, O. O. (2022). *Elite capture: How the powerful took over identity politics (and everything else)*. Pluto Press.
Venice International Film Festival. (2013). *Sacro GRA*. [Online]. Available from: http://www.labiennale.org/en/cinema/archive/70th-festival/line-up/off-sel/venezia70/sacro-gra.html
Vetter, D. (2022). Who cares about cinema? *The Film Comment Letter*. Available from: https://www.filmcomment.com/blog/who-cares-about-cinema-film-festivals-film-workers-dennis-vetter/
Vogel, A. (2022). *Cinema and the festivalization of capitalism*. Brill.
Yossman, K. J. (2021). Press conference at Cannes film festival. *Variety*. Available from: https://variety.com/2021/film/global/cannes-thierry-fremaux-talks-netflix-pandemic-challenges-in-pre-festival-press-conference-1235011781/
Žižek, S. (2000a). Class struggle or postmodernism? Yes, please! In J. Butler, E. Laclau, & S. Žižek (Eds.), *Contingency, hegemony, universality: Contemporary dialogues on the left* (pp. 91–135). Verso.
Žižek, S. (2004a). *Iraq: The borrowed kettle*. Verso.

Filmography

A Children's Story (*Certi bambini*) (2004). Frazzi, A., & Frazzi, A. dirs. Italy.
Ceasar Must Die (*Cesare deve morire*) (2012). Taviani, P., & Taviani, V. dirs. Italy.
Facing Window (*La finestra di fronte*) (2003). Özpetek, F. dir. Italy.
Fire at Sea (*Fuocoammare*) (2016). Rosi, G. dir. Italy.
Gomorrah (*Gomorra*) (2008). Garrone, M. dir. Italy.
The Great Beauty (*La grande bellezza*) (2013). Sorrentino, P. dir. Italy.
Private (2004). Costanzo, S. dir. Italy.
The Son's Room (*La stanza del figlio*) (2001). Moretti, N. dir. Italy.
Sacro GRA (2013). Rosi, G. dir. Italy.

Appendices

Appendix 1: A-List Film Festivals

This list is adapted from the most recent *FIAPF Festivals Directory* (FIAPF 2023).

Festival (est.)	Location	Dates
Berlin International Film Festival (1951)	Berlin, Germany	February 7–17
Cairo International Film Festival (1972)	Cairo, Egypt	November 20–29
Festival de Cannes (1946)	Cannes, France	May 14–25
Fajr International Film Festival (1982)	Tehran, Iran	May 26–June 2
Goa – International Film Festival of India (1952)	Goa, India	November 20–28
Karlovy Vary International Film Festival (1946)	Karlovy Vary, Czech Republic	June 28–July 6
Festival del film Locarno (1946)	Locarno, Switzerland	August 7–17
Mar del Plata International Film Festival (1954)	Mar del Plata, Argentina	November 9–18
San Sebastián International Film Festival (1953)	Donostia-San Sebastián, Basque Country, Spain	September 20–28
Shanghai International Film Festival (1933)	Shanghai, China	June 15–24
Tallinn Black Nights Film Festival (1987)	Tallinn, Estonia	November 16–December 2
Tokyo International Film Festival (1985)	Tokyo, Japan	October 28–November 5
Venice International Film Festival (1932)	Venice, Italy	August 28–September 7
Warsaw Film Festival (1985)	Warsaw, Poland	October 11–20

Johnson, R., Film Festivals, *Ideology and Italian Art Cinema: Politics, Histories and Cultural Value*.
Taylor & Francis Group, 2024
DOI 10.5117/9789463720366_APP

Appendix 2: Italian Best Picture Winners, 1946–2020

Italian films that have won Best Picture award or equivalent at a European A festival. I have included some awards given prior festivals' "A" accreditation due to their role in the formation of discourses about Italian art cinema and the development of the European A circuit.

Year	Film	Director	Festival
1946	*Rome, Open City/ Roma, città aperta*	Roberto Rossellini	Cannes
1948	*Germany Year Zero/ Germania, anno zero*	Roberto Rossellini	Locarno
1951	*Miracle in Milan/ Miracolo a Milano*	Vittorio de Sica	Cannes
1952	*Two Cents Worth of Hope/ Due soldi di speranza*	Renato Castellani	Cannes
1955	*Days of Love/ Giorni d'amore*	Giuseppe de Santis & Leopoldo Savona	San Sebastián
1956	*Man of Iron/ Il ferroviere*	Pietro Germi	San Sebastián
1957	*The Outcry/ Il grido*	Michelangelo Antonioni	Locarno
1957	*Oh! Sabella/ La nonna Sabella*	Dino Risi	San Sebastián
1959	*General Della Rovere/ Il generale della Rovere* *The Great War/ La grande guerra*	Roberto Rossellini Mario Monicelli	Venice
1960	*La Dolce Vita/ La dolce vita*	Federico Fellini	Cannes
1960	*Il Bell'Antonio/ Il bell'Antonio/*	Mauro Bolognini	Locarno
1961	*La Notte/ La notte*	Michelangelo Antonioni	Berlinale
1962	*Family Portrait/ Cronaca familiare*	Valerio Zurlini	Venice
1962	*Arthur's Island/ L'isola di Arturo*	Damiano Damiani	San Sebastián
1963	*The Leopard/ Il gattopardo*	Luchino Visconti	Cannes
1963	*Mafioso/ Mafioso*	Alberto Lattuada	San Sebastián
1963	*Hands Over the City/ Le mani sulla città*	Francesco Rosi	Venice
1963	*To Bed or Not to Bed/ Il diavolo*	Gian Luigi Polidoro	Berlinale
1964	*Red Desert/ Deserto rosso*	Michelangelo Antonioni	Venice
1965	*Sandra/ Vaghe stelle d'Orsa*	Luchino Visconti	Venice
1966	*The Birds, the Bees, and the Italians/ Signori e signore*	Pietro Germi	Cannes
1966	*The Battle of Algiers/ La battaglia di Algeri*	Gillo Pontecorvo	Venice
1967	*Blow-Up/ Blow-Up*	Michelangelo Antonioni	Cannes
1968	*The Visionaries/ I visionari*	Maurisio Ponzi	Locarno
1970	*Dead of Summer/ Ondata del colore*	Nelo Risi	San Sebastián
1971	*The Garden of the Finzi-Continis/ Il girdino dei Finzi Contini*	Vittorio de Sica	Berlinale

Year	Film	Director	Festival
1971	*They Have Changed Their Face/ Hanno cambiato faccia* *On the Point of Death/ In punto di morte*	Corrado Farina Mario Garriba	Locarno
1972	*The Mattei Affair/ Il caso Mattei* *The Working Class Goes to Heaven/ La classe operaia va in paradiso*	Francesco Rosi Elio Petri	Cannes
1972	*The Canterbury Tales/ I racconiti di Canterbury*	Pier Paolo Pasolini	Berlinale
1977	*Antonio Gramsci, the Days of Prison/ Antonio Gramsci, i giorni di carcere*	Lino Del Fra	Locarno
1977	*Padre padrone/ Padre padrone*	Paolo e Vittorio Taviani	Cannes
1978	*The Tree of Wooden Clogs/ L'albero degli zoccoli*	Ermanno Olmi	Cannes
1980	*To Love the Damned/ Maledetti vi ameró*	Marco Tullio Giordana	Locarno
1988	*The Legend of the Holy Drinker/ La leggenda del Santo Bevitore*	Ermanno Olmi	Cannes
1991	*The House of Smiles/ La casa del sorriso*	Marco Ferrari	Berlinale
1998	*Così ridevano/ Così ridevano*	Gianni Amelio	Venice
2001	*The Son's Room/ La stanza del figlio*	Nanni Moretti	Cannes
2001	*Off to the Revolution by a 2CV/ Alla rivoluzione sulla due cavalli*	Maurisio Sciarra	Locarno
2003	*Facing Window/ La finestra di fronte*	Ferzan Ozpetek	Karlovy Vary
2004	*Private/ Private*	Saverio Costanzo	Locarno
2004	*A Children's Story/ Certi bambini*	Andrea & Antonio Frazzi	Karlovy Vary
2012	*Caesar Must Die/ Cesare deve morire*	Paolo e Vittorio Taviani	Berlinale
2013	*Sacro GRA/ Sacro GRA*	Gianfranco Rosi	Venice
2013	*The Great Beauty/ La grande bellezza*	Paolo Sorrentino	Tallinn
2016	*Fire at Sea/ Fuocoammare*	Gianfranco Rosi	Berlinale

Appendix 3: Synopses of Secondary Case Studies

A3.1 *A Children's Story* (*Certi Bambini*, Andrea and Antonio Frazzi, 2004)

Eleven-year-old Rosario lives in a cheerless apartment in the suburbs with his sick grandmother who spends most of the day in bed. He and a couple of friends spend time slacking off between a dive pub and the Las Vegas gambling joint. They smoke, drink and steal, imitating the worst of the adult world they see around them. The laughter that once graced their faces as children has been replaced by a queer, ambiguous smile bearing witness to myriad painful experiences. The makers of *A Children's Story* (based upon the novel by Diego De Silva) have placed incidents from the boys' lives in extensive flashbacks, mental flights Rosario embarks upon during long subway rides. With every new abrupt closing of the train doors, the boy drags us into his recent past and presents the three most influential people in his life: the admired Santino, the feared Damiano and the alluring Caterina. This fascinating film bears cruel witness to how easy it is for a troubled child to get mixed up in the Naples camorra.

– *Karlovy Vary 2004 print and online programme*

A3.2 *Caesar Must Die* (*Cesare deve morire*, Paolo and Vittorio Taviani, 2012)

The performance of Shakespeare's *Julius Caesar* comes to an end and the performers are rewarded with rapturous applause. The lights go out; the actors leave the stage and return to their cells. They are all inmates of the Roman maximum security prison Rebibbia. One of them comments: "Ever since I discovered art this cell has truly become a prison."

Filmmakers Paolo and Vittorio Taviani spent six months following rehearsals for this stage production; their film demonstrates how the universality of Shakespeare's language helps the actors to understand their roles and immerse themselves in the bard's interplay of friendship and betrayal, power, dishonesty and violence. This documentary does not dwell on the crimes these men have committed in their "real" lives; rather, it draws parallels between this classical drama and the world of today, describes the commitment displayed by all those involved and shows how their personal hopes and fears also flow into the performance.

After the premiere the cell doors slam shut behind Caesar, Brutus and the others. These men all feel proud and strangely touched, as if the play has somehow revealed to them the depths of their own personal history.

– Berlinale 2012 print and online programme

A3.3 *Sacro Gra* (Gianfranco Rosi, 2013)

After the India of Varanasi's boatmen, the American desert of the dropouts, and the Mexico of the killers of drug trade, Gianfranco Rosi has decided to tell the tale of a part of his own country, roaming and filming for over two years in a minivan on Rome's giant ring road—the Grande Raccordo Anulare, or GRA—to discover the invisible worlds and possible futures harbored in this area of constant turmoil. Elusive characters and fleeting apparitions emerge from the background of the winding zone: a nobleman from the Piemonte region and his college student daughter sharing a one-room efficiency in a modern apartment building along the GRA; a botanist making audio recordings of the interiors of palm trees to detect and then poison the insects that are devouring them like a plague; a modern day cigar-smoking prince doing gymnastics on the roof of his castle, surrounded by the sea of new apartment buildings proliferating around him; a paramedic in an ambulance eternally on duty treating car accident victims along the vast road; and an eel fisherman living on a houseboat beneath an overpass along the Tiber River. Far from the iconic sites of Rome, the GRA is a repository of stories of those at the edges of the ever expanding universe of the capital city.

– Venice 2013 print and online programme

Bibliography

Film Synopses

Berlin International Film Festival. (2012). *Cesare deve morire.* [Online]. Available from: https://www.berlinale.de/en/archiv/jahresarchive/2012/02_programm_2012/02_Filmdatenblatt_2012_20125150.html#tab=boulevard

Berlin International Film Festival. (2016a). *Fuocoammare.* [Online]. Available from: https://www.berlinale.de/en/archiv/jahresarchive/2016/02_programm_2016/02_Filmdatenblatt_2016_201614479.php#tab=filmStills

Festival de Cannes. (2001). *La Stanza del Figlio* (*The Son's Room*). [Online]. Available from: http://www.festival-cannes.com/en/films/la-stanza-del-figlio

Festival de Cannes. (2008). *Gomorra* (*Gomorrah*). [Online]. Available from: https://www.festival-cannes.com/en/films/gomorra

Festival de Cannes. (2013). *La Grande Bellezza* (*The Great Beauty*). [Online]. Available from: http://www.festival-cannes.com/en/films/la-grande-bellezza

Karlovy Vary International Film Festival. (2003). *Facing Window/La Finestra di Fronte.* [Online]. Available from: http://www.kviff.com/en/programme/film/03383-facing-window/

Karlovy Vary International Film Festival. (2004). *A Children's Story/Certi bambini.* [Online]. Available from: https://www.kviff.com/en/programme/film/04996-a-childrens-story/

Priimägi, T. (2013). *The Great Beauty.* Tallinn Black Nights Film Festival. [Online]. Available from: http://2013.poff.ee/eng/films/programmes.p/official-competition-eurasia-1/the-great-beauty

Venice International Film Festival. (2013). *Sacro GRA.* [Online]. Available from: http://www.labiennale.org/en/cinema/archive/70th-festival/line-up/off-sel/venezia70/sacro-gra.html

Secondary Sources

Ahmed, S. (2000). *Strange encounters: Embodied others in post-coloniality.* Routledge.

Ahn, S. (2012). *The Pusan International Film Festival, South Korean cinema and globalisation.* Hong Kong University Press.

Althusser, L. (2001 [1971]). Ideology and ideological state apparatuses (notes towards an investigation). In L. Althusser, *Lenin and philosophy and other essays* (pp. 85–126). New York University Press.

Amin, S. (2018). Globalisation and its alternative. *Political Notebook #1*. Tricontinental Institute for Social Research. Available from: https://www.thetricontinental.org/wp-content/uploads/2018/10/181029_Political_Notebook_1_EN_Final_Web.pdf

Andrews, D. (2010). Art cinema as institution, redux: Art houses, film festivals, and film studies. *Scope: An Online Journal of Film and Television Studies*, *18*, 1–21.

Andrews, E. (2014). *Place, setting, perspective: Narrative space in the films of Nanni Moretti*. Fairleigh Dickinson University Press.

ANSA. (2017). Strong Venice Film Festival line-up heavy on migration. *ANSA Med*. 28 July 2019. Available from: https://www.ansamed.info/ansamed/en/news/nations/italy/2017/07/28/strong-venice-film-festival-line-up-heavy-on-migration_5c87917a-d3f2-48e6-aafc-02b1fbc6ce77.html?idPhoto=2

Antonello, P. (2011). Dispatches from hell: Matteo Garrone's *Gomorrah*. In D. Renga (Ed.), *Mafia movies: A reader* (pp. 377–385). University of Toronto Press.

Antonello, P., & Barotsi, R. (2009). The personal and the political: The cinema of Nanni Moretti. In P. Antonello & F. Mussgnug (Eds.), *Postmodern impegno: Ethics and commitment in contemporary Italian culture* (pp. 189–212). Peter Lang.

Appadurai, A. (1990). Disjuncture and difference in the global cultural economy. *Theory, Culture & Society*, *7*(2–3), 295–310.

Austin, T. (2017). *Benefaction, processing, exclusion: Documentary representations of refugees and migrants in Fortress Europ*e. European Cinema: Perspectives on Post-Democracy and the Crisis of the European Project, 19 May 2017, University of Leeds.

Balicco, D. (Ed.). (2013). Conoscere l'Italia contemporanea. Indagine sul Made in Italy. *Allegoria*, *68*.

Balicco, D. (2013). Il film in questione: *La grande bellezza* (2013). *Allegoria*, *68*, 205–212.

Barthes, R. (2012 [1957]). *Mythologies*. Hill and Wang.

Bartolo, P., & Tilotta, L. (2017). *Lampedusa: Gateway to Europe*. MacLehose Press.

Bauman, R. (2015). *Divi ambigui*: Ferzan Özpetek's starstruck gaze. *Italian Studies*, *70*(3), 389–401.

Bauman, Z. (2000). *Liquid modernity*. Polity.

Baumann, S. (2007). A general theory of artistic legitimation: How art worlds are like social movements. *Poetics*, *35*(1), 47–65.

Bayman, L., & Rigoletto, S. (2013). The fair and the museum: Framing the popular. In L. Bayman & S. Rigoletto (Eds.), *Popular Italian cinema* (pp. 1–28). Palgrave Macmillan.

Bazin, A. (2008 [1957]). De la politique des auteurs. In B. K. Grant (Ed.), *Auteurs and authorship: A film reader* (pp. 19–28). Blackwell.

BBC News. (2016). *Berlin Film Festival:* Fire at Sea *wins Golden Bear*. [Online]. 20 February. Available from: http://www.bbc.co.uk/news/entertainment-arts-35623412

Bell, K. M. (2013). Raising Africa? Celebrity and the rhetoric of the white saviour. *PORTAL Journal of Multidisciplinary International Studies, 10*(1), 1–24.

Benvenuto, S. (2001). *The Son's Room*, or: The analysis is over. *Journal of European Psychoanalysis, 12*. [Online]. Available from: http://www.psychomedia.it/jep/number12-13/benvenuto.htm

Bergfelder, T. (2005). National, transnational or supranational cinema? Rethinking European film studies. *Media, Culture & Society, 27*(3), 315–331.

Berlin International Film Festival. (2016b). Yearbook: 66th Berlin International Film Festival, 11–21 February 2016. Available from: https://www.berlinale.de/en/archive/jahresarchive/2016/01_jahresblatt_2016/01_jahresblatt_2016.html

Betz, M. (2001). The name above the (sub)title: Internationalism, coproduction, and polyglot European art cinema. *Camera Obscura, 46*, 1–45.

Bhabha, H. K. (1983). The other question. *Screen, 24*(6), 18–36.

Bhambra, G. K. et al. (2018). *Decolonising the university*. Pluto Press.

Bianchi, P. (2018). La spada di Lazzaro. *Doppiozero*. 15 May. [Online]. Available from: https://www.doppiozero.com/materiali/la-spada-di-lazzaro

Bláhová, J. (2020). Political significance of a *Butcher in Love*: The 1956 Karlovy Vary International Film Festival, *Marty* and the restoration of contact between Hollywood and Czechoslovakia during the Cold War. *Studies in European Cinema, 17*(2), 97–112.

Boase, R. (1977). *The origin and meaning of courtly love: A critical study of European scholarship*. Manchester University Press.

Bondavalli, S. (2011). Waste management: Garbage displacement and the ethics of Mafia representation in Matteo Garrone's *Gomorra*. *California Italian Studies, 2*(1), 1–17.

Bonsaver, G. (2001). The egocentric Cassandra of the left: Representations of politics in the films of Nanni Moretti. *The Italianist 21*(1), 158–183.

Bordwell, D. (1979). The art cinema as a mode of film practice. *Film Criticism, 4*(1), 56–64.

Bordwell, D., & Carroll, N. (1996). *Post-theory: Reconstructing film studies*. University of Wisconsin Press.

Bosma, P. (2015). *Film programming: Curating for cinemas, festivals, archives*. Columbia University Press.

Boutsko, A. (2021). Dieter Kosslick: Berlinale's former head publishes memoir. *Deutsche Welle*. 3 February 2021. Available from: https://www.berlinale.de/en/archive/jahresarchive/2016/01_jahresblatt_2016/01_jahresblatt_2016.html

Box Office Mojo. (2018a). *Gomorrah: International box office results*. [Online]. Available from: https://www.boxofficemojo.com/movies/?page=intl&id=gomorrah.htm

Box Office Mojo. (2018b). *The Great Beauty: International box office results*. [Online]. Available from: http://www.boxofficemojo.com/movies/?id=greatbeauty.htm

Box Office Mojo. (2019). *City of God: International box office results.* [Online]. Available from: https://www.boxofficemojo.com/movies/?id=cityofgod.htm

Breyfogle, S. (2020). Stories from the margins: The practicality and ethics of refugee film festivals. *Frames Cinema Journal.* Available from: http://framescinemajournal.com/article/stories-from-the-margins-the-practicality-and-ethics-of-refugee-film-festivals/

Brook, C. (2005.) Screening the autobiographical. In W. Hope (Ed.), *Italian Cinema: New Directions* (pp. 27–52). Peter Lang.

Brown, W. (2009). The festival syndrome: Report on the International Film Festival Workshop, University of St Andrews, 4 April 2009. In D. Iordanova & R. Rhyne (Eds.), *Film Festival Yearbook 1: The Festival Circuit* (pp. 216–225). St. Andrews Film Studies & College Gate Press.

Brunetta, G. P. (2007). *Il cinema italiano contemporaneo: da* La dolce vita *a* Centochiodi. Laterza.

Brunetta, G. P. (2009). *The history of Italian cinema: A guide to Italian film from its origins to the twenty-first century.* Princeton University Press.

Burgess, D., & Kredell, B. (2016). Positionality and film festival research: A conversation. In M. de Valck, B. Kredell, & S. Loist (Eds.), *Film festivals: History, theory, method, practice* (pp. 159–176). Routledge.

Buscombe, E. (2008 [1973]). Ideas of authorship. In B. K. Grant (Ed.), *Auteurs and authorship: A film reader* (pp. 76–83). Blackwell.

Butler, J. (2000). Restaging the universal: Hegemony and the limits of formalism. In J. Butler, E. Laclau, & S. Žižek (Eds.), *Contingency, hegemony, universality: Contemporary dialogues on the left* (pp. 11–43). Verso.

Butler, J. (2002). *Antigone's claim: Kinship between life and death.* New York: Columbia University Press.

Butler, J., Laclau, E., & Žižek, S. (Eds.). (2000). *Contingency, hegemony, universality: Contemporary dialogues on the left.* Verso.

Carroll, N. (1998). *A philosophy of mass art.* Oxford University Press.

Cavaliere, F. (2010). *Gomorrah*: Crime goes global, language stays local. *European Journal of English Studies, 14*(2), 173–188.

Chambers, I. (2008). *Mediterranean crossings: The politics of an interrupted modernity.* Duke University Press.

Chambers, I. (2015). The "Southern Question"... again. In A. Mammone, E. G. Parini, & G. A. Veltri (Eds.), *The Routledge handbook of contemporary Italy: History, politics, society* (pp. 25–34). Routledge.

Chan, F. (2011). The international film festival and the making of a national cinema. *Screen, 52*(2), 253–260.

Cheung, R. (2016). Ever-changing readjustments: The political economy of the Hong Kong International Film Festival (HKIFF). *New Review of Film and Television Studies, 14*(1), 59–75.

Ciliento, F. (2011). Saviano, Garrone, *Gomorrah*: Neorealism and noir in the land of the Camorra. *Fast Capitalism, 8*(1). [Online]. Available from: https://www.uta.edu/huma/agger/fastcapitalism/8_1/cilento8_1.html
Coladonato, V. (2021). "Mon cher Fédérico": Fellini and the Cannes Film Festival. *Journal of Italian Cinema & Media Studies, 9*(1), 117–132.
Copjec, J. (1994). *Read my desire: Lacan against the historicists*. Verso Books.
Cordoba, C. (2022). The Locarno Film Festival under the influence? Programming Eastern European movies in anti-communist Switzerland (1946–1962). *Contemporary European History: First View, 1*(1), 1–19.
Cousins, M. (2009). Widescreen on film festivals. In D. Iordanova & R. Rhyne (Eds.), *Festival yearbook 1: The festival circuit* (pp. 155–158). St Andrews Film Studies and College Gate Press.
Cucco, M. (2014). Che cosa è un film? *La grande bellezza* in una prospettiva di economia e politica di media. In M. Cucco (Ed.), *La trama dei media. Stato, imprese, pubblico nella societa dell'informazione* (pp. 101–119). Carocci editore.
Czach, L. (2004). Film festivals, programming, and the building of a national cinema. *The Moving Image, 4*(1), 76–88.
Damiens, A. (2018). The queer film ecosystem: Symbolic economy, festivals, and queer cinema's legs. *Studies in European Cinema, 15*(1), 25–40.
Damiens, A. (2020). *LGBTQ festivals: Curating queerness*. Amsterdam University Press.
Dayan, D. (2000). Looking for Sundance: The social construction of a film festival. In I. Bondebjerg (Ed.), *Moving images, culture and the mind* (pp. 43–52). University of Luton Press.
De Gaetano, R. (1999). *Il corpo e la maschera: Il grottesco nel cinema italiano*. Bulzoni.
De Lauretis, T. (1984). *Alice doesn't: Feminism, semiotics, cinema*. MacMillan.
De Marco, C. (2015). Moretti, Sorrentino, Garrone: "In it together for Italian film." *Cineuropa*. [Online]. Available from: http://cineuropa.org/nw.aspx?t=newsdetail&l=en&did=289826
De Valck, M. (2007). *Film festivals: From European geopolitics to global cinephilia*. Amsterdam University Press.
De Valck, M. (2013). Migration and film festivals. In I. Ness (Ed.), *The encyclopedia of global human migration* (Vol. 3, pp. 1502–1504). Wiley-Blackwell.
De Valck, M. (2014). Film festivals, Bourdieu, and the economisation of culture. *Canadian Journal of Film Studies, 23*(1), 74–89.
De Valck, M. (2016). Fostering art, adding value, cultivating taste: Film festivals as sites of cultural legitimisation. In M. de Valck, D. B. Kredell, & S. Loist (Eds.), *Film festivals: History, theory, method, practice* (pp. 100–116). Routledge.
De Valck, M., & Zielinski G. (2022). Greening film festivals. In M. de Valck & A. Damiens (Eds.), *Rethinking film festivals in the pandemic era and after* (pp. 307–328). Palgrave MacMillan.

Debruge, P. (2016). Berlin film review: "Fire at Sea." *Variety.* [Online]. Available from: https://variety.com/2016/film/reviews/fire-at-sea-film-review-fuocoammare-1201705492/

Diawara, M. (2010). *African film: New forms of aesthetics and politics.* Prestel Verlag.

Donadio, R. (2013). La dolce vita gone sour (and this time in color). *The New York Times.* 8 September. [Online]. Available from: https://www.nytimes.com/2013/09/09/movies/paolo-sorrentinos-great-beauty-explores-italys-decline.html

Dovey, L. 2015. *Curating Africa in the age of film festivals.* Palgrave Macmillan.

Dovey, L. et al. (2013). "From, by, for" – Nairobi's slum film festival, film festival studies, and the practices of development. *Jump Cut: A Review of Contemporary Media, 55*(1). Available from: http://ejumpcut.org/archive/jc55.2013/DoveySFFNairobi/index.html

Duncan, D. (2008). Italy's postcolonial cinema and its histories of representation. *Italian Studies 63*(2), 195–211.

Duncan, D. (2013). The geopolitics of spectatorship and screen identification: What's queer about Italian cinema? *The Italianist, 33*(2), 256–261.

Dupré, N. (2015). La "condivisione" della Shoah: Un confronto tra Perlasca, un eroe italiano e *La finestra di fronte.* In M. Jansen & M. B. Urban (Eds.), *Televisionismo: Narrazioni televisive della storia italiana negli anni della seconda Repubblica* (pp. 61–68). Edizioni Ca' Foscari.

Elgot, J., & Taylor, M. (2015). Calais Crisis: Cameron condemned for "dehumanising" description of migrants. *The Guardian.* [Online]. 30 July. Available from: https://www.theguardian.com/uk-news/2015/jul/30/david-cameron-migrant-swarm-language-condemned

Elsaesser, T. (2005). *European cinema: Face to face with Hollywood.* Amsterdam University Press.

Elsaesser, T. (2016). The global author: Control, creative constraints, and performative self-contradiction. In S. Jeong & J. Szaniawski (Eds.), *The global auteur: The politics of authorship in 21st century cinema* (pp. 21–41). Bloomsbury.

Esposito, R. (2011). *Immunitas: The protection and negation of life.* Polity Press.

Fabbri, L. (2015). Neorealism as ideology: Bazin, Deleuze, and the avoidance of fascism. *The Italianist, 35*(2), 182–201.

Falicov, T. (2010). Migrating from south to north: The role of film festivals in funding and shaping global south film and video. In T. Falicov et al. (Eds.), *Locating migrating media* (pp. 3–22). Lexington Books.

Falicov, T. (2016). The "festival film." In M. de Valck, B. D. Kredell, & S. Loist (Eds.), *Film festivals: History, theory, method, practice* (pp. 209–229). Routledge.

Fehrenbach, H. (1995). *Cinema in democratising Germany: Reconstructing of national identity after Hitler.* University of North Carolina Press.

Festival de Cannes. (2019a). *Festival de Cannes: Partners.* [Online]. Available from: https://www.festival-cannes.com/en/participer/prepare/partners

Festival de Cannes. (2019b). *Nanni Moretti.* [Online]. Available from: https://www.festival-cannes.com/en/artist/nanni-moretti-3

FIAPF (International Federation of Film Producers Associations). (2023). *Accredited festivals: Competitive feature film festivals.* [Online]. Available from: https://fiapf.org/festivals/accredited-festivals/competitive-feature-film-festivals

FIAPF (International Federation of Film Producers Associations). (2019). *FIAPF accredited festivals directory: 2016 edition.* [Online]. Available from: https://fiapf.org/festival_file/fiapf-accredited-festivals-directory-2019-edition/

FIAPF (International Federation of Film Producers Associations). (2016). *International film festivals signed FIAPF's mutual trust contract and received accreditation in 2016.* [Online]. Available from: http://www.fiapf.org/intfilmfestivals.asp

Fink, B. (1995). *The Lacanian subject: Between language and jouissance.* Princeton University Press.

Forgacs, D. (2004). Space, rhetoric, and the divided city in *Roma città aperta.* In S. Gottlieb (Ed.), *Roberto Rossellini's* Rome Open City (pp. 106–130). Cambridge University Press.

Foucault, M. (2012 [1975]). *Discipline and punish: The birth of the prison.* Vintage.

Frater, P. (2018). Pingyao festival celebrates indie spirit at opening. *Variety.* [Online]. Available from: https://variety.com/2018/film/asia/pingyao-festival-celebrates-indie-spirit-1202976792/

Freud, S. (1917). *Mourning and melancholia.* Vintage.

Frey, M. (2021). *MUBI and the curation model of video on demand.* Palgrave MacMillan.

Galt, R., & Schoonover, K. (2010). Introduction: The impurity of art cinema. In R. Galt & K. Schoonover (Eds.), *Global art cinema: New theories and histories* (pp. 3–27). Oxford University Press.

Garofalo, D. (2018). Italian cinema in the shadow of film festival crisis. *International Circulation of Italian Cinema.* [Online]. Available from: https://www.italiancinema.it/italian-cinema-in-the-shadow-of-film-festival-crisis/

Garrone, M. (2008). *Nota di regia, Gomorra.* Press pack. [Online]. Available from: http://www.archimedefilm.it/docs/gomorra_pressbook_ita.doc

Gramsci, A. (1994 [1926]). Some aspects of the Southern Question. In R. Bellamy (Ed.), *Antonio Gramsci: Pre-prison writings* (pp. 313–337). Cambridge University Press.

Gordon, R. (2012). *The Holocaust in Italian culture, 1944–2010.* Stanford University Press.

Gordon, R. (2015) Inside-out. History, beauty and the cultural currents of Italianness within and across borders. *Studi culturali, 12*(3), 325–338.

Gordon, L., & Gordon, J. (2006). Introduction: Not only the master's tools. In L. Gordon & J. A. Gordon (Eds.), *Not only the master's tools: African-American studies in theory and practice* (pp. i–xi). Paradigm.

Gray, J. (2010). *Show sold separately: Promos, spoilers, and other media paratexts.* NYU Press.

Guerini Rocco, S. (2019). Italian world cinema: Alice Rohrwacher's "Lazzaro Felice" abroad. *International Circulation of Italian Cinema.* [Online]. Available from: https://www.italiancinema.it/italian-world-cinema-alice-rohrwachers-happy-as-lazzaro-abroad/

Gundle, S. (2007). *Bellissima: Feminine beauty and the idea of Italy.* Yale University Press.

Hall, S. (2018 [1977]). Re-thinking the "base-and-superstructure" metaphor. In D. Morely (Ed.), *Essential essays, volume 1: Foundations of cultural studies* (pp. 143–171). Duke University Press.

Halle, R. (2010). Offering tales they want to hear: Transnational European film funding as neo-orientalism. In R. Galt & K. Schoonover (Eds.), *Global art cinema: New theories and histories* (pp. 303–319). Oxford University Press.

Harbord, J. (2002). *Film cultures.* Sage.

Harbord, J. (2009). Film festivals as time-event. In D. Iordanova & R. Rhyne (Eds.), *Film festival yearbook 1: The festival circuit* (pp. 40–46). St Andrews Film Studies & College Gate Press.

Hardt, M., & Negri, A. (2000). *Empire.* Harvard University Press.

Harrow, K. (2013). *Trash: African cinema from below.* Indiana University Press.

Hayward, S. (2013). *Cinema studies: The key concepts* (4th ed.). Routledge.

Higson, A. (1989). The concept of national cinema. *Screen, 30*(4), 36–47.

Higson, A. (2020). Soft power and national cinema: James Bond, Great Britain and Brexit. In R. Dwyer (Ed.), *Cinema and soft power: Configuring the national and transnational in geo-politics* (pp. 210–235). Edinburgh University Press.

Hipkins, D. (2008). Why Italian film studies needs a second take on gender. *Italian Studies, 63*(2), 213–234.

Hipkins, D., & Renga, D. (2016). A new canon? Contemporary Italian cinema and television and the role of quality in the anglophone curriculum. *Comunicazioni sociali, 1*(3), 375–397.

Hjort, M., & MacKenzie, S. (2000). *Cinema and nation.* Routledge.

Holdaway, D. (2014). Osservazioni sulla retorica di *Gomorra.* In W. Hope, S. Serra, & L. D'Arcangeli (Eds.), *Un nuovo cinema politico italiano? Il passato sociopolitica o, il potere istituzionale, la marginalizzazione* (pp. 198–210). Troubador.

hooks, b. (1992). *Black looks: Race and representation.* South End Press.

Horton, J. (1972). Combatting empiricism: Toward a practical understanding of Marxist methodology. *Insurgent Sociologist, 3*(1), 24–34.

International Documentary Association (IDA). (2017). Gianfranco Rosi on "Fire at Sea." Video interview. Available from: https://www.youtube.com/watch?v=xzNVTUziT8k

Iordanova, D. (2006). Showdown of the festivals: Clashing entrepreneurships and post-communist management of culture. *Film International, 4*(5), 25–37.

Iordanova, D. (2009). The festival circuit. In D. Iordanova & R. Rhyne (Eds.), *Film festival yearbook 1: The festival circuit* (pp. 23–39). St Andrews Film Studies and College Gate Press.

Iordanova, D. (2015). The film festival as an industry node. *Media Industries Journal, 1*(3), 7–11.

Iordanova, D., & Rhyne, R. (2009). Introduction. In D. Iordanova & R. Rhyne (Eds.), *Film festival yearbook 1: The festival circuit* (pp. 1–9). St Andrews Film Studies and College Gate Press.

Iyer, U. (2022). A pedagogy of reparations: Notes toward repairing the film and media studies curriculum. *Feminist Media Histories, 8*(1), 181–193.

Jabri, V. (2013). *The postcolonial subject: Claiming politics/governing others in late modernity.* Routledge.

Jaikumar, P. (2016). Feminist and non-Western interrogations of film authorship. In K. Hole, D. Jelača, E. Ann Kaplan, & P. Petro (Eds.), *The Routledge companion to cinema & gender* (pp. 205–214). Routledge.

Jeong, S. (2021). World cinema in a global frame. *Studies in World Cinema, 1*(1), 29–38.

Johnson, R. (2020). A brutal humanism for the new millennium? The legacy of neorealism in contemporary cinema of migration. *Journal of Italian Cinema & Media Studies, 8*(1), 61–77.

Johnson, R. (2021). Film circulation in times of coronavirus. *Curating and Exhibiting Visual Culture in Times of Coronavirus.* [Online]. Available from: https://ahc.leeds.ac.uk/downloads/download/230/sadler_blog_post_1_film_circulation_in_times_of_coronavirus

Johnson, R. (forthcoming). On studying film festivals and migration: Borderlands and beginnings. In D. Ostrowska & T. Falicov (Eds.), *Contours of film festival research and methodologies.* Amsterdam University Press.

Karakayalı, S. (2019). Solidarity with refugees. In J. Bock & S. Macdonald (Eds.), *Refugees welcome? Difference and diversity in a changing Germany* (pp. 191–214). Berghahn Books.

Karlovy Vary International Film Festival. (2019). *Programme Sections.* [Online]. Available from: https://www.kviff.com/en/about-the-festival/programe-sections

Kellner, D., & Lewis, T. (2007). Liberal humanism and the European critical tradition. In W. Outhwaite & S. P. Turner (Eds.), *The SAGE handbook of social science methodology* (pp. 405–422). SAGE.

Kennedy, D. (1999). Summer films: Indies; festival to festival, a movable marketplace. *New York Times*. 2 May. [Online]. Available from: https://www.nytimes.com/1999/05/02/movies/summer-films-indies-festival-to-festival-a-movable-marketplace.html

Kessy, R. (2014). *Decoding the donor gaze: Documentary, aid and AIDS in Africa* [PhD thesis]. University of Huddersfield.

King, G. (2022). *Positioning art cinema: Film and cultural value*. Bloomsbury.

Kristeva, J. (1982). *Powers of horror: An essay on abjection*. Columbia University Press.

La Porta, F. (2013). Il film in questione: *La grande bellezza* (2013). *Allegoria*, *68*, 213–216.

Lacan, J. (2004 [1949]). The mirror stage as formative of the *I* function as revealed in psychoanalytic experience. In J. Lacan (Ed.), *Écrits: A selection* (pp. 3–9). Norton & Co.

Lacan, J. (2004 [1964]). *The four fundamental concepts of psychoanalysis*. Norton.

Lacan, J. (2011 [1973]). Seminar XXI: Les non-dupes errant. In C. Gallagher (Ed.), *Lacan in Ireland*. Available from: http://www.lacaninireland.com/web/translations/seminars/

Laclau, E. (2014). *The rhetorical foundations of society*. Verso.

Lampel, J., Nadavulakere, S., & Rawat, A. (2013). The impact of reputational resources on event performance in international film festivals. *American Journal of Management*, *13*(2), 9–21.

Lampel, J., & Meyer, A. (2008). Field-configuring events as structuring mechanisms: How conferences, ceremonies, and trade shows constitute new technologies, industries, and markets. *Journal of Management Studies*, *45*(6), 1025–1035.

Latour, B. (1996). On actor-network theory: A few clarifications. *Soziale Welt*, *47*(4), 369–381.

Leavitt, C. (2020). *Italian neorealism: A cultural history*. University of Toronto Press.

Leavitt, C., O'Rawe, C., & Renga, D. (2015). "La polvere dei sogni." *The Italianist*, *35*(2), 171–175.

Leão, T. (2022). *Can we openly talk about precarious and voluntary work at film festivals? Reflections on the Portuguese case*. NECS annual conference, Epistemic Media: Atlas, Archive, Network, 22–26 June 2022. Politechnica University of Bucharest.

Loist, S. (2016). The film festival circuit: Networks, hierarchies and circulation. In M. de Valck, D. B. Kredell, & S. Loist (Eds.), *Film festivals: History, theory, method, practice* (pp. 49–64). Routledge.

Loist, S. (2017–2022). *Film circulation on the international film festival network and the impact on global film culture*. Project website: http://www.filmcirculation.net/

Loist, S. 2020. Film festival research workshops: Debates on methodology. In A. Vallejo & E. Winton (Eds.), *Documentary film festivals Vol. 1* (pp. 41–52). Palgrave MacMillan.

Loist, S., & Verhoeven, D. (2019). Complex not complicated: Gendered media industries in the wake of #MeToo. *Media Industries*, *6*(1), 67–71.

Lombardi Diop, C., & Romeo, C. (2015). State of the union: Survival blankets and falling stars. *Postcolonial Studies*, *18*(4), 337–352.

Lule, J. (1995). Enduring image of war: Myth and ideology in a *Newsweek* cover. *Journal of Popular Culture*, *29*(1), 199–211.

Ma, J. (2010). Tsai Ming-Liang's haunted movie theater. In R. Galt & K. Schoonover (Eds.), *Global art cinema: New theories and histories*, pp. 334–350. Oxford University Press.

MacDonald Carolan, M. A. (2013). Moretti's children: The next generation? *Quaderni d'italianistica*, *34*(2), 113–132.

MacDowell, J. (2013). *Happy endings in Hollywood cinema.* Edinburgh University Press.

MacKenzie, S. (2014). *Film manifestos and global cinema cultures: A critical anthology.* University of California Press.

Macfie, A. L. (Ed.). (2000). *Orientalism: A reader.* New York University Press.

Manzoli, G., & Minuz, A. (Eds.). (2017). *Il cinema di stato: finanziamento pubblico ed economia simbolica nel cinema italiano contemporaneo.* Mulino.

Marcus, M. (1996). *Caro Diario* and the cinematic body of Nanni Moretti. *Italica*, *73*(2), 233–247.

Marcus, M. (2002). *After Fellini: National cinema in the postmodern age.* John Hopkins University Press.

Marcus, M. (2007). *Italian film in the shadow of Auschwitz.* University of Toronto Press.

Mariani, A. (2017). The empty heterotopic (non-)space of Sorrentino's characters in *The Great Beauty* and *The Consequences of Love.* In S. G. Byer & F. Cecchini (Eds.), *Representations of female identity in Italy: From Neoclassism to the 21st Century* (pp. 170–186). Cambridge Scholars Publishing.

Marshall, L. (2008). Gomorrah (Gomorra). *Screen Daily.* [Online]. Available from: https://www.screendaily.com/gomorrah-gomorra/4038782.article

Martin, A. (2016). Refocusing authorship in women's filmmaking. In J. Levitin, J. Plessis, & V. Raoul (Eds.), *Women filmmakers: Refocusing* (pp. 29–37). Routledge.

Martini, A. (2015). Concept city: Roma ri-vista e vissuta ne *La dolce vita* e *La grande bellezza. Carte Italiane*, *2*(10), 107–119.

Maule, R. (2008). *Beyond auteurism: New directions in authorial film practices in France, Italy and Spain since the 1980s.* Intellect.

Maule, R. (2014). Women's festival 2.0 between grassroots globalisation and neoliberal feminism: The Birds Eye View Festival. *Comunicazioni sociali*, *1*(3), 368–374.

Mazdon, L. (2006). The Cannes Film Festival as transnational space. *Post Script*, *25*(2), 19–30.

Mazierska, E., & Rascaroli, L. (2004). *The cinema of Nanni Moretti: Dreams and diaries*. Wallflower.

McCarthy, T. (1999). High art pays low dividends for Cannes auds. *Variety*. [Online]. Available from: https://variety.com/1999/voices/columns/high-art-pays-low-dividends-for-cannes-auds-1117502356/

McGowan, T. (2007). *The real gaze: Film theory after Lacan*. State University of New York Press.

McGowan, T., & Kunkle, S. (2004). Introduction: Lacanian psychoanalysis in film theory. In T. McGowan, S. Kunkle, & F. L. Restuccia (Eds.), *Lacan and contemporary film*. Other Press.

Metz, C. (1982). *The imaginary signifier: Psychoanalysis and the cinema*. Indiana University Press.

Mezias, S. et al. (2008). Much ado about nothing? Untangling the impact of European premier film festivals. *Creative Encounters Research Paper Series, 14*, 1–31.

Mezias, S. et al. (2011). Transforming film product identities: The status effects of European premier film festivals, 1996–2005. In B. Moeran & J. S. Pedersen (Eds.), *Negotiating values in the creative industries: Fairs, festivals and competitive events* (pp. 169–196). Cambridge University Press.

Mignolo, W. D., & Walsh, C. E. (2018). *On decoloniality: Concepts, analytics, praxis*. Duke University Press.

Minuz, A. (2013). Il film in questione: *La grande bellezza* (2013). *Allegoria, 69*, 217–220.

Moine, C. (2013). La Fédération internationale des associations de producteurs de films: un acteur controversé de la promotion du cinéma après 1945. *Le movement social, 243*, 91–103.

Mori, G. (2016). Il cinema del godimento: lo sguardo come fattore politico da Fellini a Sorrentino. *L'avventura, 61*(1), 149–169.

Mulvey, L. (1975). Visual pleasure and narrative cinema. *Screen, 16*(3), 6–18.

Mumford, G. (2018). Cannes 2018: Cate Blanchett defends festival's failure to select more female directors. *The Guardian*. [Online]. Available from: https://www.theguardian.com/film/2018/may/08/cannes-2018-cate-blanchett-defends-festivals-failure-to-select-more-women-directors

Neale, S. (1981). Art cinema as institution. *Screen, 22*(1), 11–40.

Nichols, B. (1994). Discovering form, inferring meaning: New cinemas and the film festival circuit. *Film Quarterly, 47*(3), 16–30.

Nicolson, M., de Oliveira Andreotti, V., & Mafi, B. F. (2015). The unstated politics of stranger making in Europe: A brutal kindness. *European Journal of Cultural Studies, 19*(4), 335–351.

Nixon, M. (2005). On the couch. *October, 113*, 39–76.

Nord, L. (2016). "Fire at Sea": How Gianfranco Rosi made an anti-documentary. *No Film School.* [Online]. Available from: https://nofilmschool.com/2016/09/fire-at-sea-gianfranco-rosi-interview

Nornes, A. M. (2013). Asian film festivals, translation and the international film festival short circuits. In D. Iordanova (Ed.), *The film festival Reader* (pp. 245–262). St. Andrews Film Studies.

O'Healy, Á. (2000). Theatre and cinema: 1945–2000. In L. Panizza & S. Wood (Eds.), *History of women's writing in Italy* (pp. 254–265). Cambridge University Press.

O'Healy, Á. (2010). Mediterranean passages: Abjection and belonging in contemporary Italian cinema. *California Italian Studies, 1*(1), 1–19.

O'Healy, Á. (2019). *Migrant anxieties: Italian cinema in a transnational frame.* Indiana University Press.

O'Leary, A. (2017). What is Italian cinema? *California Italian Studies, 7*(1), 1–26.

O'Leary, A., & Johnson, R. (2022). Flow. In D. Duncan & J. Burns (Eds.), *Transnational modern languages: A handbook* (pp. 123–131). Liverpool University Press.

O'Leary, A., & O'Rawe, C. (2008). Preface. *Italian Studies, 63*(2), 171–172.

O'Leary, A., & O'Rawe, C. (2011). Against realism: On a "certain tendency" in Italian film criticism. *Journal of Modern Italian Studies, 16*(1), 107–128.

O'Rawe, C. (2008). "I padri e i maestri": Genre, auteurs, and absences in Italian film studies. *Italian Studies, 63*(2), 173–194.

O'Rawe, C. (2012). "A past that will not pass": Italian cinema and the return to the 1970s. *New Cinemas: Journal of Contemporary Film, 9*(2/3), 101–113.

O'Rawe, C. (2014). *Stars and masculinities in contemporary Italian cinema.* Palgrave Macmillan.

Ostrowska, D. (2016). Making film history at the Cannes film festival. In M. de Valck, B. D. Kredell, & S. Loist (Eds.), *Film festivals: History, theory, method, practice* (pp. 18–33). Routledge.

Ostrowska, D. (2019). "The migrant gaze" and "the migrant festive chronotope" – Programming the refugee crisis at the European human rights and documentary film festivals. The case of the One World International Human Rights Documentary Film Festival. *Studies in European Cinema, 16*(3), 266–281.

Parker, I. (2005). Lacanian discourse analysis in psychology: Seven theoretical elements. *Theory & Psychology, 15*(2), 163–182.

Parrot, L., & Stahnke, L. (2021). *Curation as research: A masterclass with the London Migration Film Festival,* 1 July, University of Leeds.

Paz Peirano, M. (2021). Between industry labs and audience formation: Film festivals and the transformation of the field of film production in Chile. *Loisir et Société/Society and Leisure, 44*(1), 47–65.

Peranson, M. (2008). First you get the power, then you get the money: Two models of film festivals. *Cineaste, 33*(3), 37–43.

Pisu, S. (2018). A transnational love-hate relationship: The FIAPF and the Venice and Cannes Film Festivals (1950–1970). In T. Jenkins (Ed.), *International film festivals. Contemporary cultures and history beyond Venice and Cannes* (pp. 109–131). Bloomsbury.

Polan, D. (2001). Auteur desire. *Screening the Past.* [Online]. Available from: http://www.screeningthepast.com/issue-12-first-release/auteur-desire/

Ponzanesi, S. (2016a). Of shipwrecks and weddings: Borders and mobilities in Europe. *Transnational Cinemas, 7*(2), 151–167.

Ponzanesi, S. (2016b). Does Italy need postcolonial theory? Intersections in Italian postcolonial studies. *English Literature, 3*, 145–161.

Ponzanesi (2016c). The point of Europe: Postcolonial entanglements. *Interventions, 18*(2), 159–164.

Powell, E. (1968). Rivers of Blood (also known as The Birmingham Speech). Address to the Conservative Political Centre, Birmingham, 20 April 1968. Transcript. *The Telegraph*. [Online]. Available from: http://www.telegraph.co.uk/comment/3643823/Enoch-Powells-Rivers-of-Blood-speech.html

Pulver, A. (2016). *Fire at Sea* review – A powerful study of migrant crisis. *The Guardian*. [Online]. Available from: https://www.theguardian.com/film/2016/feb/13/fire-at-sea-review-lampedusa-migrants-berlin-film-festival-2016

Rajaram, P. K. (2016). Europe's "Hungarian solution." *Radical Philosophy, 197*, 2–7.

Rastegar, R. (2012). Difference, aesthetics and the curatorial crisis of film festivals. *Screen, 53*(3), 310–317.

Renga, D. (2013). *Unfinished business: Screening the Italian Mafia in the new millennium*. University of Toronto Press.

Renga, D. (2014). *Mafia movies: A reader.* University of Toronto Press.

Rhyne, R. (2009). Film festivals circuits and stakeholders. In D. Iordanova & R. Rhyne (Eds.), *Film festival yearbook 1: The festival circuit* (pp. 9–22). St. Andrews Film Studies & College Gate Press.

Rich, B. R. (1998). *Chick flicks: Theories and memories of the feminist film movement.* Duke University Press.

Rich, B. R. (2003). Abstract from "Taste, fashion, and service: The ideology of film curating." In *Terms of address: The pedagogy and politics of film and video programming and curating, 7–8 March 2003, Centre for Media and Culture in Education (CMCE), Ontario Institute for Studies in Education, Toronto.* Available from: http://fcis.oise.utoronto.ca/~cmce/terms%20of%20address%20symposium.htm

Ridda, M. (2017). The siren's children: Rethinking postcolonial Naples. *Interventions, 19*(4), 467–486.

Rigoletto, S. (2014). *Masculinity and Italian cinema: Sexual politics, social conflict and male crisis in the 1970s*. Edinburgh University Press.

Robbins, P., & Saglier, V. (2015). Introduction. Other networks: Expanding film festival perspectives. *Synoptique, 3*(2), 1–8.

Romney, J. (2018). "Happy as Lazzaro": Cannes review. *Screen Daily*. [Online]. Available from: https://www.screendaily.com/reviews/happy-as-lazzaro-cannes-review/5129305.article

Rooney, D. (2001). Review: *The Son's Room*. *Variety*. [Online]. Available from: https://variety.com/2001/film/reviews/the-son-s-room-1200467299/

Rose, J. (2007). *The last resistance*. Verso.

Ross, M. (2011). The film festival as producer: Latin American films and Rotterdam's Hubert Bals Fund. *Screen, 52*(2), 261–267.

Ruberto, L. E., & Wilson, K. M. (Eds.). (2007). *Italian neorealism and global cinema*. Wayne State University Press.

Rüling, C. C. (2009). Festivals as field-configuring events: The Annecy International Animated Film Festival and Market. In D. Iordanova & R. Rhyne (Eds.), *Film festival yearbook 1: The festival circuit* (pp. 49–66). St Andrews Film Studies and College Gate Press.

Rumph, R. S. (2011). *I am African: Branding Africa through the gaze of philanthropy* [PhD thesis]. New York University.

Said, E. (1993). *Culture and imperialism*. Vintage.

Said, E. (2003 [1978]). *Orientalism: Western conceptions of the Orient*. Penguin

Saperstein, P. (2018). Kristen Stewart climbs Cannes red carpet stairs barefoot. *Variety*. [Online]. Available from: https://variety.com/2018/film/news/kristen-stewart-cannes-red-carpet-barefoot-1202810872/

Sarris, A. (1962). Notes on the *auteur* theory in 1962. *Film Culture, 27*(1), 1–8.

Saviano, R. (2008). *L'impero criminale, Gomorra*. Press pack. [Online]. Available from: http://www.archimedefilm.it/docs/gomorra_pressbook_ita.doc

Saviano, R., & Jewiss, V. (2007). *Gomorrah: A personal journey into the violent international empire of Naples' organised crime system*. Farrar, Straus and Giroux.

Scaglioni, M. et al. (2015–2020). *International Circulation of Italian Cinema*. [Online]. Available from: https://www.italiancinema.it/

Scaglioni, M. et al. (2018). International circulation of Italian cinema: About. *International Circulation of Italian Cinema*. [Online]. Available from: https://www.italiancinema.it/about/

Schich, M. et al. (2020–). *Cultural data analytics* (CUDAN). Project website: https://cudan.tlu.ee/

Schneider, J. (1998). *Italy's "Southern Question": Orientalism in one country*. Berg.

Schoonover, K. (2012). *Brutal vision: The neorealist body in postwar Italian cinema*. University of Minnesota Press.

Scott, A. O. (2016). "Fire at Sea" is not the documentary you'd expect about the migrant crisis. It's better. *New York Times*. [Online]. Available from: https://www.nytimes.com/2016/10/21/movies/fire-at-sea-review.html

Sellors, C. P. (2010). *Film authorship: Auteurs and other myths*. Columbia University Press.

Sendra, E. (2020). Dak'Art. 30 years of arts curation and reception in postcolonial African societies. *Arts Management Quarterly*, *135*(1), 65–71.

Shakespeare, W. (2008 [1599]). *Julius Caesar*. Oxford University Press.

Shambu, G. (2019). For a new cinephilia. *Film Quarterly*, *72*(3), 32–34.

Shambu, G. (2020). Rethinking film evaluation. *Quorum*. Available from: https://filmquarterly.org/2020/03/11/rethinking-film-evaluation/

Shohat, E., & Stam, R. (2014). *Unthinking Eurocentrism: Multiculturalism and the media*. Routledge.

Silverman, K. (2003 [1988]). The female authorial voice. In V. W. Wexman (Ed.), *Film and authorship* (pp. 50–75). Rutgers University Press.

Simor, E., & Sorfa, D. (2017). Irony, sexism and magic in Paolo Sorrentino's films. *Studies in European Cinema*, *14*(3), 200–215.

Smits, R., & Nikdel, E. W. (2019). Beyond Netflix and Amazon: MUBI and the curation of on-demand film. *Studies in European Cinema*, *16*(1), 22–37.

Solanas, F., & Getino, O. (1970). Toward a third cinema. *Cinéaste*, *4*(3), 1–10.

Sorlin, P. (1996). *Italian national cinema: 1896–1996*. Routledge.

Spinazzola, V. (1985). *Cinema e pubblico: lo spettacolo filmico in Italia 1945–1965*. Bulzoni.

Strandgaard Pedersen, J., & Mazza, C. (2011). International film festivals: For the benefit of whom? *Culture Unbound*, *3*, 139–165.

Stringer, J. (2001). Global cities and the international film festival economy. In T. Shiel & T. Fitzmaurice (Eds.), *Cinema and the city: Film and urban societies in a global context* (pp. 134–144). Blackwell.

Stringer, J. (2008). Genre films and festival communities: Lessons from Nottingham, 1991–2000. *Film International*, *6*(4), 53–60.

Sutton, P. (2004). "Can the man panic?": Masculinity and fatherhood in Nanni Moretti's *Aprile*. In P. Powrie, A. Davies, & B. Babington (Eds.), *The trouble with men: Masculinities in European and Hollywood cinema* (pp. 144–154). Wallflower Press.

Táíwò, O. O. (2022). *Elite capture: How the powerful took over identity politics (and everything else)*. Pluto Press.

Tarr, C. (1999). *Diane Kurys*. Manchester: Manchester University Press.

Tarrow, S. (1996). Making social science work across space and time: A critical reflection on Robert Putnam's *Making Democracy Work*. *American Political Science Review*, *90*, 389–397.

Taylor, P. (2010). *Žižek and the Media*. Polity.

Tomšič, S. (2015). Materialism between critique and speculation. In A. Hamza (Ed.), *Repeating Žižek*, (58–71). Duke University Press.

Tuck, E., & Wang, K. W. (2012). Decolonization is not a metaphor. *Decolonisation: Indigeneity, Education & Society*, *1*(1), 1–40.

Tulante, M. (2013). High fashion in film: Italian identity and global anxiety in *Valentino: The Last Emperor* and *Gomorrah*. *Journal of Italian Cinema & Media Studies*, *1*(3), 245–262.

Turan, K. (2002). *Sundance to Sarajevo: Film festivals and the world they made*. University of California Press.

UNHCR. (1951). *Protocol relating to the status of refugees*. The United Nations Refugee Agency.

UNHCR. (2015). *The sea route to Europe: The Mediterranean passage in the age of refugees*. The United Nations Refugee Agency.

Vallejo, A. (2020). Rethinking the canon: The role of film festivals in shaping film history. *Studies in European Cinema*, *17*(2), 155–169.

Venice International Film Festival. (2018). *The history of the Venice Film Festival*. [Online]. Available from: https://www.labiennale.org/en/history-venice-film-festival

Verdicchio, P. (1997). The preclusion of postcolonial discourse in Southern Italy. In B. Allen & M. Russo (Eds.), *Revisioning Italy. National culture and global culture* (pp. 191–212). University of Minnesota Press.

Verhoeven, D., Coate, B., & Zemaityte, V. (2019). Re-distributing gender in the global film industry: Beyond #MeToo and #MeThree. *Media Industries*, *6*(1), 136–155.

Vetter, D. (2022). Who cares about cinema? *The Film Comment Letter*. Available from: https://www.filmcomment.com/blog/who-cares-about-cinema-film-festivals-film-workers-dennis-vetter/

Vighi, F. (2003). Unravelling Moretti's (political) unconscious: The abyss of the subject in *La stanza del figlio*. *Journal of Romance Studies*, *3*(2), 79–94.

Vighi, F. (2005). Nanni Moretti: Trauma, hysteria, and freedom. In W. Hope (Ed.), *Italian cinema: new directions* (pp. 79–106). Peter Lang.

Vighi, F. (2010). *On Žižek's dialectics: Surplus, subtraction, sublimation*. Continuum.

Vighi, F., & Feldner, H. (2007). Ideology critique or discourse analysis? Žižek against Foucault. *European Journal of Political Theory*, *6*(2), 141–159.

Vimercati, G. (2012). Festivals: Karlovy Vary. *Film Comment*. [Online]. Available from: https://www.filmcomment.com/blog/festivals-karlovy-vary/

Vogel, A. (2022). *Cinema and the festivalisation of capitalism*. Brill.

Wagstaff, C. (2007). *Italian neorealist cinema: An aesthetic approach*. University of Toronto Press.

Waldman, P. (2015). Aylan Kurdi, and the ethics of an image that shocked the world. *The Week*. 4 September 2015. [Online]. Available from: https://theweek.com/articles/575415/aylan-kurdi-ethics-image-that-shocked-world

Wallis, E. (2019). "Beyond the Beach": Venice Film Festival spotlights migration. *InfoMigrants*. 5 September 2019. Available from: https://www.infomigrants.net/en/post/19328/beyond-the-beach-venice-film-festival-spotlights-migration

Walton, D. (2012). *Doing cultural theory*. Sage.

Wayne, M. (2002). *The politics of contemporary European cinema: Histories, borders, diasporas*. Intellect.

Weissberg, J. (2008). Gomorrah. *Variety*. [Online]. Available from: https://variety.com/2008/film/markets-festivals/gomorrah-1200522327/

White, P. (2015). *Women's cinema, world cinema: Projecting contemporary feminisms*. Duke University Press.

Wilson, E. (2018). From Lampedusa to the California desert: Gianfranco Rosi's scenes of living and dying. *Film Quarterly*, *71*(3), 10–20.

Wilson, J. (2016). The joy of inequality: The libidinal economy of compassionate consumerism. *International Journal of Žižek Studies*, *9*(2), 1–26.

Wiseman, A. (2015). Cannes: Women denied Palais entry for wearing flats. *Screen Daily*. [Online]. Available from: https://www.screendaily.com/festivals/cannes/cannes-women-denied-palais-entry-for-wearing-flats/5088395.article

Wiseman, A. (2016). Kristen Stewart, Julia Roberts kick off their heels in Cannes. *Screen Daily*. [Online]. Available from: https://www.screendaily.com/cannes/kristen-stewart-julia-roberts-kick-off-their-heels-in-cannes/5103878.article

Wong, C. H-Y. (2016). Publics and counterpublics: Rethinking film festivals as public spheres. In M. de Valck, D. B. Kredell, & S. Loist (Eds.), *Film festivals: History, theory, method, practice* (pp. 83–99). Routledge.

Wong, C. H-Y. (2011). *Film festivals: Culture, people, and power on the global screen*. Rutgers University Press.

Wood, M. P. (2005). *Italian cinema*. Bloomsbury Academic.

Yossman, K. J. (2021). Press conference at Cannes film festival. *Variety*. Available from: https://variety.com/2021/film/global/cannes-thierry-fremaux-talks-netflix-pandemic-challenges-in-pre-festival-press-conference-1235011781/

Young, L. (1996). *Fear of the dark: "Race," gender and sexuality in the cinema*. Routledge.

Zagarrio, V. (2012). L'eredità del neorealismo nel "New-new Italian Cinema." *Annali d'Italianistica*, *30*, 95–111.

Zagarrio, V. (2016). Una certa tendenza del cinema italiano. *Flinders University Languages Group Online Review*, *5*(1), 1–8.

Zambenedetti, A. (2006). Multiculturalism in New Italian Cinema. *Studies in European Cinema*, *3*(2), 105–116.

Žižek, S. (1989). *The sublime object of ideology*. Verso.

Žižek, S. (1992). *Looking awry: An introduction to Jacques Lacan through popular culture*. MIT Press.

Žižek, S. (1993). *Tarrying with the negative: Kant, Hegel, and the critique of ideology.* Duke University Press.
Žižek, S. (1997). *The plague of fantasies.* Verso.
Žižek, S. (1999). *The ticklish subject: The absent centre of political ontology.* Verso.
Žižek, S. (2000a). Class struggle or postmodernism? Yes, please! In J. Butler, E. Laclau, & S. Žižek (Eds.), *Contingency, hegemony, universality: Contemporary dialogues on the left* (pp. 91–135). Verso.
Žižek, S. (2000b). Da capo senza fine. In J. Butler, E. Laclau, & S. Žižek (Eds.), *Contingency, hegemony, universality: Contemporary dialogues on the left* (pp. 213–262). Verso.
Žižek, S. (2000c). Melancholy and the act. *Critical Inquiry, 26*(4), 657–681.
Žižek, S. (2001a). *Enjoy your symptom! Jacques Lacan in Hollywood and out* (2nd ed.). Routledge.
Žižek, S. (2001b). *The fright of real tears: Krzysztof Kieślowski between theory and post-theory.* British Film Institute.
Žižek, S. (2002). *Welcome to the desert of the Real! Five essays on September 11 and related dates.* Verso.
Žižek, S. (2003). *The puppet and the dwarf: The perverse core of Christianity.* MIT Press.
Žižek, S. (2004a). *Iraq: The borrowed kettle.* Verso.
Žižek, S. (2004b). *The reality of the virtual* [lecture]. Recorded 11 December 2003. Ben Wright Film Productions.
Žižek, S. (2005). *The metastases of enjoyment: Six essays on women and causality.* Verso.
Žižek, S. (2006). *The parallax view.* MIT Press.
Žižek, S. (2008). *Violence: Six sideways reflections.* Profile Books.
Žižek, S. (2012). *Mapping ideology.* Verso Books.
Žižek, S. (2016). *Against the double blackmail: Refugees, terror and other troubles with the neighbours.* Penguin.

Filmography

Corpus

A Children's Story (*Certi bambini*) (2004). Frazzi, A., & Frazzi, A. dirs. Italy.
Ceasar Must Die (*Cesare deve morire*) (2012). Taviani, P., & Taviani, V. dirs. Italy.
Facing Window (*La finestra di fronte*) (2003). Özpetek, F. dir. Italy.
Fire at Sea (*Fuocoammare*) (2016). Rosi, G. dir. Italy.
Gomorrah (*Gomorra*) (2008). Garrone, M. dir. Italy.
The Great Beauty (*La grande bellezza*) (2013). Sorrentino, P. dir. Italy.
Private (2004). Costanzo, S. dir. Italy.
The Son's Room (*La stanza del figlio*) (2001). Moretti, N. dir. Italy.
Sacro GRA (2013). Rosi, G. dir. Italy.

Films and Television Series Referred To

A Brighter Tomorrow (*Il sol dell'avvenire*) (2023). Moretti, N. dir. Italy.
Alcarràs (2022). Simón, C. dir. Spain.
Anatomy of a Fall (*Anatomie d'une chute*) (2023). Triet, J. dir. France.
Aprile (2007). Moretti, N. dir. Italy.
As Far as I Can Walk (*Strahinja Banović*) (2021). Arsenijević, S. dir. Serbia.
Atlantics (*Atlantique*) (2019). Diop, M. dir. Senegal, France.
The Battle of Algiers (*La battaglia di Algeri*) (1966). Pontecorvo, G. dir. Italy/Algeria.
Blade Runner (1982). Scott, R. dir. USA.
Camp de Thiaroye (1989). Sembene, O. dir. Senegal.
Chroniques des années de braise (1975). Lakhdar-Hamina, M. Algeria.
City of God (*Cidade de Deus*) (2003). Lund, K., & Meirelles, F. dirs. Brazil.
Dear Diary (*Caro diario*) (1993). Moretti, N. dir. Italy.
The Dark Sea (*Mare nero*) (2005). Torre, R. dir. Italy.
Daughter of Mine (*Figlia mia*) (2018). Bispuri, L. dir. Italy.
Dogman (2018). Garrone, M. dir. Italy.
Dolce Vita (*La dolce vita*) (1960) Fellini, F. dir. Italy.
Don't Tell (*La bestia nel cuore*) (2005). Comencini, C. dir. Italy.
Double Indemnity (1944). Wilder, B. dir. USA.
Fahrenheit 9/11 (2004). Moore, M. dir. USA.
Father and Master (*Padre Padrone*) (1977). Taviani, P., & Taviani, V. dirs. Italy.
Ecce bombo (1978). Moretti, N. dir. Italy.
Examined Life (2008). Taylor, A. dir. USA.

Euphoria (*Euforia*) (2018). Golino, V. dir. Italy.
Farenheit 9/11 (2004). Moore, M. dir. USA.
Germany Year Zero (*Germania anno zero*) (1949). Rossellini, R. dir. Italy.
Girls of the Sun (*Les filles du soleil*) (2018). Hussan, E. dir. France/USA.
The Godfather (1972). Ford Coppola, F. dir. USA.
The Godfather Part II (1974). Ford Coppola, F. dir. USA.
The Godfather Part II (1990). Ford Coppola, F. dir. USA.
Grbavica: The Land of My Dreams (*Grbavica*) (2006). Žbanić, J. dir. Bosnia and Herzegovina.
Hamam: The Turkish Bath (*Hamam Suare*) (1997). Özpetek, F. dir. Italy.
Happening (*L'Événement*) (2021). Diwan, A. France.
Happy as Lazzaro (*Lazzaro felice*) (2018). Rohrwacher, A. dir. Italy.
Harem Suare (1999). Özpetek, F. dir. Italy.
Honey (*Miele*) (2013). Golino, V. dir. Italy.
I Was Told There's Freedom Here (2021). Abdalla, A. dir. UK.
Identifying Features (*Sin señas particulares*) (2020). Valadez, F. dir. Mexico.
Ignorant Fairies (*Le fate ignoranti*) (2001). Özpetek, F. dir. Italy.
Il Divo (*Il divo: La spettacolare vita di Giulio Andreotti*) (2008). Sorrentino, P. dir. Italy.
Life Is Beautiful (*La vita è bella*) (1997). Benigni, R. dir. Italy.
Mediterranea (2015). Carpignano, J. dir. Italy/USA.
Mia madre (2015). Moretti, N. dir. Italy.
Non è giusto (2001). De Lillo, A. dir. Italy.
On the Bride's Side (*Io sto con la sposa*) (2014). Augugliaro, A., Del Grande, G., & Al Nassiry, K. S. dirs. Italy.
Obsession (*Ossessione*) (1943). Visconti, L. dir. Italy.
Padre Padrone (1977). Taviani, V., & Taviani, P. dirs. Italy.
Paisan (*Paisà*) (1948). Rossellini, R. dir. Italy.
The Piano (1993). Campion, J. dir. UK.
The Postman Always Rings Twice (1934). McCain, J. USA.
Quo Vado? (*Quo vado?*) (2016). Zalone, C. dir. Italy.
Reality (2012). Garrone, M. dir. UK.
Rome, Open City (*Roma, città aperta*) (1945). Rossellini, R. dir. Italy.
Scarface (1983). De Palma, B. dir. USA.
Shooting the Moon (*L'albero delle pere*) (1998). Archibugi, F. dir. Italy.
Shoplifters (*Manbiki kazoku*) (2018). Koreeda, H. Japan.
Still Life (*San xia hao ren*) (2006). Zhangke, J. dir. China.
Tale of Tales (*Il racconto dei racconti*) (2015). Garrone, M. dir. Italy.
La terra trema (1948). Visconti, L. dir. Italy.
Terraferma (2011). Crialese, E. dir. Italy.
Titane (2021). Ducournau, J. dir. France.

Touch Me Not (2018). Pintilie, A. dir. Romania.

Via degli specchi (*Via degli specchi*) (1983). Gagliardo, G. dir. Italy.

The Vesuvians (*I vesuviani*) (1997). Capuano, A., Corsicato, P., de Lillo, A., Incerti, S., & Martone, M. dirs. Italy.

When the Night (*Quando la notte*) (2011). Comencini, C. dir. Italy.

The Wonders (*Le meraviglie*) (2014). Rohrwacher, A. dir. USA.

The Young Pope (2016, television series). Sorrentino, P. dir. Italy/USA.

Youth (2015). Sorrentino, P. Italy.

Index of Films

Page numbers followed by "n" refer to notes.

Index of Names

Page numbers followed by "n" refer to notes.

Index of Subjects

Page numbers followed by "n" refer to notes.

For Product Safety Concerns and Information please contact our EU
representative GPSR@taylorandfrancis.com
Taylor & Francis Verlag GmbH, Kaufingerstraße 24, 80331 München, Germany

www.ingramcontent.com/pod-product-compliance
Ingram Content Group UK Ltd.
Pitfield, Milton Keynes, MK11 3LW, UK
UKHW020017200926
475702UK00014B/1924
* 9 7 8 1 0 4 1 1 7 9 3 3 7 *